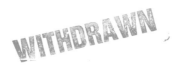
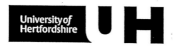
University of
Hertfordshire UH

College Lane, Hatfield, Herts. AL10 9AB
Information Hertfordshire
Services and Solutions for the University

For renewal of Standard and One Week Loans,
please visit the web site http://www.voyager.herts.ac.uk

This item must be returned or the loan renewed by the due date.
A fine will be charged for the late return of items.

South African AIDS Activism and Global Health Politics

In the early 2000s, South African AIDS activists fought corporate greed and indifferent political leaders. Mbali's remarkable book is an impassioned and convincing account that locates treatment activism in a transnational frame, and gives novel attention to its gendered politics. It is inspiring but not romantic – a rich account that deserves to be widely read by historians, activists, and healthworkers.

Mark Hunter, author of *Love in the Time of AIDS*

Global Ethics Series

Series Editor: Christien van den Anker, Reader, Department of Politics, University of the West of England, UK

Global Ethics as a field builds on longer traditions of ethical reflection about (global) society and discusses ethical approaches to global issues. These include but are not limited to issues highlighted by the process of globalisation (in the widest sense) and increasing multiculturalism. They also engage with migration, the environment, poverty and inequality, peace and conflict, human rights, global citizenship, social movements, and global governance. Despite fluid boundaries between fields, Global Ethics can be clearly marked out by its multidisciplinary approach, its interest in a strong link between theory, policy and practice and its inclusion of a range of work from strictly normative to more empirical.

Books in the series provide a specific normative approach, taxonomy, or an ethical position on a specific issue in Global Ethics through empirical work. They explicitly engage with Global Ethics as a field and position themselves in regard to existing debates even when outlining more local approaches or issues. The *Global Ethics Series* has been designed to reach beyond a liberal cosmopolitan agenda and engage with contextualism as well as structural analyses of injustice in current global politics and its disciplining discourses.

Titles include:

Carlos R. Cordourier-Real
TRANSNATIONAL SOCIAL JUSTICE

Anna Grear
REDIRECTING HUMAN RIGHTS
Facing the Challenge of Corporate Legal Humanity

Shahram Khosravi
'ILLEGAL' TRAVELLER
An Auto-Ethnography of Borders

Ivan Manokha (*editor*)
THE POLITICAL ECONOMY OF HUMAN RIGHTS ENFORCEMENT

Mandisa Mbali
SOUTH AFRICAN AIDS ACTIVISM AND GLOBAL HEALTH POLITICS

Darrel Moellendorf
GLOBAL INEQUALITY MATTERS

Michal Nahman
EXTRACTIONS
Securing Borders, Trafficking Human Ova

Derrick M. Nault and Shawn L. England (*editors*)
GLOBALIZATION AND HUMAN RIGHTS IN THE DEVELOPING WORLD

Christien van den Anker and Ilse van Liempt (*editors*)
HUMAN RIGHTS AND MIGRATION
Trafficking for Forced Labour

Global Ethics Series
Series Standing Order ISBN 978–0–230–01958–4
(outside North America only)

You can receive future titles in this series as they are published by placing a standing order. Please contact your bookseller or, in case of difficulty, write to us at the address below with your name and address, the title of the series and the ISBN quoted above.

Customer Services Department, Macmillan Distribution Ltd, Houndmills, Basingstoke, Hampshire RG21 6XS, England

South African AIDS Activism and Global Health Politics

Mandisa Mbali

Lecturer, Department of Sociology and Social Anthropology,
Stellenbosch University, South Africa

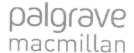

First published 2013 by
PALGRAVE MACMILLAN

Palgrave Macmillan in the UK is an imprint of Macmillan Publishers Limited, registered in England, company number 785998, of Houndmills, Basingstoke, Hampshire RG21 6XS.

Palgrave Macmillan in the US is a division of St Martin's Press LLC, 175 Fifth Avenue, New York, NY 10010.

Palgrave Macmillan is the global academic imprint of the above companies and has companies and representatives throughout the world.

Palgrave® and Macmillan® are registered trademarks in the United States, the United Kingdom, Europe and other countries.

ISBN 978–0–230–36062–4

This book is printed on paper suitable for recycling and made from fully managed and sustained forest sources. Logging, pulping and manufacturing processes are expected to conform to the environmental regulations of the country of origin.

A catalogue record for this book is available from the British Library.

A catalog record for this book is available from the Library of Congress.

10   9   8   7   6   5   4   3   2   1
22 21 20 19 18 17 16 15 14 13

Contents

Figures

Acknowledgements

This book is dedicated to the memory of Simon Tseko Nkoli, Peter Busse, Linda Ngcobo, Chris Moraka and the millions of others taken by AIDS. Ruben Sher passed away, but from other illnesses, while the book was being written – I also wish to acknowledge his contribution to the history of AIDS in South Africa.

My career as a researcher had its origins in my own voluntary AIDS activism, which began in early 1999. I would like to thank several people – in no particular order – for teaching me so much about human rights, democracy and solidarity: Samantha Willan, Annie Devenish, Andy Gibbs, David Carel, Jared Augenstein, Nick DeVito, Helen Jack, Rebecca Hodes, Claire Ichou, Vicci Tallis, Dawn Cavanagh, Ann Ntombela, Kimendhri Pillay, Richard Pithouse, Kathleen Pithouse, Xolani Tsalong and Thabo Cele.

The graduate and postdoctoral research behind this book was rendered possible because of the advice and mentorship of senior colleagues. Catherine Burns at the University of KwaZulu-Natal (UKZN) helped to cement my conviction that historical research on AIDS in South Africa was both possible and necessary. Julie Parle deftly guided me in key theoretical concepts in the history of medicine and archival research methods. I learnt a great deal from William Beinart in relation to South African political history during my time at Oxford. My postdoctoral fellowship at Yale came with the priceless gift of Naomi Rogers's mentorship.

Of course, I take full responsibility for the views expressed in all my writings, but I would like to express my appreciation for the input of numerous colleagues who read and discussed my work and, thereby, contributed to my overall thinking on the project. I am especially indebted to Shula Marks, Lucie Cluver, Adam Habib, John Daniel, Amanda Alexander, Raj Patel, Mark Gevisser, William Gumede, Hakan Thorn, Patrick Bond, Sharad Chari, Keith Breckenridge, Peris Jones, Baruti Amisi, Richard Ballard, Vasu Reddy, Julian May, David Newmarch, Kerry Chance, Marcelle Dawson, Richard McKay, Mark Hunter, Sloan Mahone, Mark Harrison, Karen Brown, Terrence Ranger, Hugh Macmillan, Margaret Pelling, Nicoli Nattrass, Ryan Irwin, Luke Messac, Elizabeth Bradley, Kaveh Khoshnood, Claire Potter, Frank Snowdon, John Warner, Theodore Brown and Steven Robins.

I would like to express my gratitude to each and every person who agreed to be interviewed. In addition to entrusting me with their precious memories, my key informants offered me directions, food, cups of tea and coffee and gave me access to their private papers. They all shared powerful insights about the workings of social justice activism which have remained with me years later.

Throughout my career as a researcher, I have experienced influential intellectual exchanges with several highly professional archivists, including Anthony Manion, Ruth Morgan, Paul Mokgethi, John Meletsi and Busisiwe Khetsi (Gay and Lesbian Memory in Action); Nandipha Miti (COSATU House Archives); Mothomang Diaho and Verne Harris (Nelson Mandela Foundation); all the staff at the ANC Archives at the University of Fort Hare; Sello Hatang, Michelle Pickover, Carol Archibald, Sam Jacob and Judy Seidman (Historical Papers and South African History Archive, University of the Witwatersrand) and Hester van den Bergh (SA Media Project, University of the Free State).

Several trusts and foundations offered me generous scholarships for research travel funding to pursue the project such as the Rhodes Trust, the Beit Fund for Commonwealth History, St Antony's College, Yale University and the South African National Research Foundation (NRF).

Christina Brian, my editor at Palgrave Macmillan, gave me a break for which I will always be grateful.

Over the years, I have particularly treasured the friendship of Priya Lall, Alex Buck, Jeri Hilt, Lina Cherfas, Rebecca Hodes, Berenike and Frank Steffens, Aaron Mertz, Asya Passinsky, Rebecca Wexler, Eva Namusoke-Nsubuga, Allison Gilder, Keon West, Julian Brown, Nick Anthis, James Linscott, Sarah Linscott, Kerry Chance, Elizabeth Dubbeld, Anslyn John, Gustavo Barros de Carvalho, Nancy Odendaal, Andreas Chasomeris, Hannah Karlsson and Michal Singer.

In order for a book to be written, its author must be fed, loved and encouraged. I would like to recognize the kindness of Juliet and Roger Blackburn and Janine Smith during my time at Oxford. Ngaere Macray and David Seeler provided me with greatly appreciated companionship and two heavenly writing retreats in New York. Thandiwe and Rocco Renaldi, Ma-Jali and Jai Henry and Nono and Bheki Twala have also loved me and believed in my ability to complete the book. I will forever cherish my parents, Charlotte and Zolile Mbali, who receive pride of place in my acknowledgements for offering me – and my scholarship – their immeasurable support.

Author's note: All net author royalties will be donated to the Treatment Action Campaign.

A Note on Racial Terms

The fields of contemporary biology and physical anthropology hold that all humans belong to the same species. Race is, rather, a complex and contested socially fashioned phenomenon, which has changed over time. This book does not centrally deal with the history of race or racial politics, in South Africa, but while writing it, I found that referring to racial categories was unavoidable. The concept of race was used by South Africa's ruling class – a matrix of state, business and social institutions – to maintain its hegemony in South Africa for most of the twentieth century. Even in post-apartheid South Africa, racial categories have been used by the state to obtain redress for historically disadvantaged groups.

In the colonial and early apartheid periods, indigenous people were frequently referred to by the state as being 'natives'. Then, the apartheid state took to calling them 'Bantus' in the 1960s to confer a veneer of anthropological credibility on their grand racist scheme. The term 'African' became favoured by African nationalists and their allies from all races from the mid-twentieth century, a development which was concurrent with the rise of the African National Congress (ANC).

South Africa's Population Registration Act of 1950 required state division of the country's populace into the racial categories of 'native', 'coloured', 'white' and 'other' (including 'Indians', a term used for descendants of immigrants from South Asia). The Act used the term 'coloured' to refer to all those who were identified as being racially mixed. From the 1970s, the state started using the term 'black' to refer to Africans. By contrast, the Black Consciousness (BC) movement used the term 'black' in a more inclusive sense from the 1970s, as an affirmative, self-defined term for African, coloured and Indian people and as an alternative to the apartheid term 'non-white'. I use the term 'black' in the book in this BC sense.

Acronyms and Abbreviations

3TC	Lamivudine
AAG	AIDS Advisory Group
ABIGALE	Association of Bisexuals, Gays and Lesbians
ACT UP	AIDS Coalition to Unleash Power
AGM	Annual General Meeting
AIDS	Acquired Immunodeficiency Syndrome
ALP	AIDS Law Project
AMFAR	American Foundation for AIDS Research
ANC	African National Congress
ANCYL	ANC Youth League
ARREPP	African Research and Education in Puppetry Programme, which was also referred to as 'Puppets Against AIDS'
ARV	Antiretroviral (drugs)
ASET	AIDS Support and Educational Trust
ASSA	Actuarial Society of South Africa
AWG	AIDS Working Group of PPHC
AZT	Zidovudine
CADRE	Centre for AIDS and Development Research
CALS	Centre for Applied Legal Studies, University of the Witwatersrand
CAPAB	Cape Town Performing Arts Board
CDC	[US] Centers for Disease Control
CHAI	Clinton Foundation HIV/AIDS Initiative
CHISA	Committee on Health in Southern Africa
CHP	Centre for Health Policy, University of the Witwatersrand
CODESA	Convention for a Democratic South Africa
COSAS	Congress of South African Students
COSATU	Congress of South African Trade Unions
CPT	Cryopreservation Technologies, the manufacturers of Virodene
CPT	Consumer Project on Technology
DA	Democratic Alliance
DNHPD	Department of National Health and Population Development
DOH	Department of Health
DramAidE	Drama in AIDS Education

ECC	End Conscription Campaign
EEC	European Economic Community
ELISA	Enzyme-Linked Immunosorbent Assay
ESG	Emergency Services Group
EU	European Union
FDA	Food and Drug Administration
GALA	Gay and Lesbian Memory in Action (formerly the Gay and Lesbian Archives)
GASA 6010	Gay Association of South Africa – 6010
GASA	Gay Association of South Africa
GCIS	Government Communication and Information System
GEAR	The Growth Employment and Redistribution Strategy
GFATM	Global Fund to Fight AIDS, Tuberculosis and Malaria
GLOW	Gays and Lesbians of the Witwatersrand
GPA	WHO Global Programme on AIDS
Health GAP	Health Global Access Project
HIV	Human Immunodeficiency Virus
HIVNET	HIV Network for Prevention Trials
HRC	Human Rights Commission
HTLVIII-LAV	Human T lymphotropic virus-III (HTLV-III) - Lymphadenopathy-associated virus, an early term for HIV
IDASA	Institute for a Democratic Alternative in South Africa
IFP	Inkatha Freedom Party
ILGA	International Lesbian and Gay Association
IMF	International Monetary Fund
LGBT	Lesbian, Gay, Bisexual and Transgender
MASA	Medical Association of South Africa
MCC	Medicines Control Council
MK	*Umkhonto we Sizwe*, the military wing of the ANC
MRC	Medical Research Council
MSF	*Médicins Sans Frontières* (Doctors Without Borders)
MWT	Marxist Workers' Tendency
NACOSA	National AIDS Convention of South Africa
NAMDA	National Medical and Dental Association
NAPWA	National Association of People living with HIV/AIDS
NIAID	National Institute of Allergy and Infectious Diseases
NIH	National Institutes of Health
NCGLE	National Coalition for Gay and Lesbian Equality
NCOP	National Council of the Provinces
NEC	National Executive Committee
NEDLAC	National Economic Development and Labour Council
NGOs	Non-governmental Organizations
NIH	National Institutes of Health
NNVAW	National Network on Violence Against Women

NPA	National Prosecuting Authority
NPPHCN	National Progressive Primary Health Care Network
NUM	National Union of Mineworkers
OASSA	Organization for Appropriate Social Services in South Africa
OLGA	Organization of Lesbian and Gay Activists
PAC	Pan-Africanist Congress
PEP	Post-Exposure Prophylaxis
PHC	Primary Health Care
PhRMA	Pharmaceutical Research and Manufacturers of America
PMA	Pharmaceutical Manufacturers' Association
PMTCT	Prevention of Mother-to-Child Transmission
PPHC	An alternate acronym for National Progressive Primary Health Care Network
PEPFAR	US President's Emergency Fund for AIDS Relief
PWAs	People living with HIV/AIDS
PWN	Positive Women's Network
RDP	The Reconstruction and Development Programme
RRA	Reproductive Rights Alliance
RSA	Republic of South Africa
SA	South Africa
SAA	South African Airways
SACP	South African Communist Party
SADC	Southern African Development Community
SAHA	South African History Archive
SAIMR	South African Institute for Medical Research
SAIRR	South African Institute for Race Relations
SAMA	South African Medical Association
SAMDC	South African Medical and Dental Council
SAMJ	South African Medical Journal
SANAC	South African National AIDS Council
SCA	Supreme Court of Appeals
SRCs	Student Representative Councils
STDs	Sexually Transmitted Diseases
STIs	Sexually Transmitted Infections
TAC	Treatment Action Campaign
TAG	Treatment Action Group
TAP	Township AIDS Project
TRIPS	Trade-Related aspects of Intellectual Property Agreement
UDF	United Democratic Front
UDHR	Universal Declaration of Human Rights
UNAIDS	Joint United Nations Program on HIV/AIDS
UNGASS	United Nations General Assembly Special Session on the Issue of AIDS

USAID	United States Agency for International Development
WHO	World Health Organization
WNC	Women's National Coalition
WTO	World Trade Organization
YPLA	Young Positive Living Ambassadors

Introduction: South African AIDS Activism and Global Health Justice

On 9 July 2000, activists assembled outside Durban's King's Park stadium, where the first International Conference on Acquired Immunodeficiency Syndrome (AIDS) to be hosted in Africa was about to begin. The sun had set and an historic occasion was coming to an end – the first demonstration for access to treatment for Human Immunodeficiency Virus (HIV) attended by activists from multiple nations. Mark Heywood, one of the leaders of South Africa's Treatment Action Campaign (TAC), addressed the crowd and said, 'Our march today demanding access to treatment is the most broad-based in the twenty year history of the epidemic.' He added that it was made up of thousands of demonstrators from different countries and walks of life, including people living with HIV/AIDS, their family members and friends. His speech urged the South African government to implement a national programme to reduce mother-to-child transmission of HIV without delay.[1] He handed a memorandum to the conference's organizers which noted that there had been 2.6 million AIDS deaths on the African continent in 1999. The memorandum also called for donor countries, the UN and pharmaceutical companies to work towards universal HIV treatment access (Health GAP and TAC 2000). Seven months before, the UN had indicated the extent of the crisis in its 1999 Epidemic Update which estimated that 33.6 million people were living with HIV globally (UNAIDS 1999, p. 3). Members of the audience, who huddled under street lamps, were wearing the South African activists' new purple and white 'HIV POSITIVE' t-shirts. Many also wore fluorescent yellow stickers demanding 'Affordable Treatment Now'!

By 2000, South Africa had undergone its globally renowned political transition which had been catalysed, in no small part, by domestic and transnational anti-apartheid activism. The country had also been reintegrated into the international community, developments which enabled such a large international conference to be held there. But as South Africa made its arresting transition from being a racially segregated, white-ruled nation to a multiracial democracy, the country faced an increasingly serious and entrenched AIDS epidemic. Government hospital wards across the country were increasingly becoming filled with children and young people who were dying from AIDS-related illnesses at a time when HIV could be treated.

Durban, the sub-tropical city hosting the conference, is situated in KwaZulu-Natal, which was at that time South Africa's most heavily AIDS-affected province. Of the total, 32.5% of pregnant women who attended public health facilities for antenatal care in 1999 had been found to be living with HIV, the virus that causes AIDS.[2] The demonstration was held at a time when effective, but expensive, drug cocktails had been available to treat HIV for four years. Due to the high cost of the drugs, combination antiretroviral (ARV) therapy was unavailable to the vast majority of people living with HIV, both within South Africa and across the globe.

The Durban march was the first large demonstration in the life of the new international HIV treatment access movement. Its demands had weighty implications in terms of global health – that is, the health of populations, considered globally. Universal access to the new drug regimens would require a fundamental restructuring of the architecture of the global health institutions and financing.[3] ARV medicines were inaccessible for the world's poor because of international trade and health-aid policies – factors which, in part, lay behind the reality that most South Africans living with HIV lacked access to treatment. Western multinational pharmaceutical companies were suing the government en masse to block it from passing a law to facilitate the domestic production of generic medicines. At the same time, the prevailing consensus among donor governments was that it was not 'cost-effective' to provide ARVs in resource-poor settings. But domestic factors were also blocking wider access to ARVs within South Africa. The country's president, Thabo Mbeki, had recently denied the basic science behind the disease and the efficacy of combination ARV therapy. Indeed, a few months before the Durban conference he had convened a panel to discuss the science on the disease which had included AIDS dissidents – a group of scientists who rejected the mainstream scientific consensus in relation to the diagnosis, causation and treatment of the disease.

At that time, I was an undergraduate student completing a Bachelor's degree in English and History and running an AIDS awareness committee at the University of Natal in Durban – activism which increasingly consumed me. Initially, our work was very basic: we handed out free condoms on campus and urged our fellow students to get tested for the virus. Through our involvement in this local AIDS activism, we started to meet people who were living openly with HIV. They were our age, they often had young children and most of them were relatively healthy-looking young people, all of whom would die an early death from AIDS-related illnesses. Then we read in the newspapers about the new medicines which could keep them alive but which they could not afford and which the government was not providing to them. HIV prevention alone could not save this vast swathe of my generation of South Africans.

For many weeks, members of our committee had been reading newspaper articles about a new social movement called the TAC which was campaigning for the multinational drug firms to drop their court case and for the government to provide the new drugs (ARVs) to prevent mother-to-child transmission of HIV. We were excited at the prospect of finally meeting up with these radical activists from Cape Town and Johannesburg who shared our vision of increased access to the new drugs at the Durban demonstration. Our committee hand-painted and sewed a banner the night before the Durban demonstration saying 'Human Need Over Corporate Greed!'

After the demonstration, once the immediate post-march exhaustion and elation had subsided, many questions occurred to me, some of which are at the heart of this book. What had brought the American, South African and European activists together to demand free AIDS drugs for the world's poor that day? How did the leaders of the South African movement know each other and their international counterparts? How did such a new movement get such a large and diverse group of people to show up for a demonstration on such a controversial issue? And, I wondered, how long had the older activists been involved in activism and how had their prior advocacy shaped their current work?

What I learnt through many years of participant observation, oral history interviews with activists and reading relevant media coverage and organizational records was that the TAC was led by seasoned social justice advocates with a history of prior involvement in various forms of anti-apartheid activism. In most cases their engagements in such activism had stretched back to the 1970s and 1980s. The participation of these activists in the TAC was crucial because it enabled it and its international allies to characterize what the drug companies were doing as a form of global medical apartheid. Within South Africa, the 'progressive' (anti-apartheid) background of some of the TAC's top leaders also enabled them to effectively frame their demand for a government ARV roll-out as motivated by humanitarian concerns rather than party-political agendas, that is, by general political opposition to the ruling African National Congress (ANC).

About this book

In this book I offer a history of AIDS activism in South Africa from its origins in gay and anti-apartheid activism to first five years of the TAC, including its formation, consolidation and central role in the international HIV treatment access movement. I start out by describing gay and lesbian and progressive healthworker non-governmental organizations' (NGOs) advocacy responses to the AIDS epidemic shortly after its emergence in South Africa in 1982. I then analyse how changes to the state following the political transition altered AIDS activism and created the political conditions necessary for South African activists to form influential alliances with their counterparts abroad: a process which I refer to as the *transnationalisation* of South African AIDS activism. The book ends in 2003 when key elements of the movement's moral authority were in place and its international influence was at a peak. I decided to focus on advocacy related to the epidemic in this 'early period' in order to understand political, social and intellectual continuities and changes between anti-apartheid and AIDS activism in South Africa. In addition, I wished to describe the ways in which South African AIDS activists formed transnational alliances over time. While South African anti-apartheid, gay rights and AIDS activism have been examined separately in scholarly texts, the book is distinctive in the longer, historical view it offers of the country's AIDS activism and also in its focus on how gender and sexuality-based anti-apartheid activism shaped the TAC's formation, consolidation and its internationally impactful moral claims.

The book's main argument is that the TAC contributed a uniquely South African form of moral legitimacy to the international HIV treatment access movement. Furthermore, I argue that the TAC's international legitimacy was based upon its leaders' past involvement in anti-apartheid activism, its popularization and defence of AIDS-related science and its strategic use of arguments based on the socio-economic right to access to health care. The TAC's legitimacy abroad matters in the political history of global health because it enabled the South African activists to effectively challenge dominant local and international policy paradigms which were hostile to universal HIV treatment access in collaboration with foreign allies such as Médecins Sans Frontières (MSF), the Health Global Access Project (Health GAP) and Oxfam. This transnationalisation of South African AIDS activism was enabled by the end of the international academic boycott against the country following its political transition and was motivated by a desire to correct global disparities in access to the new, effective HIV treatment regimens.

This book is divided into two parts: AIDS Activism and South Africa's Transition; and, The TAC and Global Health Politics. It is bisected into these two parts to reflect its dual analytic focus on

- How AIDS activists' political thinking changed across a period when the South African state was radically re-made.
- Their later cultivation of international alliances.

Part I of the book largely deals with domestic, rights-based AIDS advocacy by anti-apartheid activists, which was conducted at a time when the state was emerging from international isolation and negotiating a democratic transition. By contrast, Part II, discusses the TAC's formation and consolidation in a period where it deployed new legal strategies enabled by the state's remoulding into a constitutional democracy. It also describes the South African activists' impactful contribution to the international HIV treatment access movement, which led to a re-fashioning of critical global health policies on AIDS.

Part I AIDS Activism and South Africa's Transition

The South African state underwent fundamental changes in the first half of the 1990s, with critical implications for AIDS activism in the country. AIDS emerged in South Africa in the 1980s – a period when anti-apartheid activists' central political concern was ending the country's segregationist, authoritarian political system. Despite their competing and compelling over-arching anti-apartheid political goals, various groups of 'progressive' activists began working on AIDS from the late 1980s, including those affiliated with healthworker, gay rights and women's groups. This diverse group of activists formed an advocacy network which drafted the first National AIDS Plan (NAP) in collaboration with the government, a rights-based document which emphasized patients' autonomy and privacy. In the first half of the 1990s, the South African state underwent a transition which had critical implications for AIDS activism in the country. Its new constitution (1996) enshrined the socio-economic right to access to health care and the rights to non-discrimination on the grounds of gender and sexual orientation. South Africa's dramatic re-emergence into the 'family of nations' also laid the basis for more extensive contact and collaboration between AIDS activists from different countries.

Progressive (anti-apartheid) healthworkers saw patients living with HIV from the early 1980s. They adhered to the older idea of 'primary health care', which influenced their thinking on AIDS, as Chapter 1 describes. Exiled anti-apartheid epidemiologists based in the United States such as Mervyn Susser and Zena Stein advocated for the ANC and allied progressive organizations based within South Africa to act to prevent a major HIV epidemic at the Maputo Conference. The National Party government wanted to hold an International AIDS Conference in South Africa in the early 1990s, but progressive healthworkers vetoed this as being in violation of the academic boycott of the country. Instead, in the transition-era spirit of compromise, they co-hosted the first National AIDS Convention of South Africa (NACOSA) which led to the creation of the first National AIDS Plan (NAP). As the political transition progressed, South Africa was reintegrated into the international community, which facilitated the provision of technical assistance by the WHO in the drafting of the human rights-inclusive NAP. But a flawed plan emerged from this inclusive drafting process: it lacked clear timetables and a detailed budget, and so it proved difficult to implement.

The first two South Africans identified with AIDS were diagnosed in 1982: they were both white gay men. In the 1980s, most gay organizations in the country were white dominated, and their membership was divided on how to deal with apartheid. By contrast, in the transition era, new multiracial, anti-apartheid lesbian and gay groups effectively exploited the political opportunities presented by the country's transition to promote sexual orientation equality, as Chapter 2 describes. There was significant cross-pollination between the twin struggles for equality for gay and lesbian people and for HIV prevention and an end to unfair AIDS-related discrimination. Both involved greater openness about stigmatized identities: the first gay pride march was held, and some gay rights activists began to reveal that they were living with HIV. Many also attended Linda Ngcobo's political AIDS funeral – perhaps the first in the country. While it was human rights-based, such early gay AIDS activism focused on 'negative' rights such as the right to privacy. The Organization of Lesbian and Gay Activists (OLGA), the Gay and Lesbian Organization of the Witwatersrand (GLOW) and the Association of Bisexuals, Gays and Lesbians (ABIGALE) were successful in lobbying for the new Constitution to contain a clause outlawing discrimination on the grounds of sexual orientation. This remoulding of the South African state freed up some gay rights activists' time and energy such that they could increasingly focus on AIDS-related advocacy.

But these historic changes to the South African state did not equally empower all groups who were vulnerable to HIV-infection to challenge AIDS-related discrimination. The South African women's movement was at its apex in the early-to-mid-1990s. It was also successful in reshaping the South African state via advocacy, which led to the inclusion of the right to gender non-discrimination in the Final Constitution's equality clause and the creation of the 'gender machinery'. Yet, the South African women's movement's response to AIDS was very circumscribed, especially by comparison with that of the lesbian and gay movement, which meant that neither it nor its international allies came to play a role in the founding and consolidation of the TAC. Over the 1990s, most new infections occurred in women. Some feminist publications covered the epidemic, but most women's politicization around it was deferred because they did not identify with the issue because of their limited visibility in early AIDS-related epidemiology and mainstream media coverage of it. Moreover, what little coverage the epidemic's impact on women received in South African medical journals and newspapers in the late 1980s and early 1990s was generative of sexist AIDS-related prejudice. This meant that women such as Gugu Dlamini, Prudence Mabele and Promise Mthembu who were diagnosed as HIV-positive in the early-to-mid-1990s did not initially encounter AIDS organizations which provided safe spaces for them to discuss their gender-specific experiences as women living with the disease.

Part II The TAC and Global Health Politics

A group of radical South African AIDS activists established a new movement called the TAC which called for wider access to the new drugs. American AIDS activists assisted the TAC in developing its transnationally influential 'treatment literacy' programme. The TAC successfully deployed socio-economic rights-based arguments in court to force the pharmaceutical industry to reduce the prices of the drugs and the government to begin providing them, a strategy which was studied overseas. Its international allies expressed solidarity for the movement by replicating its demands in relation to the South African government at important venues abroad, including outside its embassies and at the international AIDS conferences. Foreign governments and intergovernmental institutions upheld several barriers to treatment access, which necessitated the TAC's collaboration with their international allies. Charismatic TAC leader Zackie Achmat's anti-apartheid background and the support of Nelson Mandela meant that the movement's international allies could credibly refer to global inequity in access to medicines using the metaphor of 'medical apartheid'. The TAC became a cause célèbre in the international media because it represented a large number of the people who lacked access to HIV medicines around the world. By the end of the period, transnational activist pressure had led to dramatic falls in the prices of first-line ARV drugs (medicines frequently used in patients' initial regimens) and unprecedented sums of development aid being distributed globally for HIV treatment.

Sexuality and science-based treatment advocacy networks played a vital role in the formation of the TAC, as I argue in Chapter 4. AIDS activists' previously warm relationships with progressive health activists who had gone into government quickly soured over the *Sarafina II*, Virodene and notification (compulsory case reporting) scandals. Achmat, of the National Coalition for Gay and Lesbian Equality (NCGLE), corresponded with other gay rights activists arguing that their lives were becoming expendable. A group of activists linked to the Coalition, the ALP and the AIDS Consortium coalesced around Achmat to collectively found the TAC as a campaign of the National Association of People Living With HIV/AIDS (NAPWA). The two organizations rapidly parted company owing to disagreements over political strategies and tactics and how to deal with the AIDS-stigma-motivated murder of NAPWA activist Gugu Dlamini. In its first two years, the TAC worked with foreign AIDS and medical humanitarian activist-allies to increase public understanding of HIV treatment, activities which were especially necessary given President Mbeki's adoption of AIDS dissidence from 1999. Its American allies helped the TAC to design its national treatment literacy programme, and it co-founded a clinic with MSF in Khayalitsha, Cape Town to save lives and demonstrate that treatment could be provided in such resource-poor settings.

In its first few years, the TAC was overwhelmingly focused on advocacy for the multinational pharmaceutical companies to drop their court case against the Mandela administration which was aimed at blocking access to both cheaper imported brand-name medicines and generics, as Chapter 5 describes. It fashioned a formidable transnational alliance for the industry association to drop its lawsuit. The TAC's Chris Moraka Defiance Campaign (2000–1) used struggle symbolism, which lent the movement moral legitimacy, especially given that many of its members had anti-apartheid backgrounds. Its media-savvy campaign was conducted in tandem with global allies, and it positioned the pharmaceutical industry as manipulating trade agreements which created a global medical apartheid in which the world's poor could not enjoy the fruits of drug research. The TAC's international allies concurrently challenged utilitarian reasoning and the singular focus on prevention, which was then dominant among governments, foundations and public health experts in the global North. South Africa's HIV treatment access movement also engaged in a sophisticated legal strategy when it applied to be made an *amicus curiae* in the case. In its legal papers, it presented arguments against the industry's litigation which were based upon the 'positive' socio-economic right to access to health care which was contained in South Africa's new Constitution.

The TAC used the law strategically yet again when it took the Mbeki administration to court to force it to provide Nevirapine for the Prevention of Mother-To-Child Transmission (PMTCT) of HIV on a universal basis, litigation described in Chapter 6. AIDS denialism lay at the core of the government's reluctance to comprehensively provide the drug in the public sector of the health system. South Africa's AIDS movement argued its case for the universal provision of Nevirapine for PMTCT on the basis of the right to access to health care. Their case's success rested on proving that the government's policy had failed the test of 'reasonableness' adopted by the Constitutional Court to assess the state's socio-economic rights obligations: expert testimony defending the science behind Nevirapine was critical to this favourable outcome.

However, some feminists argued that the TAC's counsel did not comprehensively assert women's reproductive rights. They have also subsequently criticized the movement for failing to adequately confront its internal sexism, critiques which hold some validity in relation to an issue which the movement would only fully tackle after the main period under discussion.

Mandela lent his powerful struggle symbolism to the movement when he offered it his support and, thereby, strengthened its domestic credibility. International solidarity for the TAC grew as foreign activists held vocal and colourful demonstrations in support of the movement outside South African embassies in several countries. In 2003, the movement forced the South African government to adopt a national treatment plan through its second civil disobedience campaign. The implementation of this plan was aided by the lower drug prices the TAC negotiated with two pharmaceutical companies following an anti-trust complaint at the Competition Commission, a strategy which was later copied by allies in other countries.

Before the Barcelona International AIDS Conference (2002), Achmat's refusal to take ARVs before they were readily available to all South Africans was garnering international media attention and added a sense of moral urgency to the cause of universal HIV treatment access. As Chapter 7 shows, in rich countries, the international HIV treatment access movement's campaigns were one of several factors which generated unprecedented levels of political will and foreign development aid for access to ARV medicines in developing countries. In 2001, the United Nations held its first general assembly special session on the issue of AIDS (UNGASS). A new Global Fund was created which started offering very large grants in April 2002 to dramatically expand access to HIV treatment, internationally.

Similarly, partly as a result of activist pressure on access to essential medicines, the World Trade Organisation (WTO) produced the Doha Declaration, which was aimed at clarifying wording in the TRIPS agreement. The Doha Declaration was a significant step forward in the international recognition of the impacts patent-strengthening free trade agreements could have on human health. The Declaration also strengthened the hand of middle-income, generic-ARV-producing countries like Brazil in negotiating with pharmaceutical companies for cheaper drugs.

Another major significant advance came from an entirely different – and surprising – source. In January 2003, George W. Bush announced the formation of the multi-billion dollar US President's Emergency Fund for AIDS Relief (PEPFAR), a development which emanated from advocacy by elite, conservative civil society groups. This shows that there were also sources of influence abroad other than the largely left-wing international HIV treatment access movement.

This book does not merely offer a narrative timeline of events in South African AIDS activism's past: it also reflects upon the ways in which important general principles have increasingly become central to discussions on global health among academics and in policy circles. In the sections of this introduction which follow, I identify some key terms and debates in global health which emerge in the book with reference to various bodies of relevant specialist literature. General readers may wish to skip to the conclusion of this introduction (p. 22), as I explain these concepts as they emerged in activist campaigns and discussions throughout the main part of the book.

The transnationalisation of South African AIDS activism

My analysis of the transnationalisation of South African AIDS activism sits at the intersection between literatures dealing with social movements and 'constructivist' international relations theory. In this sense, I am intellectually indebted to the work of sociologist Sidney Tarrow, and throughout the book I use the term 'transnational activists' in the way he has, that is, to describe 'individuals and groups who mobilize domestic and international resources and opportunities to advance claims on behalf of external actors [actors in another country], against external opponents [opponents abroad], or in favor of goals they hold in common with transnational allies' (2005, p. 29). I have chosen to use the terms 'transnational activism' and 'transnational activists' to describe advocacy which is conducted and coordinated in multiple countries simultaneously. This is because, like Tarrow, I deem use of the adjective 'transnational', to be more appropriate than the term 'global' to describe the work of the most cross-border activism, including that of the international treatment access movement, which cannot be said to have involved activists from all the world's countries.

In this book I use the term 'social movement' in relation to the TAC in the sense suggested by Sidney Tarrow to describe 'collective [social] challenges based on common purposes and social solidarities in sustained interaction with elites, opponents and authorities' (1998, p. 4). 'Activism' is used throughout the book to indicate ideological or policy-oriented collective political action by people in 'civil society' – that is the non-state, non-family, non-profit, partially voluntary sector of society (Cohen and Arato 1992; Habib 2003). Throughout the book I use the term 'moral capital' interchangeably with moral legitimacy. 'Moral capital' is deployed in the manner of Christopher Brown, historian of British Abolitionism, to describe how a civil society campaign framed a policy as unethical in a manner which was politically impactful and which offered ordinary individuals effective advocacy opportunities (2007, p. 29).

The South African government's opposition to the TAC stemmed from Mbeki's adoption of AIDS dissidence (which was also referred to by domestic critics as his 'denialism'). There were, however, also international barriers to the South African government widening access to treatment in the country. American and European bilateral aid agencies and the World Bank also dismissed the idea of universal access to HIV treatment, but they did so on different grounds, such as the idea that it was not a 'cost-effective' use of limited health budgets or the argument that it was culturally inappropriate in 'underdeveloped' African settings (Behrman 2004; Jones 2004). In the 1990s, American trade policy was significantly influenced by the interests of the pharmaceutical industry and, therefore, the US Trade Representative (USTR) and Vice-President Al Gore opposed demands for wider access to generic medicines (Smith and Siplon 2006; Lawson 2008).

However, the book certainly does deal with the concept of 'the global': indeed, a thread running through it is how the transnational activists came to campaign on AIDS as a global health issue. 'Global health' is a term which has been used to describe the study of the health of the population of the entire planet rather than that of particular nations (Benatar and Brock 2011). The older term 'international health' dates back to the late nineteenth century, and it has been used to describe institutions and measures which have focused on containing the cross-border spread of epidemics (Harrison 2004; Brown et al. 2006). The trend of using the term 'global health' instead of 'international health' to describe health across borders can be traced back to the late 1990s and relates to the intensified globalization which was noted by public health scholars and practitioners in the period (Brown et al. 2006). The new concept of global health aimed to take account of the overall health implications of globalization, understood as the accelerated movement of goods, people, capital and ideas through innovations in information technology and telecommunications (especially, the Internet). AIDS can be said to be a classic global health issue for two reasons. Firstly, the AIDS pandemic can be cast as global in nature because cases have been indentified in all regions of the world. Secondly, its international spread has been fundamentally influenced by globalization.

Transnational activists, such as those in the TAC, can be distinguished from their counterparts whose work was purely local in nature because the movement presented its demands in both domestic and international venues. I argue that two of the theories Tarrow puts forward, outlining how domestic and international activism can become fused in transnational activism are applicable to the TAC's cross-border work. Firstly, it 'externalized' *domestic claims* about the prices of drugs onto *international institutions* such as the World Trade Organization (WTO) and multinational pharmaceutical corporations based in the global North (2005, p. 32).[4] Secondly, there was a *cross-border* 'diffusion' of the TAC's signature forms of *collective action* such as foreign activists wearing its 'HIV POSITIVE' t-shirts abroad. This diffusion of tactics was not, however, unidirectional: the TAC also drew on, and developed, the methods of a group of Americans Steven Epstein has called AIDS 'activist-experts' to design its HIV treatment literacy programme (1996, p. 8). The South Africans, therefore, lent to, and borrowed from, the unified repertoire of the international HIV treatment access movement.

Another way of conceptualizing the transnational elements of TAC's work is that it was an example of 'activism beyond borders' (Keck and Sikkink 1998). In this sense, the international HIV treatment access movement is a classic example of a late twentieth and early twenty-first century transnational advocacy network, where activists based in different countries shared resources, information and, most importantly, expressed solidarity for one another. Margaret Keck and Kathryn Sikkink have usefully conceptualized such international solidarity as aimed at creating a 'boomerang pattern of influence', where activists facing domestic repression search for foreign (state and non-state) allies to advocate for their governments to alter the relevant, disputed policies (1998, p. 12).

TAC activism, like much popular politics, was rooted in domestic grievances: most of the movement's members were either working class, or unemployed, township-based activists who could neither purchase the drugs they needed for themselves and their families, nor obtain them at state health facilities. The pharmaceutical industry's case against the Mandela administration (1998–2001) and the TAC activists' contact with their counterparts based in the global North made them aware of some of the global phenomena behind this state of affairs. In this regard, Tarrow has noted that when activists frame their demands in global terms it can 'dignify and generalize claims that might otherwise remain narrow and parochial' (2005, p. 76).

This book's emphasis on the role of norms (ethical values) in the international system situates it within the constructivist school of international relations. Constructivism arose as a body of thought which critiqued neorealist approaches to understanding international relations, which had their heyday during the Cold War. Neorealists view the international system as being conflict prone and anarchic, in that it lacks a central authority to control states' actions (Gilpin 1986; Waltz 1986). In a neorealist account of international relations, the international system is, therefore, a 'self-help system' where states act to maximize the realization of their own material interests – that is, to amass economic and military power (Waltz 1986, p. 101). For neorealists, states do, and should, advance their own national interests; by contrast they find norms largely irrelevant to the question how states conduct, or should conduct, their foreign policy (Gilpin 1986). By contrast, constructivists hold that many of the global norms in the international system are socially fashioned (or 'constructed'). Differently put, they believe that the 'intersubjective' nature of the international system influences how states understand themselves and their interests (Klotz 1995; Finnemore 1996; Wendt 1999). For constructivists, international norms (which are social structures) influence, and are influenced by, how states see themselves (and their material interests). It also follows that in a constructivist schema, *non-state actors* – who lack the material resources of states – still matter in the international system, because norms, which civil society can influence, have an impact upon states' framing of their interests (Keck and Sikkink 1998).

The constructivist approach I adopt in the book is also revealed by my use of the term 'global health governance' to describe interconnected institutions and social sectors' roles in making and implementing international health policy since the 1990s (Hein et al. 2007; Rushton and Williams 2011). I use 'global health governance' in relation to the policy actions of intergovernmental, private sector and civil society actors. By contrast I deploy the term 'global health diplomacy' to describe the global health policy making which occurs in the interactions between states: as evident in bilateral initiatives such as the US President's Emergency Fund for AIDS Relief (PEPFAR).

But it is also important to note that transnational human rights activism is of a relatively recent historical vintage: the first modern statement comprehensively outlining them was the Universal Declaration of Human Rights (1948). Human rights should be seen as perhaps one of the last globally influential, universalistic utopian schemes, and their rise in international politics ought to be viewed against the exhaustion of Third World nationalism and socialism as internationalist projects (Moyn 2010). Amnesty International (AI) is often cited as the classic example of transnational human rights activism in that it has aimed to influence actors in the international system by means of generating, protecting and wielding its ethical authority in relation to a set of issues (Hopgood 2006). The South African activists played an important role in the global political history of AIDS because of the AI-like ethical heft they lent to the international HIV treatment access movement, which, in turn, shifted foreign governments and pharmaceutical companies' HIV treatment-related policies.

This book is not the first publication to discuss either the international HIV treatment access movement or transnational elements of the TAC's work. Indeed, it builds upon a rich and growing body of writing on the history of transnational AIDS activism. Raymond Smith and Patricia Siplon have discussed the formation and early years of Health GAP in their book *Drugs into Bodies*, which also describes elements of the international HIV treatment access movement (2006). But, by virtue of their topic – American AIDS activists – their work only briefly mentions the transnational activism of the TAC.

Eduard Grebe has mapped the TAC's 'transnational networks of influence' consisting of local and international AIDS activists, scientists and clinicians and members of South Africa's political elite and civil servants (2008). This book differs from Grebe's work because it highlights the TAC's intellectual and political contribution of 'moral capital' to the international HIV treatment access movement, a contribution which, as I show, helped to drive important changes to global health governance and diplomacy.

Jennifer Brier's *Infectious Ideas* offers a detailed history of how AIDS influenced US politics, including activism, in the late twentieth century (2009). In the book's final chapter, Brier compares the TAC's work in South Africa with American AIDS activism. She characterizes the TAC and its trade union ally, the Congress of South African Trade Unions (COSATU), as having been more effective in challenging economic injustice in relation to medicine than their American counterparts. Her work differs from this volume because it does not analyse contact and collaboration between activists in both countries – and, in a wider sense, the TAC's contribution to the international HIV treatment access movement. This is because it mostly deals with a period (the 1980s) before US AIDS activists had developed substantial links with their South African counterparts.

The book's focus on the transnationalisation of South African AIDS activism adds an important dimension to the historiography (body of written history) on AIDS in Africa, which, to date, has not focused upon how globalization affected patient-led health advocacy on the issue on the continent (Iliffe 2006; Epstein 2007; Lawson 2008). Its narration of transnational activists' influence on global health means that it wades into the waters of what has been termed as global, or transnational, history. Global, or transnational, histories offer a new approach to the writing of history, and they generally either explore transnational contact between people across borders or compare events in different countries in the same period (O'Brien 2006).

There is some debate among historians on the differences between, and relative merits of, 'global' versus 'transnational' history. While I am less concerned with the finer points of the distinctions between global and transnational history, elements of this debate can shed light on the potential benefits and pitfalls of writing cross-border histories, including those which I faced in writing this book. Since the early 1990s, proponents of 'transnational history' have argued that it can counteract the exceptionalism and isolation which they view as frequently having characterized more traditional national histories (Tyrell 1991; Saunier 2008).

The emergence of the concept of 'global history' is frequently dated back to the 1990s when economists and activists began to deliberate on the merits of globalization. For this reason critics have associated global history with an activist scholarship which they view as underemphasizing the differences between countries in the global South (Bayly et al. 2006). For these reasons, the term 'transnational history' has been favoured by some historians who study 'how people and ideas and institutions and cultures moved above, below, through and around, as well as within the nation state' (Thelen 1999, p. 967). Transnational history also often focuses heavily on themes such as: the translation, circulation and exchange of ideas; immigration; and diasporas and transnational social networks, including those composed of non-governmental organizations or activists in different countries (Hofmeyr 2004; Iriye 2004; Bayly et al. 2006; Saunier 2008).

In the light of this literature, this book has been informed by the need to be attentive to political differences between countries in the global South (as expressed, for instance, in Brazil and South Africa's divergent ARV drug policies). Like several other transnational histories it also places an emphasis on the circulation and exchange of ideas between activists based in different countries – for instance, between American and South African activists in relation to treatment literacy.

But it is also important to recognize that there are different challenges and rewards to writing transnational histories which focus on different regions of the world. Some historians who are unfamiliar with African historiographies might find my approach of merging methods taken from the disciplines of anthropology and history – as exemplified in my occasional inclusion of myself in the narrative I offer – unusual. However, it is more common among those who consider their work fall within the interdisciplinary rubric of African Studies.

Historical anthropologists of Africa have challenged older ideas in their discipline that non-Western cultures were static or closed and a tendency to overlook the impact of colonialism on these societies (Comaroff and Comaroff 1997). Scholars of Africa who produce historical anthropological studies conduct both archival research and ethnographic fieldwork – the latter of which involves testing their observations about the beliefs of those they study against their own cultural assumptions and experiences

(Comaroff and Comaroff 1992, 1997; Hunter 2010). Since the late 1960s, anthropologists, mindful of the history of their own discipline, have wrestled a great deal with the problem of 'positionality' – that is, how their own social positions and cultural backgrounds affect their interpretations of the cultures which they study (Clifford 1988; Stocking 1992). Some of these anthropologists have also fairly frequently referred to themselves in their texts (Abu-Lughod 2008). This approach can prove valuable, not least because informants sometimes frame the stories and perspectives they share, bearing in mind the person studying them. In my case, my history of volunteering as a feminist and AIDS activist on campuses where I had studied certainly helped me to gain the trust of several key informants and, also, doubtless shaped what they told me. I would, however, also like to clarify that this work is not designed as a memoir, but rather offers a narrative describing the formation of advocacy networks, some of which I participated in, as a marginal actor towards the end of the period I discuss in this book.

Likewise, historians of Africa have frequently moved beyond the archival records to seek out Africa's past by gathering and assessing oral testimony (Curtin 1969; Harms 1987; Bozzoli and Nkotsoe 1991).[5] Many have found this type of approach especially fruitful on a continent which was, until at least the precolonial era and arguably still is in the present, dominated by orality (Appiah 1992; Wiredu 1998; Draper 2003; Gunner 2004). Obtaining credible oral accounts through semi-structured interviews frequently involves building trust with key informants, something which I have found can often only be accomplished after spending time with them in various settings over time, in a manner which is virtually indistinguishable from participant observation, which is a key ethnographic method. I learned a great deal about the history of South African AIDS activism which was never written down, partly because I studied organizations and a movement which represented poor and marginalized people and dealt with a stigmatized sexually transmitted disease.

AIDS activism was certainly not the first type of transnational human rights-based advocacy in African, or South African, history. Indeed, sociologist Hakan Thorn has usefully pointed out that the anti-apartheid movements in Europe were part of an 'emerging global civil society during the post-war era' (2006, p. 5). The anti-apartheid movement was also active in campaigning against apartheid health policies (Digby 2008). Alongside the newly independent African states, European and American anti-apartheid activists used every international forum at their disposal to decry the various forms of systematic, health-related racism – indeed, they denounced segregated hospitals, the radically differing life-expectancies of Africans and whites and systematic racial discrimination against black healthworkers (as discussed in Chapter 1). Exiled South African anti-apartheid healthworkers became concerned about AIDS either by virtue of being based in heavily affected countries, or because of their professional interest in the epidemic. These exiles organized a conference for 'progressive healthworkers' in Maputo, Mozambique. South Africa was Africa's richest country in the 1990s, and it had a serious, and growing, AIDS epidemic. But anti-apartheid healthworkers were vigorous in their defence of the academic boycott of the country, and so it only became a venue for an International AIDS Conference in 2000.

Activism and ethics in global health politics

The book also contributes to an evolving literature on global health ethics by providing a case study of how activists in a middle-income developing country contributed to thinking on health norms in ways which radically changed the politics of global health, as expressed in international health governance and diplomacy. In this sense, the book describes the transnational exchange of ideas about the right to health between AIDS activists based in different countries, pharmaceutical industry representatives and international civil servants. These cross-border debates on the right to health have shaped, and been shaped by, those in academia over global health ethics: or, more precisely in this instance, what constitutes social justice in relation to global health. This global health ethics literature has generally been produced by scholars based in the global North who come from the disciplines of political philosophy and law (Pogge 2002; Benatar et al. 2003; Gostin and Taylor 2008; Lowry and Schüklenk 2009). As such, it has generally not described the contribution of activists based in middle-income countries such as South Africa to ethical thinking in relation to global health governance and diplomacy.[6] With its focus on the development of a transnational social movement in a heavily affected middle-income developing country, the book points to the agency of poor and marginalized people in advocating for their rights through a multiracial, multi-class, globally influential coalition.

Global health ethics is a comparatively new area of scholarly inquiry (Daniels 2011). This may be related to the relative novelty of institutions such as the Global Fund and the very discipline of 'global health'. David Hunter and Angus J. Dawson have provided a good working definition of global health ethics as concerned with 'global injustice in regard to health, motivated by existing historical wrongs characteristic of global trade, structural global inequalities, [and] inequalities in global power' (2011, p. 78). The term 'justice' is used in this literature to describe distributive, or social, justice; that is, fair allocations of benefits and burdens in society. The policy debates which the transnational AIDS activists participated in generally revolved around two main accounts of global health justice: a neoliberal version, emphasizing market-based delivery of medical products and health services; and a 'right to health' approach, emphasizing health equity and the decommoditization of health services.

I use the terms 'neoliberal' and 'neoliberalism' in the manner of human geographer David Harvey to describe an approach to economics which is anti-inflationary, union weakening and industry-deregulation-focused and which became globally hegemonic from the late 1970s. Harvey has crisply described the doctrine as the idea that 'human well-being can best be advanced by liberating individual entrepreneurial freedoms and skills within an institutional framework characterized by strong property rights, free markets and free trade' (2005, p. 2). Neoliberals hold that markets, when left alone, are efficient at setting prices and create the correct incentives for productivity and increased prosperity. It was in the context of the neoliberalism's rise that health-sector privatization, cost recovery and free-market-promoting health aid became dominant in international health in the 1980s (Birn et al. 2009). By contrast, older, more equity-promoting concepts such as primary health care and essential medicines fell by the wayside (Brown et al. 2006). A related development was that the patent-strengthening Trade-Related Aspects of Intellectual Property Rights (TRIPS) agreement (1994) was annexed to that which created the World Trade Organization (WTO). As the activists argued, the WTO TRIPS agreement had far-reaching implications in terms of access to medicines.

Right-wing libertarianism holds that an individual's personal liberty, including their right to private property, trumps the promotion of social justice via redistribution (Nozick 1974). This brand of libertarianism is closely allied to neoliberalism. Moreover, such libertarianism was in evidence in the Medicines Act case (1998–2001), where the pharmaceutical industry claimed that their property rights as corporate persons superseded the poor patients' rights to access to health care. But these arguments held less sway in South Africa where the right to access to health care was justiciable (a right upon which judges could rule), as the activists successfully argued, demonstrating their effective role as political advocates for global health justice. Thomas Pogge has argued for a cosmopolitan extension of John Rawls's (nation-state-focused) theory of justice: that the rules of global society should be re-structured so as to benefit the least well-off around the world (2002). Pogge's critique of Nozick's work hinges on his assumption that all private property was fairly acquired. Instead, Pogge argues, the globally unequal distribution of capital is frequently the consequence of morally tarnished and, at times illegal, past processes of resource allocation, including slavery, colonialism and plunder by dictators. He then goes on to argue that governments of industrialized countries have both positive ethical obligations to benefit others and, even stronger, negative duties not to harm others and to provide restitution in instances where they have already been malfeasant towards the world's poor (2002).

A central ethical tension in health policy is generated by the fact that the budgetary resources for its implementation are inherently limited: even in instances where the state is the only service provider, health expenditure cannot be allowed to completely 'crowd-out' governments' uses of public purses for other critical priorities such as education, social services and environmental protection. From the late 1970s, as policy makers became increasingly enamoured with neoliberal approaches to health policy, utilitarian schemes to ration health spending using cost-utility or cost-benefit analyses grew in popularity, globally. Utilitarianism has been a central idea in public health since its earliest days (Rosen 1993; Porter 1999; Harrison 2004). It is a consequentialist (consequence-focused) ethical approach which aims for the maximization of positive value (utility), which, in the earliest articulations of the theory, was initially defined in terms of happiness (Bentham 2003). Cost-effectiveness-based utilitarianism influenced the history outlined in this book, because it was a common thread in the dominant consensus among donors who were generally opposed to the provision of HIV medicines in developing countries on the grounds that it was 'unaffordable'. Chapter 6 describes AIDS activists' efforts to counteract this type of rhetoric, arguing that it failed to take into account the human right to health. There have been many critiques of such a utilitarian, cost-effectiveness approach, the most trenchant being that while it considers aggregate welfare it can lead to unfair distributions of benefits and burdens in societies (Ruger 2009). For instance, cost-effectiveness-based, utilitarian approaches often limit the poor's access to care (Beauchamp and Childress p. 348). Measures such as Disability Adjusted Life Years (DALYs) can also lead to the needs of the sickest and the disabled being overlooked (Anand and Hanson 2004; Brock 2004).

Instead, Jennifer Prah Ruger has proposed an alternative, health capabilities approach, which defends the right to health and which draws on Amartya Sen's capabilities approach to poverty reduction (2009). Sen has argued that substantive freedom consists of our capabilities to choose lives we have 'reason to value' (1999, p. 74). Development, in Sen's account, cannot be reduced to redistributing income, because it should consist of policies that enable people to be free to choose to achieve various lifestyles they have reason to value (1999, p. 75). Ruger draws on Sen's work to build a case for a policy focus on health functionings, a phenomenon which can be measured in terms of things like life expectancy, infant and child mortality and disease burden (2009, p. 77). The implementation of a health capability paradigm should address health needs, and revolve around what health (or ill health) allows us to choose and achieve in life, as opposed to our individual preferences (which we may not have reason to value) or arbitrary cost-effectiveness measures. A health capabilities approach requires the redistribution of resources in society to meet the needs of those who cannot afford health care (2009, p. 123). Such an approach was in evidence in the TAC's advocacy. The TAC activists were mindful of the fact that the realization of the right to health care services for people living with HIV would enhance their educational, workplace, social, sexual and reproductive choices – that, on a fundamental level, there was little meaningful choice or freedom for patients who experienced preventable serious illnesses or death.

AIDS activism and state transformation in South Africa

In addition to my focus on the TAC's geographic reach, I contend that in order to understand the South African movement's politics, we have to analyse it with some historical depth – i.e. in relation to the intertwined histories of anti-apartheid and AIDS activism within the country. In asserting this, I am not arguing for an intellectually unbroken line of political thinking from the liberation movement to the TAC. The epidemic's coincidental emergence in the dying days of apartheid meant that South African AIDS activists were trying to influence a changing state. Instead, I highlight the instances where activists' prior connections with each other and resonances of political morality from the past proved significant in shaping the movement's strategies and tactics.

I use the term 'networks' to discuss the TAC's intellectual and social history in a manner which draws upon an extensive sociological literature on social movements, which was developed in the global North. This literature points to the fact that networks enable movements to recruit those who identify closely with the contentious issues they are aiming to address and enable them to rapidly exploit political opportunities when they arise (McAdam 1982; Diani 2003; Passy 2003). Networks can also be pathways for 'new models, concepts and practices' to become part of a movement's repertoire (Campbell 2005, p. 61). David A. Snow has written that movements construct meaning through 'collective action frames', which focus our attention on what they view as important about an issue in the manner of picture frames (2004, p. 384). Movements do not do this in isolation from each other: indeed, they often borrow 'master-frames' from pre-existing movements (Snow 2004, p. 390). In this way, older social movements are a conduit for the passage of ideas on to newer movements.

Across the period examined, South African AIDS activists used human-rights-based language to promote normative policy responses to the epidemic, but they did so in ways which changed over time and were influenced by both advances in medicine and the remaking of the South African state. While in the early 1990s, they invoked 'classic' liberal principles such as the right to privacy, in a later period they argued for wider access to HIV treatment based upon the socio-economic right to access to health care. This change in their use of rights-based legal arguments can be attributed to the medical innovation of combination ARV therapy and the new Constitution's enshrinement of socio-economic rights. In the early 1990s, the activists cast the state's human rights obligations in relation to people living with HIV in terms of negative freedom (what Isaiah Berlin termed 'freedom from') – as encompassed in the idea of doctor-patient confidentiality, as articulated in Barry McGeary's litigation (2002, p. 169). In the early 2000s, the activists came to endorse extensive state action to ensure patient access to chronic care, calls which were grounded in positive freedom (a Berlinian 'freedom to') (2002, p. 178).

In arguing this, it is not my intention to critique socio-economic rights and I am also not making the case that the activists were opposed to them in an earlier era. I am merely highlighting the new advocacy opportunities presented by changes in the nature of the South African state, as defined in its new Constitution (of 1996). Indeed, I fully acknowledge that a Berlinian distinction between different kinds of rights is in many senses artificial. The enjoyment of civil rights through political participation requires a basic level of material well-being (Barak-Erez and Ross 2007). Similarly, political freedoms 'help promote economic security' (Sen 1999, p. 11). Finally, the example of the TAC's activism also shows that a campaign for the realization of socio-economic rights can test, and make effective use of, civil and political rights. This shift in AIDS activists' legal strategies is deserving of extensive discussion in the book because the TAC's later socio-economic rights-based litigation was among the factors which accrued moral legitimacy to the international movement.

Epoch-making alterations in South Africa's political system presented both challenges and opportunities for AIDS activism. In South Africa, *the state* was singularly able to run a national HIV-prevention strategy, but in the apartheid era it lacked credibility on sexual health and AIDS both because of its 'population control' policies and due to its racially segregated provision of health care. Then, in the early post-apartheid years, the ANC was still learning how to wield the levers of state power. From 1996, the ANC government constrained the state's capacity to implement redistributive policies to tackle the inequality by developing and implementing the neoliberal Growth, Employment and Redistribution (GEAR) strategy (Bond 2000; Klein 2007; Marais 2011). Socio-economic inequality, as expressed in the feminization of poverty, was a factor which increased women's vulnerability to HIV infection (discussed in Chapter 3). The state's capacity to implement an ARV drug programme was also limited by the fact that it was bound by the WTO's patent-strengthening international 'free trade' agreement on intellectual property rights, and, unlike Brazil, it was not prepared to aggressively exploit loopholes in the agreement to produce cheaper generic drugs.

The ANC-in-government enjoyed unparalleled domestic legitimacy across the period, not least because of the party's success in taking control of the state through a peaceful, democratic transition. South Africa may have been newly democratic, but the ANC dominated the political scene in the country during its first decade of democracy (Southall 2003; Ballard et al. 2006; Calland 2006; Gevisser 2007; Gumede 2007; Leon 2008). More bluntly, when AIDS activists challenged the ANC, they challenged the party of Mandela which had yet to fear losing a national election. Even when TAC activists challenged the government using the Constitution, their advocacy remained politically controversial. In this sense, this book can be situated among several recent histories of new social movements in South Africa, a historiographical trend which is significantly driven by the fact that such activism has been one of the few sources of effective leftist political opposition in the country (Beinart 2010).

The TAC's high-profile legal and political successes have also made it a focus of scholarship. Perhaps the most comprehensive work which had been published on the history of the TAC at the time of writing was Nathan Geffen's book *Debunking Delusions*, which offers an 'Inside Story' of the movement's history (2010). Geffen held many positions in the movement, including those of IT manager, treasurer and the leader of its policy unit. His book, which largely focuses on the domestic aspects of the TAC's work, is especially illuminating on how the TAC pressed the government to adopt and implement AIDS policies based on scientific evidence and its later litigation against Matthias Rath.

Like many other movements in history, the TAC has been led by dynamic personalities, most of whom were male, despite its mostly female membership. Many commentators on the TAC have, therefore, understandably offered accounts largely focused on the work of its most prominent (male) leaders, such as Mark Heywood and Zackie Achmat, to combat Mbeki's AIDS denialism (Fassin 2007; Nattrass 2007; Oppenheimer and Bayer 2007; Geffen 2010). But the TAC's influential human rights advocacy should not insulate it from gender-based analyses.

By contrast, when writing this book, I set out to consciously emphasize the previously under-examined experiences of activists who were lesbian or gay or female in AIDS advocacy organizations over time. Same-sex desire and practices pre-date colonialism in Southern Africa (Epprecht 2004). Since at least the mid-twentieth-century lesbians, gay men and bisexual and transgender people in South Africa have formed organizations, occupied particular spaces and adopted a range of identities around same-sex desire (Cameron and Gevisser 1994; Epprecht 2004; Keswa and Wieringa 2005; De Waal and Manion 2006). Since the 1990s, South Africa also has had a dynamic gay rights movement which has been successful in obtaining multiple pieces of law reform (Croucher 2002; Berger 2008). Similarly, the country's women's movement was successful both in 'getting women in' to the government in greater numbers and in pressing for constitutional enshrinement of gender equity and the passage of new gender-related legislation (Gouws 2005b; Hassim 2006). But while it transformed elements of the state, the women's movement failed to address what Nancy Fraser has called the 'class-like' dimensions of gender, by advocating for redistributive policies (2003, p. 21). It also barely addressed AIDS, which meant that there was no pre-existing 'safe space' for activists to develop and level feminist critiques of the TAC in numbers. This meant that while male gay rights activists were fundamental in the formation and leadership of the TAC in its early years, women only came to lead the organization after the period discussed in this book. I decided to document TAC women's experiences of sexism within the movement and their struggles to overcome it for two reasons. Firstly, I thought that it was deserving of mention in the book – especially given its focus on the movement's moral legitimacy. My thinking in this regard was influenced by the fact that the movement's lack of women-empowerment policies in the period the book discusses detracted from its standing in the eyes of some TAC women and their South African and foreign feminist allies. Secondly, the sexism within the movement points to why the TAC's subsequent, admirable women's rights programmes were necessary.

To draw out the themes of gender and sexuality in the history of South African AIDS activism I visited activist records such as those held at Gay and Lesbian Memory in Action (GALA), the South African History Archive (SAHA) and Historical Papers at the University of the Witwatersrand. I also borrowed from activists' personal papers. The material I gathered through this method enabled me to write on the links between gay rights and AIDS activism and women's activists' experiences of workplace sexism in organizations conducting advocacy on the epidemic over time.

Conclusion

The demonstration opening the 2000 Durban AIDS conference was the international HIV treatment access movement's first transnational protest. In many ways, it drew on anti-apartheid historical symbolism, framing which did not ring hollow given the TAC's leaders' past involvement in 'progressive' activism. South African AIDS activism emerged when small groups of anti-apartheid activists – from gay rights, healthworker and women's organizations – formed advocacy networks on the epidemic in the early 1990s. The re-making of the South African state, as transcribed in South Africa's constitution, facilitated the TAC's innovative socio-economic rights litigation, which also conferred international legitimacy on the domestic movement. Viewing the emergence of the TAC in historical context can help to shed light on under-examined issues in the scholarship on South African AIDS activism such as activists' changing human rights litigation strategies and how the politics of gender and sexuality in AIDS activism have evolved over time.

Transnational South African AIDS activism, as evident in the TAC, was only possible with the end of the academic boycott following the state's transition to a constitutional democracy. The TAC offered the international HIV treatment access movement moral legitimacy, but it also drew on foreign activists' expertise in designing its treatment literacy programme. South African AIDS activists' contributions to thinking on global health justice have been under-analysed in the literature on global health ethics.

The international HIV treatment access movement evolved in ways which shifted global health governance and diplomacy: this was in no small part, due to the contribution of its developing-country activists, including those from South Africa. In the pandemic's fourth decade, such developing-country histories of transnational AIDS activism remain especially worthy of retrieval given the persistence of global disparities in HIV treatment access.

Part I

AIDS Activism and South Africa's Transition

1
Health for All? Healthworker AIDS Activism, 1982–1994

Introduction

In July 1990, Mervyn Susser gave the keynote address at a gathering of anti-apartheid physicians in Durban just over five months after struggle-icon Nelson Mandela had made history in Cape Town by taking his first steps as a free man in 27 years. The South African anti-apartheid physician and epidemiologist was in his element: he had been a long-time supporter of desegregated social medicine, and he and his wife Zena Stein had left the country in the mid-1950s shortly after he had been fired from Alexandra Clinic because of his association with the African National Congress (ANC). He was now a professor at Columbia University in New York, but he knew Durban well as he and Stein had visited it on a number of occasions in the late 1940s and early 1950s. Susser's elation at the possibility of a democratic transition in South Africa was tempered, however, by his awareness of a disturbing new trend: the continent of Africa was being ravaged by the epidemic of AIDS, a new, lethal sexually transmitted disease (STD). In Uganda it had been referred to as 'Slim disease', and it was obvious that most new cases were among heterosexual people in African countries, where it had been identified. A terrifying vision lay in his mind's eye: AIDS was going to be a 'conflagration' on the continent of Africa, one which would be on a par with the syphilis epidemic in sixteenth-century Europe, and South Africa lay as dry kindling before its flames (Interview 7 August 2003).

These calculations lay behind his warning to the assembled anti-apartheid healthworkers that South Africa's AIDS epidemic could turn into a catastrophe and that there was 'little time to act'.[1] While antenatal clinic surveys had shown an infection rate of under 1%, this was not an indication of things to come: the rate of infections was doubling every 8.4 months, and within four years infection rates in Johannesburg would exceed Kampala's, where one in four adults were infected with the virus.[2] Susser said that a combination of biological and behavioural changes would eventually 'bring the pandemic into a steady balanced state', but at that time epidemiologists did not 'have long enough experience' to predict what levels infection rates would reach before this would happen.[3] So, Susser pronounced, with 'professional deliberation as an epidemiologist', that the epidemic was an emergency for the country, which needed to be politically prioritized.[4] Indeed, nothing short of 'a social movement on a national scale' could hope to stem the tide of the advancing epidemic.[5]

This chapter traces how anti-apartheid healthworker activists such as Susser – who commonly referred to themselves as 'progressive' healthworker activists – took up the issue of AIDS in the early 1990s. It describes how the first National AIDS Plan (NAP) was shaped by two groups of healthworker activists: those who were internally based, and externally based anti-apartheid physicians, such as Susser, who had seen and learnt about the disease abroad. It then focuses on their engagements with internally based gay AIDS activists, such as Edwin Cameron, who demanded human rights-based policies in relation to the epidemic.

In this chapter, I argue that 'progressive healthworkers' were central to the development of AIDS activism from an early period, by virtue of their professional experiences and expertise in relation to the disease. But it is also important not to overstate healthworker activists' prioritization of AIDS in the period. While AIDS was a small, but growing, issue for some healthworker activists, ending apartheid and ensuring that there would be a desegregated post-apartheid national health system remained their primary projects.

The chapter opens with an analysis of how internally based healthworker activists' responses to the epidemic were shaped by both their early professional engagement with the epidemic and their adherence to the old idea of community-orientated primary health care (PHC). It shows how their political orientation as *progressive* healthworkers meant that they supported the older idea of PHC, which motivated them to disseminate their knowledge about AIDS more widely in 'communities'. The chapter's second section analyses how the return of ANC exiles and the end of South Africa's international isolation facilitated greater contact between anti-apartheid physicians who had been trained abroad and those who had remained in the country, and enabled them to share ideas about how to tackle AIDS. Its third section then looks at how the political transition and the concomitant reintegration of South Africa into the international community enabled the government and ANC to collaborate on developing the first NAP with technical inputs from WHO. The final section of the chapter explores how the first NAP included human rights language at the insistence of the AIDS Consortium, an approach supported by the ANC which had an interest in combatting calls for returning exiles to undergo mandatory testing. This chapter will now turn to an analysis of how internally based progressive healthworker AIDS activism drew on the social medicine-related idea of PHC.

Primary health care in healthworker AIDS activism

Like many healthworker activists, Mervyn Susser's thinking on AIDS-related planning – and health policy in general – was profoundly influenced by the concept of PHC, which, in a South African context, could be traced back to the work of Sidney and Emily Kark in the 1930s. In 1939, the union government established three experimental health centres in the 'Native Reserves' focused on health education and the prevention and treatment of disease (Kark and Kark 1999). The South African government's thinking in this regard doubtlessly drew on that of their British counterparts who were in the earliest stages of planning to introduce a unified national health service (NHS). Sidney and Emily Kark's Pholela Health Unit was the first of the South African health centres in the country's native reserves. At this health unit they pioneered a new model of community-orientated PHC. They aimed to provide an alternative to medicine that was solely hospital-based and curative in focus by emphasizing disease prevention and the local provision of health care. Their programmes in Pholela were also implemented by ordinary community members who were trained as health assistants.

PHC, as implemented by the Karks, drew on 'social medicine', a body of thought that dated back to the late nineteenth century. The concept originated in the thinking of Rudolf Virchow, a physician, anthropologist and politician, who worked in Biskmarck's Germany. He held that diseases were never purely biological in nature: instead, they emerged from the social context in which patients lived (McNeely 2002). Simply put, for Virchow there were firm causal links between poverty and ill health. Virchow's social medicine, therefore, positioned physicians as the ideal advocates for the well-being of the poor. He also called for state funding so that they could provide free medical services to the disadvantaged (Harrison 2004).

Over the next few years, the Karks' model of community-orientated PHC exercised an increasing influence over government policy. In 1944, the Gluckman Commission recommended that more local health centres be established and that they be combined with hospitals into a nationalized hospital system to comprise a health service along the same lines as that being proposed in Britain (Porter 1999; Susser 1999; Susser 2006). A year later, the Karks moved to Durban to head up a new Institute for Family and Community Health to train health assistants for newly established health centres. But the proposal for a South African NHS faded into the distance after the National Party's 1948 ascension to power, which enabled it to implement its apartheid ideology (Susser 1999). For decades thereafter, hospitals remained segregated and 'diseases of poverty' became ever more entrenched among Africans (Digby 2008).

Despite these setbacks, the dream of free health care for all, with special emphases on disease prevention and maternal and child health care, continued to animate the anti-apartheid struggle within South Africa. In 1955, the

Freedom Charter was adopted at the Congress of the People, which included representatives of the ANC, the South African Indian Congress, the Coloured People's Congress and the Congress of Democrats. The charter had no less than three clauses dealing with health in a post-apartheid South Africa, in a section entitled 'There Shall Be Houses, Security and Comfort!'[6]

The Natal University Medical School (founded in 1950) became an important space for the politicization of a younger generation of black anti-apartheid activists despite the fact that only Africans, coloureds and Indians could attend it. It attracted a distinguished, mostly white staff and a high concentration of the young black intellectual elite. This was a combination that made the medical school a critical space in terms of the politicization of the young, black intelligentsia (Ramphele 1995; Noble 2005). Durban's Medical School was one of the incubators of the Black Consciousness (BC) movement, and Stephen Bantu Biko, the movement's founder, was a student there. Doctors opposed to apartheid decried two physicians' collusion in the activist's torture and mistreatment which led to his death in detention in 1977 (Baldwin-Ragaven et al. 1999). Biko's death also deepened anti-apartheid physicians' antipathy towards the Medical Association of South Africa (MASA), which like the South African Medical and Dental Council (SAMDC), did not censure Biko's doctors for their failure to carry out their ethical and professional duties while attending to him (Baldwin-Ragaven et al. 1999).

All of this occurred at a time when the idea of community-orientated PHC was gaining increasing traction at WHO (Kark and Kark 1999). While the Karks had been early developers of this idea and had also promoted it during their time at WHO, it was also shaped by the 'barefoot doctors' of China and NGOs and medical missionaries across the 'Third World' (Brown et al. 2006). PHC was the focus of the Declaration of Alma-Ata, which was unanimously adopted by WHO member states in September 1978. The declaration emphasized the importance of community participation in health planning, disease prevention and health promotion, collaboration between health and development programmes and local provision of health care. It also, famously, called for 'Health for All' by the year 2000 (WHO 1978). Needless to say, the goals of Alma-Ata were not met. This was due to a number of factors, which included the global rise of the Washington Consensus approach to economics from the late 1970s and the successful promotion of market-based health care provision by the Rockefeller Foundation and a much reduced set of technical interventions by UNICEF, the World Bank and WHO. This approach was referred to as 'Selective Primary Health Care' (Hall and Taylor 2003; Brown et al. 2006). South African health policy was also influenced by these international developments, and from the late 1970s, the government promoted private sector provision of health care to contain costs to the state. However, such privatization barely dented racial disparities in access to quality health care: by 1986, while between 70% and 75% of the white population benefitted from medical aid membership (health insurance coverage), just under 4% of Africans enjoyed such privileges (Price 1989, p. 126). Indeed, most Africans continued to use drastically overcrowded state facilities designated for 'non-whites'. In this context, health activists in the country continued to refer to the Declaration of Alma-Ata in a positive light, as is evident in an early leaflet outlining the goals and activities of the PPHC network which alluded to its goal of 'Health Care for All by 2000'.[7]

In the eyes of doctors who were opposed to apartheid, MASA and the SAMDC had failed to address human rights abuses in the provision of health care, so they set up their own alternative association called the National Medical and Dental Association (NAMDA) in 1982 (Baldwin-Ragaven et al. 1999). NAMDA members researched and publicized the effects of apartheid on health, pressed for the desegregation of the health system and provided health services and first aid training through affiliated entities such as the Emergency Services Group (ESG). Throughout this period, PHC continued to be one of healthworker activism's guiding ideas. Indeed, in 1987 NAMDA convened meetings of healthworker activists and organizations which culminated in the formation of the PPHC network in September of that year.

So when AIDS entered their professional lives, South African healthworker activists were politically focused on an end to apartheid and 'health for all'. For instance, in this period, Hoosen 'Jerry' Coovadia, a Natal University-trained paediatrician was a firm NAMDA supporter. The Durban-based doctor saw his first AIDS patients in 1989. For most of the 1980s, he knew about AIDS 'academically' by virtue of his profession, but he told me that he thought of it as a 'white male epidemic mostly in Johannesburg' (Interview 3 September 2003). In the late 1980s and early 1990s, he was engrossed in the more quotidian diseases seen by a paediatrician in the public sector of the health system: diarrhoea, tuberculosis and malnutrition. In this period, he saw 'a few patients' and gained a 'nodding acquaintance' with the disease, and his colleagues 'spent a lot of time, maybe a whole five years until the mid-90s trying to become familiar with the symptoms'. By contrast, at the 1987 NAMDA conference he was voluble on the topic of the need for a desegregated, equitable NHS in South Africa: for a 'transition from racist, capitalist, exploitative medicine into socialized health care' and from a hospital-based, cure-centred heath system to a community-based preventive-focused one (Coovadia 1988, p. 11).

By the end of the 1980s, some healthworker activists were, however, starting to hold informal, regional meetings on AIDS. For example, on 30 October 1988 an ad hoc Southern Transvaal PPHC AIDS forum met for the first time at the Centre for the Study of Health Policy at Wits University. Representatives from 16 different organizations attended the meeting which PPHC activists set up so that they could share information on their 'AIDS work' with each other.[8] They were also told about 'AIDS efforts in [the rest of]

Africa and among minority groups in the United States' and discussed 'which policy issues needed to be addressed'.[9] AIDS was only one of the issues the PPHC network addressed at the group's second meeting, held on 8 April 1989, and it was by no means the most prominent: in the Southern Transvaal it also held workshops on the 'relationship between health and politics' and 'informal settlements'.[10]

Meanwhile, according to Thoko Makhanya, a nurse-educator at King Edward VIII hospital, a PPHC AIDS-related network was also created in Natal in 1988 (Interview 13 September 2007). Similarly, a network was formed in the Western Cape in August 1989 which aimed to 'pull together organizations who support the PPHC [network]' and to 'lobby the state and challenge their AIDS strategy'.[11] The Western Cape PPHC AIDS Forum was very actively involved in both advocacy and awareness raising. On the advocacy front, it wrote a letter to the Ministry of Health critiquing their pamphlets and their newspaper campaigns.[12] It was also in negotiations with the Congress of South African Trade Unions (COSATU) and the United Democratic Front (UDF) to collaborate with them on AIDS.[13] To raise awareness, they produced a pamphlet for the 1989 World AIDS Day and gave talks at schools.

In August 1990, a US congressman, Jim McDermott, visited South Africa to explore which AIDS projects he wanted to recommend for USAID funding. PPHC assisted the ANC in preparing a submission for the Democrat on its position on the epidemic and its recommendations for new programmes which could be developed with US funding. In the document, PPHC claimed that its AIDS forums involved 'more or less 80% of AIDS activists'.[14] This was a deeply significant development in that anti-apartheid activists of various types discussed in this book had previously referred to themselves as gay or progressive health activists interested in, or working on, AIDS. Their new self-definition as 'AIDS activists' indicated that they saw their political goals and identities as crucially linked to their efforts to limit new HIV infections and improve the well-being of those who were already living with the virus.

By September 1990, these voluntary AIDS forums organized by healthworker activists had crystallized into the PPHC's AIDS Working Group.[15] The PPHC network developed an AIDS programme driven by community AIDS workers. These were frequently not health professionals but rather people who lived in the areas where they worked or who had experience with political education or community organizing (Schaay 1992, p. 1). This was in-line with the PHC doctrine which held that ordinary 'lay' people had an important role to play in disease prevention and health promotion and that they should have a meaningful say in health policy formulation and implementation.

In this period, Shan Ramburuth worked at the AIDS centre at the South African Institute for Medical Research (SAIMR) and he was also a member of PPHC. When I met him he recounted, 'We produced thousands of pamphlets – Judy [Seidman] helped with that' (Interview 28 February 2007).

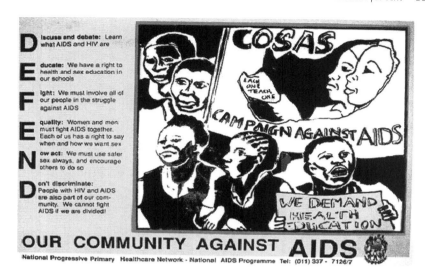

Figure 1.1 An early PPHC AIDS programme poster. Many young people did not see AIDS as a serious issue in the period
Source: © Judy Seideman; Warren Paker's personal collection.

Seidman was an activist and artist who had also produced a number of anti-apartheid posters while in exile in Botswana. One of Seidman's early posters for PPHC is reproduced in Figure 1.1. PPHC also gave talks to churches and youth clubs. At the time, he felt that their distribution of condoms was 'risqué stuff', especially in Hillbrow in inner-city Johannesburg – a gay-friendly, increasingly racially mixed area known for its sex workers and drug peddlers.

Such activist efforts seldom had the intended effects in the early 1990s. Thoko Makhanya, who volunteered with the PPHC AIDS group in Durban, told me that when she gave talks to young people in Durban 'they would laugh about it' (Interview 13 September 2007). Young, black South Africans' day-to-day existence was blighted by the immediate problems of drastic shortages of formal housing, inferior schools and rife unemployment. De Klerk had only desegregated hospitals in October 1990, and teenage pregnancy, established sexually transmitted diseases, tuberculosis and malnutrition remained very common among Africans (Digby 2008). By contrast, Makhanya found that AIDS was invisible to many young people because they'd 'never seen a person with AIDS' and lacked 'visual proof' of the disease.

Yet AIDS activists' work was not confined to educating the public about the disease and epidemic. In 1992, PPHC activist Nikki Schaay wrote that patients frequently received inadequate counselling before and after HIV tests and, therefore, workers in non-governmental groups such as the PPHC AIDS programme often had to 'witness the trauma' of someone being diagnosed with the disease (1992, p. 4). AIDS service organizations, such as GASA 6010 and Body Positive, were limited in number and scope, and many of them had been established to support white gay men living with the disease. This meant that the new community AIDS workers had to be 'social workers, lawyers, teachers and counsellors' (1992, p. 2).

Healthworker activists based within South Africa were growing increasingly concerned about the emerging issue of AIDS, a concern which largely stemmed from their early professional engagements with the disease. Their adherence to the social medicine-based idea of PHC enabled them to encourage community-based and lay activists' efforts to educate the public about the new disease. South Africa's political transition was also underway, which brought new intellectual and political influences into AIDS activism via the return of the exiles and the end of international isolation.

The return of the exiled doctors

South Africa was seldom far from Susser's thoughts during his time in exile in the United States. He was a founding member of the Committee for Health in Southern Africa (CHISA), a group which he co-founded in solidarity with NAMDA. In the 1980s, CHISA invited NAMDA representatives such as Jerry Coovadia to the United States to speak on medicine and apartheid. Susser told me that CHISA was affiliated with the American Public Health Association and that many of its members were liberal or left-wing public health specialists (Interview 7 August 2003). When AIDS emerged in South Africa, the ANC was banned and most of its leaders had been exiled or imprisoned. These exiled doctors gained important insights on AIDS in other African countries with more advanced epidemics, which they then applied to their work in South Africa after their transition-era return to the country.[16] Those who were in exile in the United States and Western Europe often gained relatively privileged, early access to, or participation in, the AIDS research which was being conducted at well-resourced universities or medical research facilities. Others who worked with the exiled ANC in neighbouring states also gained insights into the threat AIDS posed to South Africa by observing their host countries' burgeoning epidemics.

Zena Stein and Mervyn Susser had been aware of AIDS from the earliest days following its identification. Stein told me that the exiled couple knew about the emergence of the epidemic in San Francisco and New York 'almost as soon as anybody else did' (Interview 18 October 2007). By the time the new disease emerged, Susser held the Chair of Epidemiology at Columbia. He had worked as a consultant on a study searching for a vaccine for hepatitis B with a Polish-American epidemiologist. According to Susser, 'bloods that were taken from men in San Francisco on that study turned out to be one of the key bits of information about the epidemiology of HIV infection and AIDS' (Interview 7 August 2003). His wife also had an important professional interest in the epidemic and was an early advocate of greater research into AIDS in women (as discussed in Chapter 3). She became the co-director of Columbia's NIH-funded Center for HIV/AIDS Research. Stein and Susser also used their positions at Columbia to attract Fogharty fellowships to train South African epidemiologists, many of whom subsequently went on to produce significant AIDS research in the country.

Durban-born Salim Abdool Karim, a founder member of NAMDA and later its secretary-general, was the second recipient of one of these Fogharty fellowships. During his time as a student at Natal University's Medical School, he had been heavily involved in NAMDA's 'backroom' work: maintaining its membership lists, printing its pamphlets and managing its documentation (Interview 15 September 2003). AIDS first entered his professional life when, in the early 1980s, a patient with Kaposi's Sarcoma (KS) was admitted to Durban's King Edward VIII teaching hospital. Abdool Karim remembered that 'the word was out' at the medical school and that many of its students were keen to see the patient because KS was a rare disease which they did not want to encounter 'for the first time during exams'. He never saw the patient but later realized that he probably had AIDS.

Abdool Karim's deeper intellectual interest in AIDS was only sparked when he went to New York in 1988 to study at Columbia. He used his time at Columbia to continue his research into hepatitis B, and during his time in New York he also became aware of its epidemiological similarity to AIDS. By the late 1980s, he was deeply concerned about the lack of epidemiological data on AIDS in South Africa. In Abdool Karim's opinion, most of the pieces published in *SAMJ* in the period provided little more than generic 'continuing medical education updates on AIDS' which focused on how to diagnose the disease; by contrast there was almost no data on the country's epidemic.

Abdool Karim married Quarraisha during the time he was studying in New York. She was a microbiologist by training and was the next recipient of a Fogharty fellowship to study epidemiology under Susser and Stein at Columbia. Her research squarely addressed the paucity of data on the country's epidemic and contained important insights on what was driving the growth in new HIV infections in South Africa, particularly among women (as discussed in Chapter 3). On their return to South Africa in 1989, Quarraisha Abdool Karim headed the AIDS Research Unit at the Medical Research Council (MRC) in Durban and Salim Abdool Karim took a job as a registrar at King Edward VIII hospital.

Another South African doctor whose thinking on AIDS was influenced by his time abroad was William Malegapuru Makgoba. He had been born to a poor family in rural Sekhukhuneland and was the first in his family to attend university. Following a stint at boarding school, he attended the Natal University Medical School in the 1970s when BC was in its ascendancy.

While Makgoba did not consider himself to have been a BC 'activist' at that time, he was a 'follower' of its ideals and 'a very careful reader of the literature' (Interview 7 September 2007). After his internship at McCord's hospital and a stint at King Edward VIII hospital, he won a Nuffield Dominion Scholarship to study for a doctorate in human immunogenetics at Oxford University. After his move to Oxford, his interest in AIDS was stimulated from very early on by virtue of his being an immunologist.

In 1981, Harold Jaffe, an epidemiologist based at the US Centers for Disease Control (CDC) in Atlanta, came to Oxford to give a seminar on a new, poorly understood epidemic of a syndrome caused by immune malfunction which had been recently identified among gay men in New York and San Francisco. Makgoba recounted that at the end of the seminar he stood up and said to those assembled that he thought that 'this problem is much more common in Africa than people are making us believe' (Interview 7 September 2007). The basis for his assertion was that in two years he had seen close to ten young, male patients with KS at King Edward VIII hospital in Durban in 1974–5.

After completing his doctorate at Oxford in 1983, Makgoba then went on to do post-doctoral studies at the Hammersmith Hospital in London with a haematologist looking at disorders of lymphoid cells, including their relationship with the new immune deficiency disease. The following year he went to Birmingham Hospital where he encountered his first definite AIDS patient: the young man told him that he had a partner in New York and he had 'all the characteristics of HIV/AIDS'. He recalled that an AIDS case was 'such a unique thing' in those days that he was invited to present the case at the Department of Medicine's Friday Grand Round.

By 1985, he had heard about the many cases which had been identified in Uganda and, like Susser and Stein, became gravely concerned that a similar, widespread epidemic could occur in South Africa. In this period he corresponded on AIDS with Walter Prozesky, whom he would later succeed as head of the MRC. He also wrote to Ruben Sher at SAIMR about the issue. But Sher reassured him that they had done surveys with the new HIV tests and had not identified any black South African heterosexual cases.[17] Makgoba continued to follow AIDS in South Africa from the periphery but was not a significant player in progressive healthworker organizations in the period. Indeed, he only played a significant role in the politics of AIDS in South Africa after his return in late 1994, as considered in Chapter 4.

In 1990, exiles were allowed to return to the country. AIDS had been an issue addressed by the ANC health section in its camps in Southern and Eastern African countries. Many exiled progressive healthworker activists had been based in countries with more advanced AIDS epidemics. Nkosazana Zuma, for one, had recognized the threat AIDS posed to ANC cadres in exile in the late 1980s while she was working as Director of the Health Refugee

Trust in England. She also worked for the ANC health desk in Lusaka for a year before returning to South Africa in 1990 (Harnbridge 1995, p. 3).

Having seen how the epidemics developed in other African countries, and with the advantage of links to advanced and well-funded AIDS research institutes in wealthy countries such as the United States and the United Kingdom, exiled activists such as Susser, Stein and Nkosazana Zuma were well aware of the threat the disease posed. They were, therefore, keen to push for UDF-aligned progressive health organizations based within the country and senior figures in the ANC to add planning for AIDS to the post-apartheid health policy agenda. For them, the rapid growth of the epidemic meant that it was an urgent issue which could not wait until after the transition: in the interim, progressive healthworker organizations needed to develop programmes to arrest new infections.

In April 1990, CHISA held the Maputo Conference on Health in Southern Africa, which it also funded. CHISA had arranged four workshops on health in South Africa over the course of its existence: the first three, consecutively, were on nursing, women and unions. AIDS was firmly on the agenda of its fourth meeting, which indicated to some commentators that the ANC 'had woken up to the threat of AIDS' (*AIDS Analysis Africa*, August/September 1990, p. 1). Stein told me that Maputo was chosen as the venue for CHISA's fourth conference to enable exiled South African progressive healthworkers, those based within the country, and their supporters from other Southern African countries and the United States to meet to discuss plans for the development of a post-apartheid health system, including, as a matter of urgency, how to address the rapidly expanding HIV epidemic (Interview 18 October 2007). According to Stein, it was jointly planned in New York, London and Durban, by herself, Mervyn Susser, Anthony Zwi, Johnny Sachs (a South African immunologist with an interest in AIDS) and Kamy Chetty. ANC representatives at the conference included Manto Tshabalala, Chris Hani and Nkosazana Zuma (Interview 18 October 2007). Manto Tshabalala was to become a very controversial figure, as discussed in chapters 6 and 7.

A 'Declaration on Health in Southern Africa' was produced at the Maputo meeting, a gathering of activists from anti-apartheid health and social welfare organizations based within South Africa and their counterparts from across Southern Africa, including the exiled ANC.[18] Delegates' deliberations largely focused on how to develop an equitable post-apartheid national health service and, as such, they discussed specific policy proposals for the structure and financing of health and welfare policies in a democratic South Africa. Activists at the conference incorporated ideas taken from social medicine into the conference's declaration, which stated that 'progressive primary care strategy' would form the basis of health and welfare policies in a new South Africa.[19]

Stein and Anthony Zwi organized the conference's special session on AIDS. According to Stein, nearly all the delegates attended the session, which aimed to make sure that the domestically based South Africans left with the knowledge that AIDS was 'a terrible disease because they came not understanding that' (Interview 18 October 2007). To underscore the disease's horror, they also invited established black physicians from more heavily affected African countries to address delegates on how they had dealt with the epidemic – one was from Uganda and the other from Nairobi. The domestically based South Africans were not, however, uniformly under-informed about the epidemic: Stein recalled that there were some who had a good grasp of the epidemic and who gave excellent presentations on it, such as the representative from the National Union of Mineworkers (NUM).

But she also told me that tensions emerged at the conference between exiles and the activists based within the country. Some delegates who were based within the country, such as Ivan Toms and Liz Floyd, apparently felt that some of the exiles, particularly 'the Americans', were dominating the proceedings. These representatives who had come from South Africa told Stein that they had not come to 'be lectured to' and wanted to 'set their own agenda' (Interview 18 October 2007). Manto Tshabalala was among the group who contested Stein's position on AIDS because 'Health-workers in South Africa were really focused on developing a national network of primary care, grassroots care for people, so they didn't want that issue – the HIV issue – to confuse their commitment to getting health services on the ground across the country' (Interview 18 October 2007). By contrast, Stein and Zwi had different priorities: they viewed AIDS as 'a conflagration' and building the health system was 'a slow business'. Stein thought that the fire of AIDS needed to be attended to, but the internally based activists' 'revolt' came to dominate the session.

A representative from the ANC Health Department presented a paper at the session on 'Strategies for the Control of AIDS in the African National Congress'. It contained standard recommendations such as condom promotion, case detection and treatment of STDs, and better access to termination of pregnancy services to prevent mother-to-child transmission of HIV. The ANC saw that it could not 'escape' the epidemic, since many of its exile communities were 'in countries with established epidemics' (ANC Health Department 1990, p. 115). South Africa's epidemic was at an early stage, so it was critical that a national campaign should 'take root' urgently, and there were 'compelling reasons' for the ANC to start working on AIDS control (ANC Health Department 1990, p. 115).

The paper provides an interesting snapshot of the challenges ANC-in-exile faced in preventing new cases of HIV among its cadres in camps in neighbouring states. It stated that there was a need for a separate ANC programme because 'ANC communities... [were] unique in a number of ways': the ANC exiles could rarely speak their hosts' first languages, which meant that local education campaigns were of limited benefit. They were also 'highly mobile', which meant that they were frequently separated from their families (ANC Health Department 1990, pp. 115–16). While ANC communities were 'close-knit' there was 'a great deal of mixing in terms of relationships', which created a potential for high rates of transmission even though the 'reservoir' was small (1990, p. 116). The ANC Health Department had an ongoing programme to strengthen primary health care and increase its community's understanding of STDs and HIV. This programme was divided into two parts: education and information, and strengthening of laboratory resources. Beginning in May 1989, workshops had taken place at regional and national levels, talks had been given to cadres, and the movement had distributed videos, posters and leaflets to its members. It concluded by declaring that owing to the credibility deficit of the apartheid government on the issue, the ANC and progressive groups had to 'take a lead in the campaign in order to prevent a catastrophic HIV epidemic' (ANC Health Department 1990, p. 117).

The Maputo Statement on HIV and AIDS in Southern Africa emerged from the session. It emphasized that the epidemic was a political issue and that any attempt to deal with it had to be 'situated within the broader struggle for socio-political change' in the region.[20] It was imperative that 'senior political leadership within and outside South Africa', particularly the ANC, got involved with the issue since they were best placed to 'overcome the suspicion and mistrust created by the South African state'.[21] It was hoped that this would raise the epidemic's public profile and stimulate appropriate action.

The Maputo Statement also recognized that networking between different sectors was vital to the development of a successful progressive strategy: 'worker, youth, women's, gay, religious, political and other community-based organizations' had to be involved 'at all levels of work on HIV infection and AIDS'.[22] Such a 'multi-sectoral community-based approach' was deemed to be needed to effectively tackle HIV infection because it would ensure local accountability and activity around the issue.[23] Among the Maputo Statement's recommendations was the creation of an AIDS task force which would 'coordinate and promote HIV and AIDS work nationally in the progressive movement'.[24]

In May 1990, the ANC held a seminar on AIDS in Lusaka entitled 'Towards Comprehensive Intervention Strategies for the Prevention and Control of AIDS/HIV Infection'. Alan Whiteside and Jack van Niftrik published an article in *AIDS Analysis Africa* which cited reports that 'up to 25 per cent of Lusaka-based ANC operatives' were HIV positive: this was in line with the number of cases among young adults in the Zambian capital, so such an infection rate was 'hardly surprising' (1990, p. 1). They said that the ANC reiterated its commitment to prioritize the problem and create an AIDS task force at the May 1990 seminar. ANC activists apparently admitted at the Lusaka seminar that there was a lack of clarity 'about the disease and its sexual nature', which meant that the movement's response had been 'delayed' and which had caused it to 'pay a high price' (Whiteside and van Niftrik 1990, p. 1).

The negotiations, WHO and the making of the NAP

Healthworker AIDS activists played a substantial role in developing the first NAP. Their decision to work with the government in forging the NAP in the transition era was motivated by the perceived urgency of the issue and facilitated by the wider political negotiations for constitutional reform and free and fair elections. South Africa's transition was also smoothing the way for its readmission to the 'family of nations'. WHO's Global Programme on AIDS (GPA) offered technical advice on the development of the plan. Internationally, Jonathan Mann had championed non-discriminatory approaches to the epidemic during his time at WHO's GPA (described in Chapter 2). Mann's thinking doubtless also influenced the human rights approach advocated for in the NAP. But such technical advice was not uniformly well-received by the NAP's authors: in particular, some activists critiqued WHO's GPA as having slowed the plan's development and failed to create a nationally uniform approach to the epidemic.

The state's Department of National Health and Population Development (DNHPD) increasingly embraced the concept of community involvement in AIDS programmes, at least at the level of rhetoric, and, therefore, it began to work with the ANC health desk on the issue. One of the state's main proposals was to organize a large AIDS conference in South Africa, and it consulted the ANC on this idea. Salim Abdool Karim remembered that the idea of holding a big AIDS conference came from the DNHPD's Amanda Holmshaw (Interview 15 September 2003). Initially she had wanted to organize an international AIDS conference, but her efforts were stymied by the ANC because of the academic boycott which was then in operation.

Holmshaw decided that the best way around this impasse was to create a committee on the issue, with about half its members coming from the ANC and progressive organizations and half from the government.[25] ANC representatives included Quarraisha Abdool Karim and Nkosazana Zuma. At its first meeting, the new committee decided that the international conference would not be held, and according to Salim Abdool Karim this was in view of the broader political 'fights that were going on at that stage between the government and the ANC' (Interview 15 September 2003). Instead, the ANC and DPHD would co-arrange a National AIDS Convention of South Africa (NACOSA). The ANC Health Department's Cheryl Carolus was quoted in the first edition of the MRC's *AIDS Bulletin* as having described the movement's decision to work together with the government to tackle the epidemic as based on its understanding that the epidemic was an 'issue of survival' where 'political differences' had to be 'put aside'.[26] It was also driven by pragmatism: the government had more resources and funding to 'make a difference' to the issue and had not up to that point.[27]

The MRC established *AIDS Bulletin* because the multifaceted nature of the AIDS field made exchange of 'reliable, authoritative and current' information crucial.[28] It was a quarterly publication explicitly aimed at 'facilitating networking' among the target audience of 'AIDS educationalists', healthworkers and counsellors, community workers, human resource specialists, NGOs and policy makers.[29] Malcolm Steinberg wrote an article on the NACOSA conference, held on 23 and 24 October, in one of the publication's early issues. According to Steinberg, there were 442 delegates from 102 organizations.[30] It was funded by the European Economic Community (EEC) through the Kagiso Trust.[31] Steinberg described the conference as 'a tribute to commitment to overcome individual and political differences in order to pool ideas for a national AIDS strategy for South Africa'.[32]

Considering the wider political events in the country at that time, it is remarkable that a conference jointly organized by the ANC and the government on such a controversial topic went ahead. In June 1992, Inkatha Freedom Party-aligned hostel dwellers viciously attacked the residents of Boipatong township on the East Vaal. The ANC saw this violence as having been state-backed and so withdrew from the second plenary of the Convention for a Democratic South Africa (CODESA) negotiations between June and September of that year. It was only in September, a month before the NACOSA conference, that Mandela and De Klerk had resumed constitutional negotiations following the Bisho massacre where the Ciskei homeland's security forces had opened fire on ANC protest marchers, carnage which made both sides see that there was no tolerable alternative to resuming negotiations.

It was in this spirit of conciliation that Mandela opened the conference, calling for a 'non-partisan approach' to HIV/AIDS control and prevention.[33] Mandela followed the ANC Health Department's social medicine line that AIDS – like health in general – could not be viewed in a narrowly medical sense, and factors such as the migrant labour system with its single-sex hostels were shaping the epidemic. Similarly, he stated that a politically effective approach to AIDS could only be adopted by a democratic government in a non-violent society.

Alan Fleming, a professor of pathology at Wits and SAIMR and who was also based at Baragwanath Hospital, shared Steinberg's positive reception of Mandela's speech. As he put it, 'Mr Nelson Mandela opened with the eternally true and moving words of John Donne that no man is an island to himself'.[34] In common with Steinberg's account of Mandela's speech, Fleming mentioned that he had argued for a socio-economic approach to AIDS. Fleming's final assessment of the speech was that it was 'conciliatory and impressive'.[35] He optimistically believed that its publication would 'go far to making the majority population of South Africa believe in the reality of the pandemic'.[36]

At the end of the conference, a steering committee was elected to develop regional structures and establish a NACOSA Council, which wrote the first NAP. The council's steering committee members included Manto Tshabalala, Ralph Mgijima and Nkosazana Zuma from the ANC and Nathalie Stockton from the DNHPD.[37] It also included representatives from the Chamber of Mines, the South African Chamber of Business (SACOB), the National African Federated Chamber of Commerce (NAFCOC), the South African Council of Churches (SACC), COSATU and the BC-aligned National Council of Trade Unions (NACTU).[38]

Around the same time, NACOSA was renamed the National AIDS Coordinating Committee of South Africa (NACOSA).[39] Regional NACOSA meetings were held in KwaZulu/Natal, Kimberley, Pietersburg, the Western Cape and East London: these meetings were aimed at developing a national AIDS strategy.[40] The starting point for these regional meetings had already been agreed to at the national meeting, where it had been decided that the strategy had to be broad and cover issues such as

- education and training
- counselling
- preventive strategies
- care
- welfare
- research
- human rights
- socio-political and economic issues

South Africa's political transition enabled NACOSA to draw upon the international expertise of WHO on AIDS. This represented an important break from the past. In the 1980s, the South African state had been a pariah on the international stage, and it was also unwelcome at WHO, which was frequently used by exiled activists and African governments as a platform to decry the health impacts of apartheid (WHO 1983). The extent of WHO's antipathy towards the country's government became especially apparent in 1982, when the international body terminated its relationship with the World Medical Association (WMA) over its decision to readmit the government-aligned Medical Association of South Africa (MASA) as a member organization. By contrast, in the 1990s the wider political transition enabled greater collaboration between the government and ANC on AIDS, which, in turn, facilitated WHO giving the NACOSA-drafters advice on the first post-apartheid AIDS policy.

Peter Piot, a Belgian physician, microbiologist and public health expert, visited the country twice to discuss AIDS before its first democratic elections in 1994. In the 1970s, Piot had co-discovered the Ebola virus in Zaire. He was invited to Johannesburg in 1983 by a group of infectious disease specialists. Piot's first trip to the country was to speak on his international collaborative research examining cases of AIDS in Kinshasa. At this stage, there were only a few recognized South African cases, all white gay men who had visited the United States, something that he remembered made him 'kind of puzzled' (Interview 1 October 2011). When Piot returned to South Africa just under a decade later he was an international civil servant working for WHO's GPA. During this later trip to the country in August 1992, he was confronted with a very different scenario: AIDS was becoming a 'major issue'. There was still 'some ambivalence about whether to work in South Africa', he told me, but he was in the country on important business, to share his expertise to help it to develop a post-apartheid AIDS strategy – a process in which, as we have seen, the ANC was also centrally involved.

Mary Crewe, who was a co-drafter of the NAP along with Nkosasana Zuma and Quarraisha Abdool Karim, remembered the GPA's role in drafting the NAP slightly differently. Having spent 'months' drafting the plan, and having modelled it on Namibia's, the South African drafters were invited by the GPA to a workshop in September 1993 where its 'experts' recommended revisions. The international health civil servants wanted the South Africans to plan within a framework they could understand: classifying its elements in terms of 'activities, education, care and mobilization'. With WHO now on board 'there were months and months of diving things into planning, implementation and timeframes' (Interview 18 October 2006). Crewe told me that in her view this 'straight-jacketing' of the NAP did not prevent 'internecine fighting between the provinces'. The activists, government and international bureaucrats spent two years writing an 'unrealistic' plan, but the South Africans felt obliged to defer to the visitors from Geneva because 'we were so delighted to join the family of nations'.

The plan's 'unrealistic' nature may have related to when it was developed. The ANC was only elected into office in April 1994, so it could not develop a detailed, itemized budget. Instead, an external consultant estimated the cost of implementing the NAP at R256.77 million.[41] A budget developed in this manner could only serve as a 'guide,' as the plan acknowledged.[42] NACOSA National Council met on 27 January 1994 and approved the creation of an AIDS task team to draw up an implementation plan, which was finalized in June 1994. The final plan included sections on education and prevention, counselling, care for people with HIV and AIDS, welfare services, human rights and law reform, and research. Noticeably absent were specific time-lines, and the plan was ambitious considering that it only officially covered a single year – particularly since the main implementing entity, the Department of Health of the new Government of National Unity, simultaneously had to desegregate itself into being one national and nine provincial bureaucracies serving all races.

The ANC health desk, HIV testing and human rights

Gay AIDS activists worked hard in the early 1990s to ensure that the NAP placed a strong emphasis on human rights. This rights-based framing of the issue proved influential on healthworker activists' because it meshed well with their general opposition to unfair discrimination in health care, and it also advanced the ANC's interest in ensuring that HIV testing of its returning exiles remained voluntary and confidential. But while there was a consensus among 'progressive' activists working on the epidemic that post-apartheid policy on the epidemic had to be human rights-based, there were tensions as to which group – gay or healthworker AIDS activists – best represented 'civil society' as a whole.

The very real tensions between these two groups became evident both during and after the NACOSA conference. At the conference, Shaun Mellors and an unidentified African man spoke on the need to end AIDS-related discrimination and move in favour of the adoption of the AIDS Consortium's Charter of Rights on AIDS and HIV (discussed in Chapter 2). Alan Fleming was very critical of Mellors's speech, which he viewed as 'an exercise in self-pity' that 'diverted attention to the lesser problem (homosexual transmission) and away from the consequences of heterosexual and vertical transmission'.[43] He and others at the conference did not trust the AIDS Consortium because it was 'perceived to be dominated by white homosexuals and to be concerned with issues related more to gay rights than to an AIDS campaign'.[44] He contrasted the gay men of the AIDS Consortium, whom he regarded as purely interested in AIDS to promote their own rights, with 'several admitted gay men' who 'expressed their disapproval of this confusing of two issues [gay rights and AIDS] and their personal commitment to the campaign in response to the heterosexual epidemic'.[45]

These tensions between healthworker and gay AIDS activists were also evident in the NACOSA process: Steinberg reported at the time that there were initially disputes among NGOs about whether the PPHC network or AIDS Consortium should represent the civil society sector as a whole on the new body's steering committee.[46] Shan Ramburuth of the PPHC told me that 'there were different influences and strands then' and recalled conflict between those who spoke 'from the gay experience' and the 'progressives' side [PPHC]'. He perceived the gay activists as having been 'better-resourced, middle class' and 'more articulate and intelligent on the medical side of things' (Interview 28 February 2007). By contrast, PHC activists such as himself were more focused on 'organizing people around clinics'. These differences were, however, overcome. In January 1993, Ramburuth and Edwin Cameron, of the AIDS Consortium, were elected at a meeting of NGOs involved in the AIDS field as the sector's representatives on the NACOSA steering committee.

But the fact that different elements of civil society represented different constituencies did not mean that some of their interests were not aligned. AIDS rapidly became a hook for pre-existing homophobic prejudice, as discussed in Chapter 2. Returning ANC operatives were also stigmatized by the country's extreme right-wing political parties and press as being 'AIDS carriers'. As we have seen, the ANC was well aware that AIDS was a very real problem, with the disease affecting its camps in Southern Africa; it also faced a public relations problem around the issue of how to deal with the illness as it affected 'returnees'.

There was contradictory media coverage on whether or not the ANC would test returning exiles for HIV. For instance, on 23 August 1990, *The Herald*, a Port Elizabeth-based newspaper published an article headed 'Aids test for exiles returning to SA'. The article claimed that Mr. Benson Fihla, the 'national chairman of ex-political prisoners', said that a subcommittee on health had been established to 'deal with returning exiles' and that it would 'check each person for Aids and other diseases'. A fortnight later the same newspaper reported that a conference of the ESG – a NAMDA and ANC-aligned group – rejected any compulsory testing of exiles (*The Herald* 23 August 1990). This article also quoted a spokesperson for the group, Dr Mbengashe, as having said that the returnees 'must be looked upon as being a healthy group', and they did not need 'a specific Aids programme' and would not be 'subjected to an Aids test or any questions purely related to the disease'. AIDS could not be framed as 'a certain race's or group's problem', he went on, as to do so would 'derail the entire programme of awareness and the fact that it is a national problem'.

Right-wing groups were also conducting an AIDS-based disinformation campaign against the returnees. In October 1990, the *Weekly Mail* reported that a fake ANC pamphlet on AIDS addressed to 'all parents of returning exiles' was being widely circulated (*Weekly Mail* 5 October 1990–11 October 1990). The pamphlet, bearing the false signature of movement leader Walter Sisulu, warned parents of exiles that their children would have to go into quarantine and be tested for the 'dreadful disease' prior to their return. ANC spokesperson Joel Netshitenzhe denounced the document as a 'spurious hoax' and declared that the liberation movement was utterly opposed to the policy of testing retuning exiles: whether or not they were tested for HIV was 'a private matter' not 'something to be ordered by decree'. The liberal Institute for a Democratic Alternative in South Africa (IDASA) similarly alleged in its publication *Democracy in Action* that right-wingers had dropped pamphlets from planes that depicted returning exiles as 'AIDS carriers' (15 July 1994).

In 1991, the right-wing Conservative Party (CP) called for the mandatory testing of returning exiles, a proposal the ANC continued to resist because it would have constituted 'an infringement of human rights' (Citizen 16 January 1991). The liberation movement had researched the matter abroad and held that 'tests should not be randomly imposed on anyone'; the epidemic had no reverence for where a person resided, which made the focus on exiles and immigrants, in general, 'illogical'. Instead, the ANC supported cohesive AIDS projects and called on 'individuals to act responsibly regarding the contracting and the spread of the disease'.

It had good grounds to view such calls as motivated by racism: the CP used AIDS to oppose segregation, and some white people saw no point in tackling AIDS among black people because they cynically viewed it as a solution to 'overpopulation'. 'Aids is a blessing in disguise,' a white businessman told a writer for IDASA's *Democracy in Action* in July 1994 (15 July 1994). 'Isn't it going to solve the problems of overpopulation and unemployment in this country?', he added. This sort of attitude created a knee-jerk reaction among many Africans who saw AIDS as a white gay disease: the same article quoted Refiloe Serote of Alexander AIDS Action as saying that she had heard some Africans state that the 'Immorality Act (which outlawed sex across the colour line) was scrapped in the late 1980s... to spread Aids to the black population.'

The ANC's reluctance to implement mandatory, or even routine, testing of its exiles is entirely understandable, since it presented a legal threat to their successful repatriation to South Africa. Regulations had been in force since 1987 stipulating that the Medical Officer of Health could force individuals to undergo HIV tests and which made foreigners living with the disease prohibited people who could be deported.[47]

ANC health activists, such as Zuma, were caught between the Scylla of government and right-wing racism on AIDS among exiles and the Charybdis of the defensiveness about testing this catalysed among their comrades. Indeed, Alan Whiteside's publication *AIDS Analysis Africa* reported that the movement had faced 'considerable criticism' for 'refusing to face up to the problem of HIV-positivity within its ranks' (August/September 1991). But an SACP activist had died in London at the age of 35, which had 'strengthened the hands of those within the ANC who... [were] pressing for the movement to face up to reality'. The same article said that a 'prominent medical researcher' was, therefore, going to go to ANC camps in Zambia and Tanzania to test cadres there before they returned to South Africa. This development, however, does not undercut my argument that the ANC supported voluntary, confidential HIV testing: in my research I could find no evidence that this programme was either mandatory or that it violated the privacy of those tested.

Different constituencies within 'progressive' civil society had overlapping interests in ensuring post-apartheid AIDS policy was human rights-based. They had come together with the government to draft the final NAP, and they were confident that it would be implemented by the new Government of National Unity. They also predicted that NACOSA would still be able to both collaborate with the government and hold it accountable in terms of policy implementation.[48] The activists' confidence was anchored in their support for the ideals guiding new dispensation and the reality that human rights continued to be incorporated into the new government's AIDS policy documents: a 1995 Department of Health position paper on the health system stated – under the heading 'Non-discrimination and Legal Rights' – that in the new South Africa 'informed consent' had to be obtained before testing and that results had to remain 'confidential'.[49] But the AIDS activists who remained in NACOSA found it difficult to maintain both roles in the post-apartheid period – as shall be seen in Chapter 4, from the *Sarafina II* scandal onwards they increasingly became watchdogs and engaged in less collaboration with the new government.

Conclusion

The professional experience and expertise of progressive healthworker activists such as Susser meant that they played a vital role in South African AIDS activism from an early period. Their relatively rapid involvement in advocacy on the new disease is indicated by the fact that in August 1990, some progressive healthworkers affiliated to the PPHC network self-identified as AIDS activists for the first time. Although the disease was new, some of the ideas they used to develop responses to it were much older, such as the social medicine-related idea of PHC, which provided a conceptual basis for early community-based AIDS activism. Exiled South African progressive healthworkers played a key role in sounding the alarm about the growing epidemic. They gained early insights into the new disease by conducting, or having access to, early AIDS research at well-funded universities in Europe or the United States, or because they had worked in other parts of Africa which, unlike their own country, had already-recognized, serious and entrenched epidemics. South Africa's political transition and reintegration into the international community enabled the government and ANC to work together on the first NAP, with technical advice from WHO. This NAP included human rights principles: both gay rights activists and the ANC were united in their opposition to mandatory testing of groups deemed to be 'AIDS carriers', a position which also fitted with the ANC's general anti-apartheid opposition to unfair discrimination in health care provision.

The ANC and the government collaborated in holding NACOSA – South Africa's first national AIDS conference – an amazing feat given the political turmoil in the country at the time. This conference led to the development of the first NAP. AIDS activists were optimistic that the new plan would be implemented, especially as one of its drafters was Nkosasana Zuma, the Minister of Health in Mandela's new cabinet. On closer inspection, despite an elaborate and inclusive drafting process with WHO input, the plan contained the seeds of its own destruction – it lacked clear timetables for implementation and a detailed budget and only covered one year. These flaws in the NAP lay behind the abrupt end to the honeymoon period between the new government and civil society on AIDS in the post-1994 period (as discussed in Chapter 4).

Nevertheless, healthworker AIDS activists played significant roles in the creation of a new NAP in the transition era: a notable political achievement when viewed in the context of a rapidly changing South Africa. The book now turns to analysing the advocacy of gay AIDS activists, a group which also significantly influenced the NAP in this period.

2
From Pride to Political Funeral: Gay AIDS Activism, 1990–1994

Introduction

On an overcast October morning in 1990, a multiracial crowd had assembled at the Johannesburg offices of the South African Institute for Race Relations. They were about to embark on South Africa's first lesbian and gay pride march. Nelson Mandela had been released from his 27-year incarceration only eight months earlier, and the country's political leaders were in the midst of complex deliberations to create a democratic constitutional order. The political transition which was underway enabled a demonstration like pride to be held. Unprecedented opportunities were also becoming available for advocacy for gay rights to be recognized in a new South African constitution which was then under negotiation.

Simon Tseko Nkoli, who had been detained for anti-apartheid activity two years before, addressed the crowd: 'In South Africa I am oppressed because I am a black man, and I am oppressed because I am gay. So when I fight for my freedom I must fight against both oppressions' (Nkoli 2006, p. 37). Nkoli was one of the black leaders of the Gay and Lesbian Organization of the Witwatersrand (GLOW), one of the new South African, multiracial, anti-apartheid lesbian and gay organizations (Figure 2.1). He was determined to situate gay rights activism within wider anti-apartheid activism, and he decried homophobic oppression using the language of human rights. Nkoli argued that through embarking on the pride march, gays and lesbians were 'entering the struggle for a democratic South Africa where everyone has equal rights and everyone is protected by the law' (2006, p. 37).

South Africa's first pride march symbolized a new gay liberation politics in South Africa. A substantial number of the participants in pride were black and almost half were women – a dramatic change from the male-dominated and almost totally white GASA events of a few years before (Luirink 2000). After the speeches the marchers set out. Some put brown paper bags over their heads for fear of being recognized. They walked through the rain from Braamfontein to Hillbrow with drag queens at the head of the parade. A key

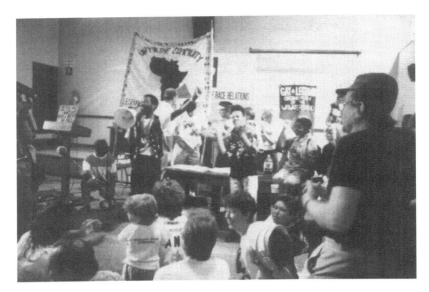

Figure 2.1   Simon Nkoli uses a megaphone to address a crowd assembled to embark on South Africa's first lesbian and gay pride demonstration in 1990. His hand is raised in a black power salute – a gesture characteristic in South African anti-apartheid activism. The banner in the background reads 'Unity in the Community' and contains an image of Africa painted in black, further emphasizing the movement's assertion that gay men and lesbians existed and had a rightful place on the continent
Source: © GALA; de Waal and Manion (2006, p. 18).

chant throughout the march was 'We're here! We're queer! We're everywhere.' At the end of the march there were more speeches including one where Nkoli urged each participant to kiss the marcher to their left. This was a daring display of same-sex sexual openness, especially considering that the oppressive laws in relation to sodomy (a common-law offense) and the Immorality Amendment Act of 1969 – which criminalized such social gatherings – remained in place.

This chapter argues that gay rights activists conducted vocal advocacy on AIDS from the 1980s onwards and increasingly viewed the two struggles for non-discrimination on the grounds of sexual orientation and HIV status as being intertwined. As the first section of this chapter shows, AIDS had been identified among gay men in the 1980s at a time when most gay organizations in the country were white-dominated, 'apolitical' and divided on the issue of how to deal with apartheid. By contrast, as its second section discusses, this new, black-led, multi-racial gay rights activism was more radical and it developed hand-in-hand with gay AIDS activism. The two struggles for equality for gay and lesbian people and those living with HIV were increasingly seen by many gay rights activists as interrelated and demanding the use of similar human rights-based language and advocacy tactics. Gay AIDS activists made human rights the dominant normative policy framework invoked by South African AIDS activists, in general, albeit one which evolved over time. A sister organization to GLOW, the Township AIDS Project (TAP), was formed in late 1989, and its AIDS educational activities were hindered by homophobic laws.

Gay AIDS activists such as Edwin Cameron used the language of human rights to develop a Charter of Rights for people living with HIV, a process shaped by similar documents abroad, despite it having predated the development of substantial transnational advocacy networks around the pandemic. Cameron and other gay rights activists deemed this AIDS charter to be complimentary to the gay and lesbian charter which was written in the same period – developments which are described in the third section of the chapter. Its fourth section then highlights their advocacy for the enshrinement of sexual orientation equality into the new Constitution's Bill of Rights – advocacy which was stunningly successful. In this transition era, (1990–4), Cameron and his AIDS activist colleagues also used 'classically liberal' rights-based arguments to emphasize the ethical value of respect for HIV patients' rights to privacy in both clinical settings and public health policy. They did so through the drafting of the AIDS Charter and civil litigation, such as that which was brought by gay AIDS patient Barry McGeary, whom Cameron represented. Cameron also founded the AIDS Consortium in this period, which in 1998 provided an important social and political basis for the formation of the Treatment Action Campaign (TAC) (see Chapter 4).

For some of the pride marchers in 1990, such as Cameron and Nkoli, underneath the feelings of exhilaration which were stirred by their open and proud displays of their sexual identities lay a deep secret laced with apprehension – they were living with HIV, which was then an incurable, stigmatized terminal illness. But the freer political climate which made the pride march possible also gradually proved more conducive to HIV-positive gay men being open for the first time about their diagnosis to fight AIDS-related discrimination. By 1992, at least two gay AIDS activists – Peter Busse and Shaun Mellors – had publicly revealed that they were living with HIV. Their thinking about using openness as a tool to promote the AIDS Charter drew directly on their political experience as gay rights activists during the democratization period.

The final section of the chapter recounts the story of GLOW activist Linda Ngcobo's burial in 1993, which was perhaps the first political AIDS funeral in the country. In the 1980s, in the midst of harsh state repression, the political funeral had developed into a powerful form of anti-apartheid protest in many black townships. Gay AIDS activists can be seen as having held such a political funeral to draw on 'struggle symbolism' to advance their rights-based vision for equality for lesbian and gay people and those living with

HIV. Nkoli and his colleagues obtained their desired Constitutional reform – making the country's constitution the first in the world to include gay rights (Thoreson 2008). This important breakthrough enabled them to focus more on AIDS activism after 1994. It also legalized same-sex, AIDS-related speech, which had important ramifications for AIDS educational projects. While the case for human rights-based AIDS policies had already been made internationally by Jonathan Mann, these constitutional law reform achievements of gay rights activists within the country can be said to be uniquely *South African*. Nkoli's success, however, would be tinged with a tragic historical irony, as we shall see in Chapter 4, the next major political AIDS funeral would be Nkoli's own in 1998. It was during that event that Zackie Achmat called for the creation of the Treatment Action Campaign (TAC).

AIDS and gay organizations in the 1980s

The novelty of Nkoli's brand of gay rights and AIDS activism can only be appreciated if one adopts a long view. Indeed, to truly understand its significance we have to situate it in the broader history of South African gay and lesbian organizations and the first years of AIDS in the country. The first two known cases of AIDS in South Africa were two South African Airways (SAA) stewards diagnosed with the disease in 1982 (Malan 1986, p. 119). Almost as soon as the epidemic emerged in the country, gay activists were forced to respond as it was framed in the media as being a 'gay plague' which generated homophobic prejudice and discrimination. But AIDS emerged at a time when gay organizations were riven by divisions over how to deal with apartheid, which meant that there was little in the way of a nationally coherent gay political response to the issue. In sum, early gay AIDS activism, like most South African lesbian and gay activism in general, was non-radical, regionally based and focused on the provision of social support.

Ruben Sher was a white South African doctor who played a key role in identifying these two earliest cases of the disease (Interview 20 January 2007). When AIDS emerged in the United States, Sher was a middle-aged immunologist. His son fell ill with another disease, and so he had to go to the United States to seek treatment for him towards to end of 1982. During his visit to the United States, he started to read about the strange new disease causing immune malfunction which seemed to mainly afflict young gay men, and it triggered his interest. The South African doctor also visited the Centers for Disease Control (CDC) in Atlanta during his stay in the United States, where he met inspiring and determined young virologists and immunologists working in the field. At this stage, the cause of AIDS had not yet been identified.

When I interviewed him at his home in Johannesburg, Sher recalled that during that trip he told the scientists he met at the CDC that lots of gay men worked for SAA. Sher's thinking may have been influenced by the fact that scientists at the CDC had already identified a gay Canadian air steward called Gaeten Dugas as an important early case, and he quickly became labelled 'patient zero' (Shilts 1987). Moreover, reasoned Sher, these young South African air stewards were mobile and may have had American sexual partners in the course of their travels. This prompted him to study this group to see whether any of them had AIDS. On his return to South Africa, he met with some gay doctors including Dennis Sifris to discuss the possibilities of doing research into the issue. In the months surrounding Sher's return to the country in late 1982, the two young gay airline stewards died of unusual chest infections. Journalists heard about the story and rang Sher to find out what he knew about the men's deaths. Based upon the clinical evidence he had heard, Sher 'put two and two together and figured out that they had died of AIDS'.

The newspaper headlines which followed in early January 1983 could not have been worse for gay men in South Africa. On 4 January 1983, *The Cape Argus* reported in an article headed ' "Homosexual" disease kills SAA staff' that 'Two South African Airways stewards have died after apparently becoming the first South African victims of a rare disease which is believed to affect mainly homosexuals and drug addicts.'[1] The *Sunday Times* coverage was even more shrill: an article entitled ' "Gay" plague: More victims?' announced in a horrified tone that 'Seven months before he became the first South African to die of the newly discovered disease Ralph Kretzen – a self-confessed homosexual – still handled food on overseas flights.'[2]

Some gay men were very aware of, and concerned about, this negative media coverage. Leon Eksteen, for instance, who was the fifth Capetonian to die of AIDS (in 1986), kept both articles in a scrap book along with all the other AIDS coverage he saw in newspapers up until his death.[3]

SAA further fanned the flames of the hysteria by telling *The Citizen* that it disapproved of homosexuality (8 January 1983). Yet, according to its spokesman, it did not want to include ' "sexual questions" ' on staff application forms since no other company did this as it was ' "a sensitive issue" '. The airline eventually decided to test all its cabin crew for 'lowered immunity' in conjunction with the Department of Health; however, it emphasized that this would be discreet as they were ' "dealing with human beings not cattle" ' (Sunday Express 9 January 1983).

Part of the panic around the new disease related to the fact that its cause still remained in question in the early 1980s. The virus causing AIDS was only publicly identified in May 1983 (by scientists in France, who named it LAV), and in April 1984 (by US scientists in the United States, who named it HTLVIII) (Safai et al. 1984; Vilmer et al. 1984). An antibody test for HTLVIII/LAV was only licensed by the American Food and Drug Administration (FDA) in 1985. HTLVIII/LAV was renamed HIV in 1986.

In this period, the South African Institute of Medical Research (SAIMR) was a key site of early AIDS research and Sher set up an AIDS department there. According to Sher, the institute had bled over 200 gay men for another study and stored their serum. When Sher decided to test this stored serum for HTLVIII/LAV (HIV) with the newly developed tests in 1985, he found that 11.8% of the samples tested positive (Interview 20 January 2007). All the patients initially diagnosed with the new disease in South Africa were white gay men. While heterosexuals were increasingly infected during the 1980s, as late as 1990 less than 1% of the country's sexually active population was estimated by the government to be infected (Department of Health 2005, p. 13).

Indeed, for much of the 1980s, AIDS was seen by South African epidemiologists as primarily affecting gay men. By 1989, of the 98 cases voluntarily reported to the government's main AIDS policy-making body the AIDS Advisory Group (AAG), 81% were recorded to have fallen into the 'homosexual/bisexual category' (Sher 1989). Similarly, in the mid-1980s it was estimated that 10–15% of gay men in Johannesburg were infected with HIV (Sher 1989). The male/female ratio was 24:1 and of the reported cases only seven were black patients who had 'heterosexually acquired African AIDS' (Schoub et al. 1988, p. 153).

The Gay Association of South Africa 6010 (GASA 6010) in Cape Town was one of the most active non-governmental groups involved in AIDS work in the 1980s. It was founded in 1981 as a gay social support group.[4] In the organization's first year, it started a volunteer-run sexually transmitted disease (STD) clinic for gay men, a clinic which was used that same year by its first client living with AIDS.[5] In 1982, the Cape-based group became affiliated with the newly formed national Gay Association of South Africa (GASA, which is discussed in more detail below) and established its first 24-hour helpline staffed by volunteers.[6]

Gay and lesbian organizations such as GASA 6010 were part of a mosaic of identities and spaces adopted by same-sex practising people in late twentieth-century South Africa. Historian Marc Epprecht has shown that same-sex sexual desire and practices predated European arrival in Southern Africa (2004). In South Africa, same-sex sexual activity was historically associated with institutions and spaces which only contained members of a single sex. So, for instance, men living and working on mines engaged in sexual practices with one another (Moodie et al. 1988; Harries 1994; Epprecht 2004). While same-sex activity always took place in a number of different spaces, some – such as prisons, ports, bars, taverns and nightclubs – were particularly known as venues where men and women engaged in same-sex practices (Epprecht 2004). But only a minority of those who engaged in same-sex sexual practices identified themselves using terms of Western origin such as 'lesbian' or 'gay'. The use of the term 'gay' only dates back to the mid-twentieth century even in the United States (Chauncey 1995). Furthermore, in South Africa, 'Lesbian' and 'gay' were only two of a diverse number of terms used for persons who engaged in same-sex sexuality. Some of these indigenous terms were derogatory, such as commonly used terms such as '*moffie*' (an Afrikaans term), *isitabane* and *ungqingili* (isiZulu terms) (Louw 2001; Keswa and Wieringa 2005).[7]

GASA was not the first gay organization in the country. The first gay law reform movement was formed in 1967; it was ephemeral, white dominated and non-radical (Gevisser 1994). In 1972, a South African gay rights movement was formed at the University of Natal in Durban (Epprecht 2004). This group was also short-lived, because it was fairly radical in political orientation, which meant that the state forced its founder to disband the movement by threatening to charge him for inciting people to sodomy, which was then a common-law offence. Discreet, mostly 'whites-only' gay and lesbian night clubs and social groups (such as supper clubs, sports clubs and religious groups) opened up in the 1970s. The first truly national gay and lesbian organization – GASA – was only formed in January 1982. The organization grew rapidly and by May 1983 it had over 1,000 signed-up members and affiliated sports clubs, religious societies, a social support and counselling service and a newsletter called *Link/Skakel* (Gevisser 1994).

GASA's social functions shared much of the petty racism of the gay social scene from which the organization emerged. In the mid-1980s, there were some gay nightclubs where black patrons were refused entry on the grounds of their skin colour (Luirink 2000). Nkoli joined GASA and formed a black gay 'Saturday Group' which initially met at the Association's offices in Hillbrow, Johannesburg. But GASA quickly prevented Nkoli's new group from meeting there by imposing a limit on the number of black people allowed to enter the building at any given time (Gevisser 1994). The Saturday Group collapsed in 1984 when Nkoli was sent to prison with other anti-apartheid activists allied to the United Democratic Front (UDF) on trumped-up treason charges linked to their role in the incendiary Vaal townships uprising of the period. While Nkoli's imprisonment became a cause célèbre for anti-apartheid gay rights activists around the world, GASA refused to condemn apartheid or support Nkoli, which led to its expulsion from the International Lesbian and Gay Association (ILGA) (Gevisser 1994). GASA then splintered, and several new anti-apartheid gay organizations were formed, such as the Organization of Lesbian and Gay Activists (OLGA) and GLOW.

Nevertheless AIDS rapidly became an issue for South African gay and lesbian organizations in the 1980s, racially and politically divided as they were. This was because they were forced to respond to AIDS-related prejudice and discrimination from an early period. For instance, in 1986 posters were put up by the Blood Transfusion Service in Natal asking those who were gay or 'moffies' not to give blood.[8] The names of gay men living with AIDS were also freely published in newspapers such as The Cape Times in violation of their desire for privacy (Pegge 1994).

From 1985, the main nationwide gay organization – GASA – published basic information about AIDS in its newsletter and arranged talks and seminars on the topic.[9] But for much of the 1980s, there appears to have been some disagreement among participants within the gay social scene and related organizations about how serious the issue was. For instance, while GASA 6010 was very active around AIDS, the national organization's newsletter *Link/Skakel*'s first headline on the topic was 'AIDS PANIC OVERSTRESSED' (Gevisser 1994, p. 59). Moreover, for much of the 1980s gay men trying to raise awareness of AIDS in gay night clubs were initially ridiculed by most other patrons as paranoid kill-joys (Pegge 1994).

GASA certainly circulated information about AIDS through its publications and at its meetings, but it was not prepared to address the issue politically. As we have seen, Gevisser argued that the organization aimed to be 'apolitical' and was nonmilitant (1994, pp. 50–1). This meant that even when GASA was denied representation on the AIDS Advisory Group (AAG), a committee of experts which was the main AIDS policy-making body in the period, it made no protest. Moreover, at a time when anti-apartheid organizations generally eschewed any collaboration with the state, GASA was content to be recognized by the minister of health in 1985 as the 'official mouthpiece of the gay community'.[10]

Nevertheless, however limited their initial response, gay men in organizations such as GASA did at least engage with the issue, because it affected them personally; by comparison, for most of the 1980s it was almost totally neglected by most other non-governmental organizations (NGOs). This engagement was evident at a 1985 meeting of GASA's Natal Coastal branch, when its chairman said 'Individually, some of us will be brought close to the reality of long term suffering and death, and collectively we will all be faced with caring for, and dealing with, people who are lonely and perhaps deserted by those closest to them. This is the kind of true gay spirit which I see developing out of the AIDS crisis.'[11]

Edwin Cameron, a human rights lawyer and activist, was among the gay men who were forced to personally confront AIDS in the 1980s. He has described his experience of being diagnosed as infected with the virus which causes AIDS in this period in his autobiography *Witness to AIDS* (2005). At the time of his diagnosis, the Rhodes Scholar was working as a public interest lawyer at Wits University's Centre for Applied Legal Studies (CALS). On Friday 19 December 1986 the then 33 year-old's doctor rang him and told him that his blood had tested positive for the virus which caused AIDS. For him, 'The shock was double. Apart from the blow of learning that I was infected, most immediately I felt as though I had experienced a stunning bereavement – the impending loss of my own life' (2005, pp. 47–8). Cameron only told a very small circle of people about his diagnosis: a close friend, a lover, a counsellor and Ruben Sher, the AIDS specialist whose work we have already noted.

AIDS was thus first identified among gay men in the 1980s: a social group which responded early but was deeply divided along the lines of race and political views. In the epidemic's early years it was by no means inevitable that a politically impactful lesbian and gay social movement would subsequently emerge in the next decade, one which would also fundamentally shape future AIDS activism.

AIDS education in the townships in the 1990s

In the 1990s, gay AIDS activists campaigned against discrimination related to the disease partly because it hindered their efforts to educate the public about the epidemic. Many early community-based AIDS and gay rights campaigns involved the same activists, relied on the same donors and used similar tactics: they were, in many senses, twin struggles. The TAP was founded by Nkoli and Peter Busse in 1989, several months before the first pride march. It was based in Soweto, one of Johannesburg's populous African townships, which were racially segregated areas surrounding the city designated for black people. Soweto was associated with the student uprising of 1976 and remained a key site of activist resistance to apartheid in the 1980s and early 1990s. By virtue of its location in a township, the TAP was one of the first AIDS organizations which primarily addressed a black, urban audience. The TAP was also innovative in its provision of AIDS-related information to lesbian and gay people in the township and its founders and first employees were all members of GLOW.

Busse, who worked as a law librarian, also volunteered as an AIDS counsellor at the SAIMR. In 1985 he was diagnosed as HIV-positive. He had decided to volunteer as an AIDS counsellor in 1989, because he did not want others to be 'diagnosed in a vacuum... with no information, no counselling and no support', as he had been (Busse 2006, p. 38). It was important for him to disclose his HIV status because he disliked presenting only some parts of himself and 'having to hide away other parts' (2006, p. 38). He viewed openness about being gay as similar to a person disclosing that they had been diagnosed as HIV-positive because 'In both cases you are disclosing something about yourself that society doesn't like or sees as taboo' (2006, 38). Busse disclosed that he was living with HIV at a tree-planting ceremony during the 1991 pride march. The ceremony commemorated those who had died from the disease and expressed solidarity for those who were AIDS-ill. He found that accepting his HIV-status helped him to disclose it to others.

The TAP's first two employees were Nkoli and lesbian activist Bev Ditsie. They gave talks on AIDS at schools, in clinics and for community-based organizations. Lesbians like Bev Ditsie who were affiliated with GLOW decided to get involved because some of their gay male friends were living with HIV and dying from AIDS-related causes, and they felt that they needed to take care of them (Interview 14 September 2006).

Ditsie told me that she found that the TAP was very influential in developing her political skills and confidence in talking publicly about sexual and medical issues. In an interview, she recounted that 'We had to learn about HIV, the virus, its transmission and we knew how to articulate what was going on. We were groomed to be leaders' (14 September 2006). The TAP activists would tailor their messaging depending on which audience they were addressing, so while they gave talks to young children in crèches about sexual abuse, they also spoke to 'gangster-type boys', using 'all the lingo about penises, vaginas and fluids'.

But lesbians such as Ditsie were still 'trying to work out where do we, or I, fit in'. In her opinion, insufficient research had been conducted on the sexual transmission of HIV between women. Without such research all she could do was 'speculate', and when she ran safer sex workshops for girls and women she would urge them to take heed of blood and open sores and be mindful of the fact that, if it was not practised with caution, sado-masochism could lead to new infections. Phumzile Mthethwa was a lesbian activist and GLOW member from KwaThema township in this period. She recalled that GLOW's early safer sex workshops were 'very masculinised' and involved demonstrating condom use on a broom stick (Interview 15 April 2008). In the same period, activist Vicci Tallis noted that the paucity of research on AIDS among lesbians was a barrier to holding education workshops among them (1992). This problem was not unique to South Africa: Paula Treichler has pointed out that in the United States in this period there was next-to-no surveillance or reporting of the risk HIV posed to lesbians and bisexual women (1999).

Tallis also found that many lesbians in South Africa were unaware that dental dams could prevent HIV transmission and were unfamiliar with how to use or obtain them (1992). Mthethwa recounted a similar sense of complacency among lesbians about same-sex transmission of HIV in this period: a popular idea among them then was that sex between women entailed 'no risk' because there was 'no penetration'. Indeed, she confessed that her own understanding of AIDS among same-sex-practising women changed in a later period when a bisexual female friend disclosed to her that she was living with HIV, which brought the issue 'closer to home'.

'Corrective' rape was chief among factors which placed lesbians at risk of infection. This homophobic hate crime involved men sexually assaulting lesbians in order to render them heterosexual. Ditsie recounted in an interview that she found it hard to encourage gay men in GLOW/TAP to 'care' about the issue of corrective rape.[12] In her experience, gay men and lesbians often had different gendered experiences of rape, and whereas most lesbians experienced deep trauma following a 'corrective' rape, some gay men experienced some physical pleasure from rape and so saw it as 'just sex' or even 'fell in love' with their assailants afterwards (Interview 14 September 2006).

Lesbians in South Africa were not alone in experiencing male activists' sexist behaviour and attitudes in gay and lesbian organizations. Discussing the early history of gay rights activism in the United States and Europe, Dennis Altman has argued that lesbians faced a 'dual oppression' of unfair discrimination within *both* the women's movement where they faced homophobia *and* the gay rights movement where they faced sexism (Altman 1973, p. 216). While lesbians were expected to care for gay activists with AIDS some were dismayed at their male colleagues' seeming disinterest in assisting in campaigning against gendered social injustices which placed same-sex-practising women at risk of HIV infection.

Gender tensions were far from the only problems that TAP faced in the early years of its existence – it was also underfunded and socially marginalized. It had limited funds in the early days and had to overcome legal barriers imposed by the sodomy laws. Its earliest offices at the Anglican Ipelegeng Centre were in 'a ramshackle Wendy House [a small wooden house] behind the church, full of posters encouraging safer sex (Luirink 2000, p. 7)'. The discriminatory and sexually conservative laws which remained in place also hindered effective AIDS educational work. For example, the laws that made gay and lesbian people 'unapprehended felons' outlawed dildoes which were used in safer sex workshops (Cameron 1994). In this political and legal context, the TAP did not receive government funding. Simon Nkoli attributed the government's initial failure to fund organizations such as the TAP – which was based in a black township – to racial perceptions of that the disease only affected white gay men. He also thought that when it later came to be perceived as a 'black peril', it was treated as irrelevant by the government since it did not affect the ruling National Party's white constituency (Luirink 2000, p. 7).

Not only did black gay rights activists see advocacy for non-discrimination on the grounds of sexual orientation and HIV-status as mutually reinforcing and interlinked struggles, but some foreign donors shared their vision. GLOW and the TAP were formed shortly after Nkoli's release from prison in 1988, and both received funding from the same Swedish and Norwegian lesbian and gay groups.[13] The TAP's ties with Scandinavian donors such as LLH Norway were deep and lasted for several years.[14] Cecil Nyati, then president of GLOW, told the feminist magazine SPEAK in 1992 that GLOW had been formed 'because other gay and lesbian organizations did not really have a place for blacks. They were dominated by white, middle-class men. Many of us did not feel comfortable in these organizations' (Panda 1992, p. 11).

According to Ditsie, the TAP also strengthened GLOW's early activism. This was because the TAP attracted gay men in numbers, and when they came together on the issue of AIDS, they perceived that there was a need for organizing around lesbian and gay issues. For Ditsie 'it was simply that it was the right time and there were the numbers' (Interview 14 September 2006). Black gay men were threatened by AIDS and the TAP provided space for concurrent gay rights organizing. Therefore, Ditsie observed 'the struggles came hand-in-hand.'

GLOW's belief in racial integration was reflected in TAP's safer sex promotional materials. Nkoli himself is shown in a TAP poster (Figure 2.2),

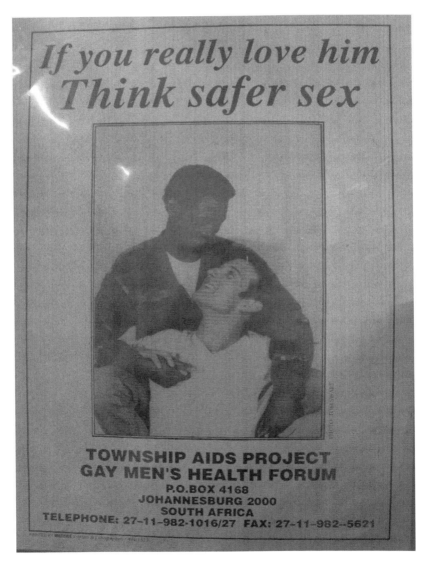

Figure 2.2   Undated early TAP safer sex promotion poster
Source: © GALA, GLOW posters: AM2560.

in an affectionate pose with an unidentified white man. This TAP poster clearly represents GLOW's dual vision of racial integration and gay pride.

Edwin Cameron thought that GLOW was much more politically powerful than any previous gay organization and had greater legitimacy because the fact that its membership was mostly black could undercut the popular notion that being gay or lesbian was 'unAfrican.'[15] He also argued that it was more politically empowered by virtue of Nkoli's close links with key activists in the ANC.[16] When GLOW started in 1989 it had a 100 members; by 1992 it had a thousand (Panda 1992, p. 11). The only impediment to its further growth was the fact that many same-sex-practising Africans did not want to be open about their sexual orientation (Panda 1992).

As we have seen, GLOW was instrumental in organizing the country's first gay and lesbian pride march. The holding of protest marches in South Africa had just become legal again, and it is no coincidence that the march was organized soon after the lifting of the five-year state of emergency which had limited civil liberties and *habeas corpus* rights (Gevisser 1994, p. 67). The organization of the march drew on (and was tied into) Johannesburg's urban black lesbian and gay social scene. Indeed, the night before the pride march Nkoli advertised it at Skyline Bar in Hillbrow; this gay venue – also known as 'Mandela's' – was by this stage multiracial, with a mostly black clientele (Luirink 2000). Nkoli made his announcement by switching off the jukebox and encouraging patrons to attend what he referred to as South Africa's first 'Pink Saturday' (Luirink 2000, p. 5).

While a new more radical form of gay and lesbian activism led by black people was taking hold in Johannesburg, in Cape Town, two coloured siblings, Zackie and Midi Achmat founded the black-led Association for Bisexuals, Gays and Lesbians (ABIGALE) in 1992. Like Nkoli, Zackie Achmat had had a history of prior involvement in anti-apartheid activism. Achmat later played a critical role in founding the TAC and was the movement's main spokesperson for most of the first decade of its existence. As we shall see, his HIV treatment fast later lent a critical measure of moral urgency to the work of the international movement. Moreover, the domestic and international HIV treatment movements' abilities to credibly invoke anti-apartheid rhetoric rested on his history of prior anti-segregationist advocacy, which is, therefore, worth recounting in some detail.

Abdurazzack ('Zackie') Achmat, of 'Cape Malay' heritage, was born in 1962 in Johannesburg, and he grew up in Salt River in Cape Town. He came from a family of anti-apartheid activists. His father Suleiman Achmat was a member of the South African Communist Party (SACP) and his mother Mymoena Adams was a trade union shop steward. Zackie decided to demonstrate his support for the 1976 Soweto Uprising when, at the age of 14, he burnt down his high school in Salt River. He spent the period from October 1978 to July 1979 in prison for this act of defiance against apartheid. After his release from prison he joined the Inter-School Magazine Committee – an organization of coloured anti-apartheid high school students. He was critical in helping the group to establish links with African students who opposed apartheid, since he had organized and been imprisoned with a group of them. In this same period, he started reading the works of Karl Marx and Leon Trotsky and *Work in Progress*, a 'progressive' journal whose editors were based at the University of the Witwatersrand. In the late 1970s and early 1980s, Achmat worked with other student activists to support strike-related boycotts (such as those of Fattis and Monis and Wilson Rowntree products) (Carson 2008). He was recruited into the ANC in 1980, while he was in prison. According to his friend and fellow activist Mark Heywood, in the 1980s and early 1990s, Achmat worked with the Marxist Workers' Tendency (MWT) – a Trotskyite group – which aimed to make the UDF and ANC in exile adopt a more explicitly socialist programme (Interview 15 April 2008). In 1990, Achmat was diagnosed as being HIV-positive following a routine medical examination. He has recounted that ' "First I went into denial . . . . Then I fell into the most profound depression. We had just won our freedom – it was the most exciting time in our country's history – and I was preparing for death" .'[17] Achmat's depression flowed from his doctor having informed him that he only had another six months to live. He returned home to Cape Town from Johannesburg where he had been living, to address the personal trauma that was caused by this diagnosis (The New Yorker 19 May 2003). Six months after his diagnosis, Achmat rebounded and decided to focus on gay rights activism, a decision which would have very important implications for the subsequent history of AIDS activism in South Africa.

In 1992, the same year that Achmat obtained a Bachelor of Arts (Honours) degree in English Literature from the University of the Western Cape, the young activist co-founded ABIGALE. It aimed to provide a networking space for bisexuals, lesbians and gay men to meet for 'social, educational and civic purposes'.[18] ABIGALE also strived for greater acceptance of gay, lesbian, bisexual and transgendered people and '[t]o fight for complete legal equality for bisexuals, gays and lesbians in all areas' affecting them.[19] As with their Johannesburg-based colleagues in GLOW, Cape-based ABIGALE organized AIDS workshops and educational initiatives.[20]

Like GLOW, and unlike GASA, the organization was explicitly political and anti-racist. Whereas GASA's social functions had been racially segregated, ABIGALE had organized a picket of 40 of its members outside the gay night club *Strawbs* which it accused of having had a racist admissions policy that excluded black patrons.[21] Likewise, while GASA was white dominated, ABIGALE claimed that of its 150 members, 99% were black and 1% white.[22]

Litigation and charters of rights

As we have seen, there was a new constellation of opportunities for freer inter-racial, gay and lesbian socializing and political organizing. This constellation's Pole Star was the newly multiracial gay rights movement which used the representational strategies of defiant openness in public displays of same-sex sexuality and the symbolic linking of the liberation of black and same-sex practising people. But this advocacy went beyond efforts to change the dominant symbolism attached to same-sex sexuality as an 'immoral' white import; it also sought to change laws for the realization of the grand goal of sexual orientation equality which would enable freer HIV prevention education. Edwin Cameron, the lawyer who had struggled with being open about his own diagnosis, was central to the movement's efforts at law reform through strategic lobbying and litigation.

This newly assertive gay rights activism was also evident in the civil litigation of Barry McGeary, a businessman living with HIV from Brakpan in the Transvaal. Shortly after moving to Nylstrom, in 1990, he went to his doctor in Brakpan where he still retained many links. During his medical appointment he obtained an HIV test because it was required by his insurance company. On 10 March 1990, he was told by his doctor that he was HIV-positive. His doctor then disclosed to two of his golfing friends that McGeary was HIV-positive, and within a week this business man's HIV-status was widely known (Dancaster and Dancaster 1995). This placed McGeary at a significant level of disadvantage because of the high degree of AIDS-related stigma and discrimination in this period when HIV-positive people faced automatic rejections to their visa applications, job termination and refusal of insurance coverage.

McGeary decided to launch civil litigation against his doctor for invasion of his right to privacy. He phoned Cameron and asked him to be his lawyer, as by this stage the human rights advocate had developed a public profile around AIDS: but all the while the advocate's own battle with the disease remained secret (Interview 4 October 2004). Cameron has written that what drew him into AIDS work was 'Not my own condition, but a condition on the outside, graphically linked to apartheid injustice. It was easy to throw myself into AIDS activism in this guise' (2005, p. 52).

McGeary instituted the court proceedings in the Witwatersrand Local Division in October 1990.[23] Cameron told me that he thought that it was 'the right case to bring before the public because the breach [of doctor-patient confidentiality] was so egregious, with no justification at all'. The case was very difficult as McGeary collapsed due to ill-health while giving evidence and died of AIDS-related illnesses before the end of the trial. His health had deteriorated rapidly, partly due to trial-related stresses. After his death, the executors of his estate continued with the case on his behalf, but ultimately the judgement went against them. In Cameron's view, this was because the judge was homophobic and unsympathetic to the needs of people living with HIV (Interview 4 October 2004). The case was subsequently taken by the executors of McGeary's estate to the Appellate Division (now the Supreme Court of Appeal) in Bloemfontein. In early 1993, when the appeal was heard, McGeary's attorney Mervyn Joseph told the *Sunday Times* that his client had decided to sue because 'he felt control had been removed from his hands.'[24] The Appeal Court found that the doctor had acted wrongly, and he was ordered to pay R5,000 in damages as well as the legal costs of the matter. In its judgement, the Court reaffirmed the principle of doctor-patient confidentiality based upon common-law 'right to privacy'.[25]

The trial also showed what legal AIDS activism could achieve, an avenue which would only widen when the final (1996) democratic constitution was enacted recognizing the rights to access to health care and non-discrimination on the grounds of sexual orientation.[26] The trial was but one of Cameron's efforts at promoting non-discriminatory approaches to the epidemic, and he was also an important driving force behind the drafting of a charter on the rights of people living with HIV and AIDS.

The interrelated nature of gay rights and AIDS advocacy can also be seen in the way that the idea of an AIDS-related charter of rights was influenced by the 'Charter of Gay and Lesbian Rights', which was drafted by the Organization of Lesbian and Gay Activists (OLGA) and endorsed by all the lesbian and gay groups in the country.[27] It was decided that HIV would not be included in this gay and lesbian charter, as the needs of same-sex practising people living with HIV were to be met by the AIDS Charter.[28] Both charters were used by gay rights and AIDS activists to advocate for relevant changes to policy and the law. In South Africa the idea of writing a charter to clarify political goals went back to anti-apartheid organizations' drafting of the Freedom Charter as a statement of principles in 1955. The concurrent drafting of the two charters is an indication of the way in which activists saw them as interrelated political documents.

The AIDS Consortium emerged as an outcome of the process of drafting the Charter of Rights on AIDS and HIV. The initial decision to draft the Charter was prompted by Cameron's feeling that the judge in the McGeary trial had not behaved with propriety or dignity, and he came out of the trial 'convinced that the notion of the dignity of people with HIV and AIDS had to be asserted through some formal statement, some encapsulation of their entitlements to non-discrimination in the epidemic'.[29] McGeary's trial was far from the only instance of AIDS-related discrimination in the early 1990s. The AIDS Consortium's newsletter also reported that the Boksburg town council wanted to close down St Francis Home, a church-run house for terminally ill and indigent AIDS patients. The town council wanted to do so on the grounds that its neighbours feared it would devalue their property, allegations that the patients there were mentally unstable and the council's anxiety that the influx of 'other racial groups' caused by the Home posed a 'security risk'.[30] The Home appealed the council's order that it close and took up the services of famous anti-apartheid lawyer George Bizos to fight their case.

In this context, Cameron saw that there was a need to draft a South African AIDS Charter because, while other similar documents had been produced elsewhere, such as a British statement of people's rights in the context of the AIDS epidemic, Cameron regarded them as too long and unfocused. So Cameron convened a meeting of 'a few... activists in South Africa who were already known to be involved in AIDS policy making and about 20 or 30 people got together I remember in the old seminar room at Kel's [sic – CALS]'.[31] He hoped that the document-drafting process would be as inclusive as possible. Mary Crewe, who was by then the head of Johannesburg's AIDS Training Testing and Counselling Centre (ATTIC) apparently suggested to Cameron that CALS start a loose affiliation of AIDS organizations which could meet more often.[32] After the meeting, Edward Swanson (an American intern at CALS), Mahendra Chetty (of the Legal Resources Centre) and Cameron circulated various drafts amongst themselves which were later approved (with several amendments) by the AIDS Consortium as a whole.[33] The final Charter was formally launched at the end of 1992.[34]

The Charter was a classically liberal document in that it placed a strong emphasis on respect for HIV positive individuals' rights to privacy and autonomy. For instance, the Charter's first three subheadings were: 'Liberty, autonomy, security of the person and freedom of movement'; 'Confidentiality and privacy' and 'Testing' (The AIDS Consortium 1992). The importance of confidentiality was again asserted in the section on the media.

Access to health care was only dealt with in section 6 (of 12 sections). It stated that people living with HIV had the right to equal 'medical assistance' and 'reasonable accommodation' in public health facilities (The AIDS Consortium 1992). They were also entitled to 'non-discrimination in the provision of health services, facilities and medication' and health insurance (medical aid) coverage (The AIDS Consortium 1992).

The AIDS charter can also be described as classically liberal in that it foregrounded the principle of liberty. The liberal notion of human rights is often traced back to the work of the Enlightenment philosopher John Locke, who held that state power should be limited and have 'the preservation of society' as its primary goal (2003, p. 198). John Stuart Mill, another important figure in the history of liberalism held that the right to privacy rested upon the ideal of a self-limiting state where individuals would enjoy self-rule (sovereignty) which could be breached 'only in respect of those actions of each [person] that concern the interest of other people' (2003, p. 95).

The rights to privacy and autonomy fall under the liberal rubric of what Isaiah Berlin termed 'negative freedom', that is, a person being 'left to do or be what he is able to do or be, without interference by other persons' (Berlin 2002, p. 169). While he offered a clear definition of negative freedom, his concept of positive freedom was less brightly demarcated and folded in both political participation and the realization of collective goals, through various means, including social policy. Berlin feared that when it was not subordinated to negative freedom, positive freedom could result in coercive action by states or social groups to promote a 'higher' form of freedom and group self-actualization (Berlin 2002, p. 179). In other words, he held that positive freedom ought to be subordinated to negative freedom to promote pluralism and guard against authoritarianism. But it is also important to note that he was not completely opposed to the idea of positive freedom, he simply felt that the contest of ideas enabled by negative freedom would result in a beneficial degree of pluralism.

A Berlinian distinction between negative and positive freedom is especially useful for analysing ethical disputes over public health policy, which have often hinged around the tension between the state and individuals' sovereignty: between the freedom of individuals and the rights and interests of groups. For ease of expression, such 'negative' freedom will hereafter be referred to as a 'classic' conception of liberty.

South African AIDS activists' emphasis on a classic conception of liberty in this period was hardly surprising given the lack of effective HIV treatment in the period: compulsory testing or disclosure of living with HIV made little sense from the perspective of patients, and there were fears it would merely hinder people from seeking testing to ascertain whether they had contracted the virus.

A major emphasis on classic liberty also meshed well with the work of the wider gay rights movement to decriminalize consensual adult same-sex sexual acts. The emphasis on privacy doubtless related to the fact that outing a person as living with HIV could also reveal that they were gay. AIDS activism shared with gay rights advocacy the paradox of being a public movement for the right to privacy. This paradox stemmed from the reality that rights must be demanded by a visible constituency of affected people: as in the gay rights movement, some AIDS activists had to 'come out' as living with HIV for their campaigns to be effective.

These demands for AIDS policy to protect and promote human rights were far from singularly South African. At the global level, Jonathan Mann was a critical champion of human rights-based approaches to AIDS during his tenure (1987–90) as head of the World Health Organization's Global Program on AIDS (WHO GPA). Mann, who had called for a dramatically increased global response to AIDS from the late 1980s, also proposed a new paradigm which posited that human rights and public health were not inherently opposed. Rather, he argued, it was social marginalization itself which rendered people vulnerable to HIV infection. This meant that policies like mandatory testing and quarantine would not work to combat AIDS, because they would push ostracized groups such as men who had sex with other men, sex workers and injecting drug users further to the margins of society and away from HIV testing and related medical assistance. In 1990, Mann asserted his scepticism towards coercive AIDS policies for there was scant evidence that they had reduced risk behaviours (1990, p. S249). For

Mann, while the protection of rights could not guarantee 'effective' AIDS programmes 'denial of human rights was incompatible with effective AIDS prevention and control' (1990, p. S250). But Mann fell out with the Japanese head of WHO, Hiroshi Nakajima, because he thought that the organization was offering inadequate support to WHO's GPA, and he moved to Harvard University. Consequently, WHO's GPA remained substantially less effective for much of the rest of the 1990s (Behrman 2004).

Mann's voice was a relatively lonely one in the late 1980s and early 1990s. Moreover, prior to 1996 Northern countries had few governmental or civil society advocates for increases in aid to combat AIDS in Africa. After the fall of the Berlin Wall, Africa was deemed by the US State Department to be 'strategically irrelevant' and the prevailing view in the Senate, aggressively promoted by influential representatives such as Jesse Helms, was that most foreign aid merely fed corruption and did not help those in need (Behrman 2004, p. 71). Activists such as Eric Sawyer of the Global AIDS Action Committee of the AIDS Coalition to Unleash Power (ACT UP) and Paul Boneberg of Global AIDS Action Network (GAAN) were early advocates of treatment access in developing countries. However, in this period where there were no effective treatment options 'international' AIDS activism largely consisted of interactions between activists based in developed nations and their exchanges focused on comparing their own domestic AIDS crises (Smith and Siplon 2006, pp. 53–4). Indeed, in the early 1990s, AIDS activist movements in most countries can be seen to have largely operated in parallel.

In this period, Gregg Gonsalves was one such domestically focused American activist and a member of the ACT UP and its Treatment and Data Committee. Members of this committee, including Gonsalves, broke off from ACT UP and formed the Treatment Action Group (TAG). As Stephen Epstein has demonstrated, TAG permanently altered the way that drugs were approved in America, not least by pressing for greater patient and community involvement in the operations of the US Food and Drug Administration (FDA) (1996). They were also successful in pressing for community members to participate in all research committees and sites of the National Institute of Allergy and Infectious Diseases (NIAID) at the National Institutes of Health (NIH). Gonsalves was heavily involved in this advocacy for more rapid and inclusive HIV drug development and approval for much of the 1990s. Later, in the early 2000s, Gonsalves came to embody the internationalization of AIDS activism, and he assisted the TAC in designing its treatment literacy programme (as discussed in Chapter 4). But he had other domestically focused advocacy priorities in the 1990s (Interview 19 May 2011).

By international comparison, activist calls for human rights in AIDS policy were not unique to South Africa. What was more uniquely *South African* about the gay AIDS activism which evolved in the country in this period was that the spectacular law reform achievements of the gay rights movement created space for the more candid HIV prevention education and the provision of social support to those affected by the disease.

Gay activists were absolutely central to the AIDS Consortium's consolidation of civil society alliances on the epidemic. Like gay rights activism, AIDS activism as expressed in the Consortium also had a clear focus on individual rights. Professor Alan Fleming, a pathologist at the South African Institute of Medical Research (SAIMR) and Baragwanath Hospital, noted that as in the United States, South African AIDS activism had 'its roots in the gay liberation movement' (Fleming 1992, p. 426). He thought that this explained the 'great emphasis that has been given to issues of the rights of all individuals to receive pre-test counselling and to give informed consent before testing' (1992, p. 426). By contrast, Fleming saw black heterosexual patients as more concerned with their immediate needs for food and shelter, but he thought that they too would benefit from the rights contained in the AIDS charter.

The pressing need for law reform for non-discrimination on the grounds of sexual orientation was also revealed by a controversy about apartheid government censorship of two HIV-prevention videos. In 1993, the government Committee on Publications banned two safer sex videos made in South Africa called *For Men who have Sex with Men* and *A Lover's Guide*. The films were produced by Reel Communications, a production company based in Cape Town (Weekly Mail 28 October 1993). The ban was confirmed when it was taken on appeal to the Publications Appeal Board which reported that the films featured 'long, drawn out scenes of sexual activity' which the committee saw as not contributing to 'information about Aids or safe sex' but as aimed, instead, at 'provocation of lust and sexual stimulation'.[35] Nathalie Stockton of the Department of National Health and Population Development's AIDS Unit was opposed to an outright ban but supported restriction of the circulation of the videos.[36]

The Publications Act 42 of 1974 gave such censors broad powers to ban 'undesirable material', legislation that was only replaced in 1996. The censors fastidiously adhered to the dictates of Calvinist Christian Nationalist apartheid ideology: they were notoriously prudish and banned anything that could be interpreted as primarily aimed at sexual stimulation. For example, stars were placed on the nipples of topless women depicted in a 'soft-core' pornographic magazine called 'Scope' which was aimed at a heterosexual male readership. These censors also routinely confiscated publications from booksellers catering to the lesbian and gay market (Retief 1994).

Ruben Sher was in favour of the videos' distribution because they served a public health purpose in that they provided people with information to protect themselves. Gay activists were totally outraged by the banning of the videos. ABIGALE covered the issue extensively in its newsletter which included a press clipping of an article by Mark Gevisser, a gay activist and journalist at the *Weekly Mail*. The organization argued that it should challenge the ban because it amounted to 'self-appointed moral watchdogs' prescribing to gays and lesbians what they could 'read, view and do'.[37] ABIGALE held that lesbians and gays were 'major victims of the censorship system' which banned 'Informative and quite tame magazines like the ADVOCATE [an American gay and lesbian magazine]'.[38]

The South African branch of ACT UP went even further, arguing that, in the face of 500 infections a day, 'to deprive people of this kind of information is no different from infecting them; preserving the archaic, hypermoralistic attitudes of a handful of people is no excuse for genocide'.[39]

Petty censorship of this kind must have been particularly irritating for gay activists who were increasingly plugged into global networks. While dildoes and gay safer sex videos were banned in South Africa, sexual paraphernalia were readily available in predominantly gay areas in the United States. For instance, when Simon Nkoli visited the Castro district of San Francisco in 1988 as part of a 13-city US tour in his honour after his release from prison, *The Sowetan* reported that he had 'gaped in amazement at the window displays of condoms, colour photos of unclothed male bodybuilders, a telephone in the shape of a high-heel shoe, and a [sic] black leather gear' (28 August 1988). He reportedly told the local newspaper ' "There's nothing like this in my country".'

By the same token, not all Western countries were equally progressive in allowing free speech around same-sex sexuality. In Britain, section 28 of the Local Government Act of 1988 prohibited councils from 'promoting' homosexuality as a 'pretended family relationship', and it was only repealed in 2003. Moreover, even in the United States, gay sex remained illegal in many states and in its 1986 *Bowers v. Hardwick* opinion the Supreme Court rejected the argument that the right to privacy guaranteed that of two adult males to engage in consensual sex. This ruling remained in place at a federal level until it was overturned by *Lawrence and Garner v. Texas*, which invalidated all state sodomy laws in 2003. Similarly, in 1987 conservative Republican Senator Jesse Helms successfully proposed an amendment to a spending bill which prohibited any federally funded AIDS education efforts from depicting homosexual sex (Treichler 1999).

In South Africa, the outcry among gay rights activists and their supporters over the banning of the videos intensified. The increasing links between South African and American AIDS NGOs were indicated in a *Weekly Mail* article which reported that the American Foundation for AIDS Research (AMFAR) had written to the Publications Appeal Board protesting its decision to uphold the ban.[40] AMFAR reportedly had a board packed with Hollywood stars, including members such as director Woody Allen and actors Barbara Streisand, Warren Beatty, Raquel Welch and Elizabeth Taylor.[41] In response to the letter, Dr Bram Coetzee, Director of Publications, bizarrely claimed that the directorate of publications had ' "nothing to do with the 'banning' or 'unbanning' of films" ', and that the decision was made by committees appointed on an *ad hoc* basis from a panel of people (Weekly Mail 28 October 1993).

While there certainly were links between South African and American gay AIDS activists in this period, it is also important to note that the two were different in many critical respects. There was clearly some cross-pollination in that the ACT UP briefly had a branch in South Africa from 1993–5, but it was more radical than most South African AIDS NGOs in the period. Indeed, the South African ACT UP branch's focus on encouraging accountability among 'defunct, money guzzling organizations' in the AIDS sector was seen by many activists in the country as possibly 'angering people without results'.[42] After returning from a US trip representing the AIDS Consortium, Edwin Cameron noted that in comparison to their South African counterparts, American activists were using more radical methods such as high-profile lobbying and street protests.[43] But even after the ANC government had come to power in May 1994, the Consortium recognized that the new government had competing priorities and wanted to give it a chance to deliver on its election promises. Indeed, as late as 1995, when an ACT UP activist used a Consortium meeting to attack most AIDS NGOs as being on the 'gravy train', Achmat who was by then working at the ALP pointed out that AIDS posed different issues in South Africa and, therefore, activists needed to engage in tactics using a less 'strident tone', which was more fitting when addressing the former National Party government.[44]

Constitutional advocacy for gay rights and AIDS activism

While gay rights activists were devising these charters of rights, they were also closely following the constitutional negotiations, which were important because they led to the outlawing of discrimination on the grounds of sexual orientation in both the Interim and the Final Constitutions. The success of this advocacy had important implications for AIDS activism, and it is worth describing in some detail.

Gay rights activists such as Ivan Toms and Peter Tatchell (a British campaigner) had successfully lobbied Thabo Mbeki and other ANC leaders such as Ruth Mompati on the importance of sexual orientation equality, while the liberation movement was still in exile. Simon Nkoli had persuaded his co-defendants who were key UDF leaders to accept his sexual orientation. In September 1990, activists affiliated with OLGA, such as Sheila Lapinsky and Julia Nichol, made a submission on gay rights to the ANC's Constitutional Drafting Committee, which included legal scholars such as Albie Sachs. Sachs was a member of the ANCs National Executive Committee (NEC), and he had delivered a message in support of pride which stated that many people in his organization wanted to see a new Constitution in South Africa that guaranteed 'members of the lesbian and gay community full protection against any form of discrimination, harassment and abuse'

(Sachs 2006, p. 14). According to Sachs, the issue was 'on the ANC's agenda', and to demonstrate its acceptance of gay and lesbian people, he pointed to the example of stalwart Cecil Williams 'a well loved personality in the struggle in the 1940s and 1950s, whose homosexuality was well-known to [ANC] comrades' (Sachs 2006, p. 14). Edwin Cameron recounted that they urged gay rights activists to present their concerns to the ANC.[45] In November 1990, non-discrimination on the grounds of sexual orientation was included in the ANC's draft Constitution under the subheading of gender rights (Hoad et al. 2005, p. 92). At Cameron's own 1992 inaugural lecture as a full professor of law at the University of the Witwatersrand, he presented the legal case for full equality for gay and lesbian people to an audience including members of the ANC's Constitutional drafting committee, such as Sachs, Arthur Chaskalson and George Bizos.[46]

In Cape Town, ABIGALE followed all these developments closely and gave input on campaigning efforts.[47] The Charter of Lesbian and Gay Rights was drawn up by OLGA from 1992 to 1993, and it was endorsed by all South African gay and lesbian organizations at a national conference held in Cape Town in 1993. It asserted that same-sex-practising couples and individuals had rights to adopt children and to privacy, public expression, and freedom of speech and association. The Charter also discussed rights in terms of relationships, children, education, employment, housing, health and welfare services, immigration, media, prisons, religion, policing and the courts. OLGA had also started lobbying the political parties involved in drawing up the constitution. The ANC and the Democratic Party had committed themselves to gay and lesbian equality, but there were fears that other parties could be opposed to the idea, so the feeling was that the pressure had to be maintained in order for the lobbying to be successful.[48]

Gay rights activists and organizations such as GLOW, OLGA and ABIGALE were closely engaged in efforts to have non-discrimination on the grounds of sexual orientation included in the country's new constitution, which by 1993 was being negotiated at Kempton Park. Gay and lesbian activists in ABIGALE felt that 'It's now or never. As South Africa moves towards a democratic government, we have the chance to make sure that lesbian, gay and bisexual rights are included in the new constitution.'[49]

Funds left over from pre-emptive fundraising in the 1980s for advocacy against former President P. W. Botha's never-realized proposals for further anti-gay law reform were converted into an Equality Foundation. This money was then used to employ Kevin Botha, a lawyer, to be a full-time lobbyist at the constitutional negotiations. Botha was formerly the chairman of GASA, but he had come to see the importance of a multiracial lesbian and gay movement. He produced memoranda, submissions and draft reports for the lesbian and gay movement on debates relevant to the sexual orientation clause in the constitutional negotiations, which Cameron revised. Cameron has reflected that having a full-time gay rights lobbyist who was a qualified lawyer present at the negotiating forums at Kempton Park proved invaluable in keeping the sexual orientation clause in the various drafts of the Constitution, despite stiff opposition from the ruling National Party at various points. Cameron recalled that Botha 'got to know the people, he got to know the bureaucrats who were responsible for making the submissions' and 'he kept a very close eye on behalf of the NASANT [sic – nascent] gay movement.'[50] Through these coordinated, nationwide advocacy efforts of individual gay rights activists and organizations, the sexual orientation clause was included in the new constitution.

The inclusion of the sexual orientation clause in the country's interim (1993) and final (1996) constitutions was remarkable, since South African society remained deeply homophobic. Sheila Croucher has argued that this constitutional campaign's success hinged on gay rights activists' successful use of a new political opportunity structure created by the negotiations (2002). She holds that this opportunity structure consisted of the new accessibility of the government to activists, fresh possibilities to build alliances with sympathetic rising elites and the centrality of human rights in political discourse in the period (2002).

After 1994, the constitutional clause would facilitate extensive law reform aimed at securing equality for lesbians and gay men, including the repeal of the sodomy laws (Berger 2008). This law reform would be driven by the National Coalition for Gay and Lesbian Equality (NCGLE), co-founded by Zackie Achmat and other activists which was one of the organizations later involved in co-founding the TAC. That year Achmat also became an employee of the AIDS Law Project, where his friendship with Edwin Cameron began. While Cameron left the ALP shortly afterwards, like Achmat, he later became an important advocate for wider access to combination antiretroviral (ARV) therapy (as discussed in Chapter 4).

The success of this gay rights activism was significant in the history of AIDS activism for three reasons. Firstly, the clause enabled the repeal of laws which had inhibited activist work seeking to foster greater AIDS awareness, because they had inhibited freedom of gay and lesbian speech and expression. Secondly, the constitutional clause paved the way for the rapid post-apartheid success of the gay rights law reform agenda and freed up gay rights activists' time to focus on other issues of importance to lesbians and gay men, such as AIDS. Thirdly, in a later period, the success of legal activism following, and based upon, the constitutional clause provided wider lessons about legal activism which would be applied to later struggles such as that for universal access to Nevirapine to prevent mother-to-child transmission of HIV.

The clause can also be said to be superior to appeals to the right to privacy in terms of both gender and sexual orientation equality. Philosopher Martha C. Nussbaum has illuminated the flaws of defending sexual rights based upon a traditional reading of the right to privacy. She has argued that it is a vague concept in law because 'It includes ideas of informational secrecy, modesty, seclusion and decisional autonomy, in a potentially confusing way' (2010, pp. 74–5). Nussbaum has offered a feminist critique of 'the appeal to the privacy of the home' as expressed in the *Lawrence and Garner v. Texas* opinion as 'all too frequently been used to protect child abuse, domestic violence, and marital rape from the law's scrutiny' (2010, p. 75). Instead, she proposes that privacy be regarded in the sense suggested by Mill: as 'self-regarding conduct' by individuals with no adverse affect on others; as acts over which the state should have no control (2010, p. 89). In a similar vein, legal theorist Courtenay Daum has noted that in the United States 'private' non-governmental organizations have invoked the right to defend their exclusion of lesbians and gay men (2009). By contrast, the gay rights clause in the South African Constitution places sexual orientation alongside sex, race and disability-related discrimination (s9.3). It obliges the state to pass legislation to prohibit and prevent sexual-orientation-related discrimination. The Bill of Rights also states that 'Equality includes the full and equal enjoyment of all rights and freedoms' (s9.2).

Greater public openness about being lesbian or gay, as evident in the pride march, was also vital in achieving these gains and was mirrored in some gay activists' decisions to emerge from a 'second closet' by disclosing that they were also living with HIV. White gay activists such as Shaun Mellors began to be open about their HIV status at big conferences debating the future shape of post-apartheid AIDS policy. Mellors had been 'outed' as living with HIV in the media by the Department of Health's AIDS Unit in 1988. Mellors disclosed his HIV status again at the 1992 National AIDS Convention of South Africa (NACOSA), and he made an impassioned plea for delegates to endorse the AIDS Consortium's Charter. He told them that he was 'tired of being treated like an object; an object without any identity; without feelings and emotions, an object who has no place in society and is generally referred to as an AIDS victim, or an AIDS sufferer'.[51]

These emotional revelations were personal and had political impacts in that they meant that discussions about AIDS policy could no longer be discussed in the abstract, without those most directly affected being present and vocal in expressing their interests in relation to it. They also added an emotional intensity to arguments for AIDS policy to be human rights-based, as set out in the AIDS Charter.

Political funerals

In the early 1990s, the new, more radical, black-led gay rights activism would start to draw upon anti-apartheid iconography and repertoires to combat homophobia and develop public awareness about AIDS. A case in point was the political funeral of Linda Ngcobo, who had been a founding member of GLOW and the organizer of the annual Miss GLOW drag show in Soweto.

Ngcobo's political funeral was held on 13 February 1993 at Soweto's Phiri Hall. He had died of AIDS-related renal failure at the age of 28. Mark Gevisser has described Ngcobo's funeral as perhaps the first AIDS activist's political funeral in the country, noting that 'Ngcobo was one of the first black men to declare his homosexuality publicly and draw others around him; he was also the first black gay leader to [publicly] die an AIDS-related death' (1994, p. 16).

Simon Nkoli addressed the mourners standing in front of Ngcobo's coffin with the GLOW banner – a pink triangle framing a raised, clenched black power fist – placed strategically behind him. The pink triangle was a badge homosexual men were forced to wear in Nazi concentration camps during the Second World War. It had been an international gay rights symbol since the late 1970s. This symbol is shown emblazoned on a 1990 pride t-shirt depicted in Figure 2.3.

Gevisser has described Ngcobo's burial as a political funeral because it was 'as much a memorial to a dead comrade as an impassioned plea for tolerance and a call-to-arms for rights' (1994, p. 16). According to Gevisser, 't-shirt clad

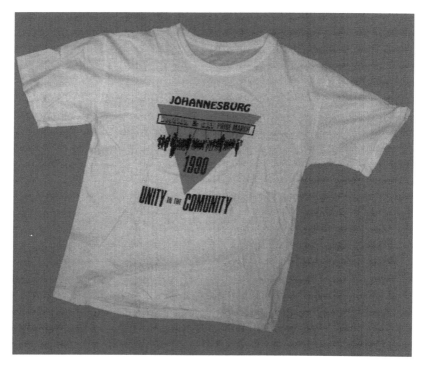

Figure 2.3   1990 pride t-shirt with pink triangle
Source: © GALA, From the GALA t-shirt collection (GALA, GLOW t-shirts, AM 2560).

comrades' *toyi-toyi*-ed (performed a political protest dance) in front of the funeral procession as it moved to Soweto's Avalon cemetery (1994, p. 16). They sang conventional anti-apartheid songs interspersed with chants of 'hey, hey, ho, ho, homophobia's got to go' (1994, p. 16). Five years on, Zackie Achmat would call for the launch of the TAC at Nkoli's own political AIDS funeral. This new, radical black-led gay rights activism laid the foundation for the later development of more assertive AIDS activism which was driven by people living with HIV.

In highlighting the political nature of Ngcobo's funeral, Gevisser was situating it as a traditional South African anti-apartheid organizing tactic which was creatively re-fashioned by gay rights and AIDS activists. Funerals of slain anti-apartheid activists had grown increasingly militant and politically important in the 1980s, as almost all other forms of black protest were banned. Mamphela Ramphele has argued that these political 'struggle' funerals afforded an opportunity for history to be 'reinterpreted, reenacted, and represented in a manner ... intended to shape social memory in the[ir] political speeches and other ceremonial acts' (1996, p. 107). The large political funerals of ANC and United Democratic Front (UDF) activists sometimes involved mass burials of scores of young activists who had been killed by the security forces. They became symbolically elaborate pieces of political theatre with thousands of mourners and were arranged to obtain maximum international media coverage, as domestic censorship remained in place. Posters and flags of the banned ANC were often prominently displayed at such funerals. The political funerals of the 1980s often became violent as armed 'young lions' clashed with security forces.

In the early 1990s, gay rights activists used the political space created by the transition to hold a peaceful political AIDS funeral for Linda Ngcobo. While its scale may not have been as grand as some of the political funerals of the 1980s and early 1990s, it was, nevertheless, an important statement of the social and political status gay rights activists were demanding. These demands would be met in the new South Africa which was being negotiated and that would shortly come into existence with the first democratic elections on 27 April 1994.

Conclusion

By the eve of the 1994 elections, gay AIDS activism had undergone many critical developments. Efforts to generate AIDS awareness and provide social support to gay men living with, and vulnerable to, HIV infection had been sustained over many years. AIDS had emerged in 1983 at a time when many lesbian and gay organizations were white-dominated and divided over the issue of how to deal with apartheid. But by the end of the transition era (1990–4), new strings had been added to the AIDS activist's bow. In particular, activists who focused on gay rights work and those who focused on AIDS both came to use human rights-based discourse to combat homophobic and AIDS-related discrimination. They did so assertively in new spaces which had been created by the political liberalization which accompanied the transition. The country's first pride march had ushered in a new, more defiant, black-led gay and lesbian politics. Gay AIDS activists were increasingly radical in their tactics to push for human rights-based approaches to the epidemic, as was evinced in Linda Ngcobo's political AIDS funeral. This was partly because there was more political space for the holding of demonstrations and political meetings.

Charters of rights for gay and lesbian people and those living with HIV had been drafted. The lesbian and gay charter had provided a powerful basis for advocacy at constitutional negotiations. Similarly the AIDS-related charter was an influential rhetorical tool at key AIDS-policy-making forums such as the NACOSA conference. In addition, gay AIDS activists had facilitated the formation of coalitions such as the AIDS Consortium and later the National Coalition for Gay and Lesbian Equality (as discussed in Chapter 4).

The idea that AIDS policies should respect and promote human rights was nothing new internationally – Jonathan Mann had already asserted this. But the Constitutional clause outlawing sexual-orientation-based discrimination was a singularly *South African* human rights achievement, because it was a direct, far-reaching legally binding statement of equality obtained during the country's political transition. This accomplishment provided a rich legacy for AIDS activism as it liberated the time and energies of gay rights activists such as Edwin Cameron and Zackie Achmat to focus on AIDS and it also afforded them the freedom of speech to promote safer sex and combat AIDS-related prejudice.

This chapter has shown that gay rights activists actively and publicly owned the issue of AIDS, and from the late 1980s onwards, saw it as central to their increasingly vocal struggle for equal rights and dignity. Indeed, for activists such as Bev Ditsie, gay rights and AIDS activism grew so intertwined over the period that it is hard to understand the history of the one without reference to that of the other.

3
Women, Science and Sexism in AIDS Activism in the 1990s

Introduction

Gugu Dlamini was a young woman who was diagnosed as HIV-positive at KwaMashu polyclinic in October 1998. At the time, the National Association of People Living with HIV/AIDS (NAPWA) had a Disclosure Campaign which urged people living with HIV to publicly reveal their status – a call she answered by speaking openly about her diagnosis on Radio Zulu in November 1998.[1] She was subsequently assaulted by four men behind a friend's shack. Following the assault, one of the suspects was heard to accuse her of being a prostitute who had infected people with HIV.[2] She was later taken to a clinic and then a hospital where she died from her injuries. According to AIDS activist Mark Heywood, the police investigated her murder but their inquiries proved inconclusive and at the AIDS Law Project's request an inquest was later held into her death (Interview 15 April 2008). No suspects were ever prosecuted for the activist's murder.

This chapter documents South African women's involvement in AIDS activism in the 1990s, a period when studies found that most new HIV infections were occurring in women: this was a significant departure from the 1980s, when cases had been concentrated in men who had sex with men. In 1990, the government instituted the first national survey of pregnant women attending public-sector antenatal clinics – a method which was used to estimate HIV prevalence in the general population. The first national antenatal clinic survey found an infection rate of 0.7% in expectant mothers tested (Department of Health 2011, p. 38). By contrast, in 1998, the survey found that just over one-in-five (22.8%) of the pregnant women tested were living with the virus (Department of Health 2011, p. 38).

In this chapter, I describe the social and political marginalization of women living with HIV and also how certain groups of women worked to counter sexism in AIDS-related science, in the media and within civil society groups working on the epidemic. This feminist work was necessary because some early scientific hypotheses of the epidemic's spread in women lacked sociological detail, and these explanations were frequently amplified by the media. In the late 1980s, and early 1990s, much of the epidemiological literature produced on the country's epidemic posited that most women affected by the disease were sex workers. Consequently, the few South African newspaper articles that dealt with the issue minimized its impact on most women. This meant that women's organizations were often late to engage with AIDS, which was paradoxical given that the South Africa's women's movement was at its zenith in the early-to-mid-1990s. Indeed, in this period, it was using the rhetoric of rights and deftly forming alliances which were pivotal to the achievement of several substantive pieces of gender-equality-promoting law reform and, after 1994, unprecedented numbers of women entered government. However, neither established women's NGOs nor the government were developing programmes addressing the psychological and socio-economic needs of (the mostly young) women who were being diagnosed as HIV-positive in increasing numbers. Women like Gugu Dlamini, Prudence Mabele and Promise Mthembu who were diagnosed as living with the virus in the early-to-mid-1990s, therefore, found that male-dominated AIDS-related civil society groups were the only avenue to obtain counselling and social support from other people who were living with the disease. But these entities did not provide them with safe spaces to discuss their gender-specific experiences of living with the disease *as women*.

Although such women AIDS activists felt disempowered by science, the media and civil society, it is important to emphasize that they exercised their agency in tackling sexism in these spheres in the 1990s. Moreover, amplifying women's voices on organizing around AIDS as an issue which affected them *as women* is particularly imperative given the existence of relevant written sources and that the recentness of the period itself, which readily facilitates the gathering of oral histories. The political dimensions of women's AIDS activism in South Africa's past have been under-examined in existing literature on the phenomenon which has mostly been contemporaneous and ethnographic in nature and has tended to focus on their intimate relationships and roles as caregivers and support group members (Akintola 2004; Susser 2009; MacGregor and Mills 2011). In this chapter, I identify three groups of women who challenged sexism in AIDS-related science and popular representations of the epidemic: women epidemiologists; women writer-activists and women living with HIV.

By the end of the 1990s, these three groups of women had shaped AIDS epidemiology, media portrayals of the epidemic and AIDS activism itself. Epidemiologist Quarraisha Abdool Karim and psychologist Catherine Campbell had described the social and cultural factors which placed women at greater risk of infection than men with increasing sociological sophistication. In the early-to-mid-1990s, feminist writers were publishing articles in *SPEAK* magazine documenting women's experiences of gendered barriers to condom use. Journalist Charlene Smith's newspaper articles on her efforts to prevent herself from contracting HIV after she was raped brought to the fore the ways in which violence against women made them vulnerable to infection with the virus. Women AIDS activists living with HIV such as Dlamini, Mthembu and Mabele increasingly disclosed their status. But their increased visibility carried risks in a society where violence against women was endemic – risks which were not fully acknowledged by NAPWA, a mixed-gender organization. The murder of NAPWA activist Gugu Dlamini following her public revelation that she was living with HIV radicalized many AIDS activists and led to the development of a feminist critique of gender-blind disclosure campaigns. In 1998–9, some of these feminist AIDS activists moved across to support the newly formed TAC. While the new movement provided a political 'home' for some individual feminist AIDS activists its formation was not primarily driven by established South African women's organizations, in the same way as it was associated with the country's gay rights movement (an association I describe in Chapter 4). This also contributed to the fact that foreign and international women's organizations were not, initially, prominent among the fledgling TAC's international allies (listed in chapters 4 and 5).

Women in AIDS-related epidemiology

In 1990, the epidemiology surrounding the epidemic in women remained in its infancy. Many women's organizations only substantively engaged with AIDS more recently (in the 2000s) compared to gay rights or healthworker organizations, and this can be linked to two phenomena. Firstly, women who were living with HIV were stigmatized as being sex workers. Secondly, evidence-based epidemiological studies of factors driving HIV transmission to women only emerged in the 1990s. Some of the first few South African scientific articles on the issue in the late 1980s offered the untested hypothesis that the epidemic's spread was being driven by prostitutes. By contrast, in the 1990s, female academics published evidence-based work showing the complex interplay between women's socio-economic status, mobility, age and their engagement in risky sexual behaviours.

Many of the earliest epidemiological articles on AIDS in South Africa framed the disease as a problem which mainly afflicted gay men and a few foreign 'heterosexual' men. For example, a 1986 letter to the editor of the *South African Medical Journal* asserted that no black South African woman had been diagnosed with HIV (Malan 1986). That same year, Ruben Sher conducted a study which tested 1,200 women 'providing companionship' to miners for infection and none was found to be HIV-positive (Sher cited in Zwi and Bachmayer 1990, p. 318). The first few South African women were diagnosed as HIV-positive in 1987 (Van Harmelen et al. 1997).

In the 1980s, South African epidemiologists were far from internationally singular in being slow to recognize that women were at risk of infection and to identify the factors which made them vulnerable to contracting HIV. As we have seen, in the early 1980s, American physicians first recognized AIDS in gay men. Anthropologist Ida Susser has noted that although poor women in the United States were diagnosed with the disease, shortly thereafter, they were 'swiftly classified according to other characteristics, as Haitians, or as partners of drug users' and 'not seen collectively as women' (2002, p. 45).

By the mid-1980s, Zena Stein was an exiled South African physician and epidemiologist based at Columbia University in New York. She and her student Robynn Flan were among the first to recognize that women's risk of infection had been understudied. Stein told me in an interview that they started talking to each other and questioned 'Why do only men get it?' They pondered this because they knew it was sexually transmitted, and so they wondered about the risk faced by women who had sex with infected men (Interview 17 October 2007). At the time it was viewed as a disease that only affected men, so they were unsuccessful in applying to the National Institutes of Health (NIH) and American Foundation for AIDS Research (AMFAR) for grants. In 1987, Stein and Flann wrote a paper which called for more research into which factors in women's sexuality were placing them at risk of infection, the creation of a microbicide (which they then called a vaginal virucide) and the development of female condoms (Susser 2002). This paper was declined for publication by several journals before finally being accepted by the *American Journal of Public Health* in 1990.

In South Africa, with the identification of HIV in women in the late 1980s, epidemiologists put forward a two-stage theory of the epidemic. They projected that most new infections in the country would be part of a 'heterosexual' epidemic following an 'African pattern' (Schoub et al. 1988, p. 156). This 'two epidemics' theory had originated at the WHO. The WHO had described 'Pattern One' AIDS as 'homosexual' and concentrated in Europe and the United States and used the term 'Pattern Two' to describe 'African' epidemics which were seen to be concentrated among heterosexuals and injecting drug users (Patton 1990, p. 61). In 1990, anthropologist Cindy Patton documented how epidemiologists deemed heterosexual African-Americans and injecting drug users to have been living in social conditions which they viewed as equivalent to 'African' urban social disequilibrium (1990, p. 61). By the end of the 1980s they were describing the demography of the epidemic in various US cities as conforming to Pattern Two, or as being akin to African AIDS. Patton characterized this lumping together of the epidemics among African-Americans and black Africans as having been racially essentializing: they operated in very different social contexts, and so their chief commonality was racial (1990).

South African epidemiologists feared that the country would develop an epidemic much like its neighbours to the North, and they set prostitution at the centre of their explanations for the spread of HIV in women. In a

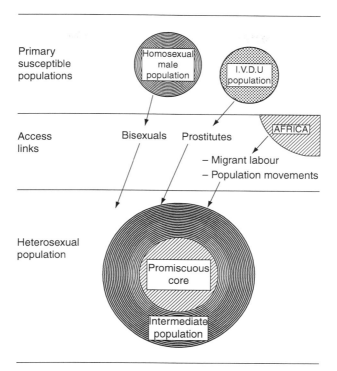

Figure 3.1 Diagram showing model of how HIV came into the country
Source: © Health and Medical Publishing Group; Schoub et al. (1988, p. 156).

1988 article, virologist Barry Schoub and his colleagues argued that 'Once established in the heterosexual population, the epidemic will be sustained, as in other part of Africa and, indeed, as with all epidemics of STDs, by a promiscuous core consisting largely of female prostitutes' (1988, p. 156). This hypothesis for how HIV would spread in the heterosexual population was illustrated by a diagram reproduced in Figure 3.1: in this diagram the heterosexual population was represented as resembling a cell with a nucleus-like 'Promiscuous core'. This cell-resembling heterosexual population was shown as being threatened by the 'viruses' of the 'Homosexual male population', Intravenous Drug Users ('I.V.D.U.') and the rest of 'Africa'. The article's authors went on to argue that because sex workers were regarded as a threat to the 'intermediate population', serious consideration needed to be given to 'efforts to shrink the promiscuous core of prostitution, irrespective of the guise under which it is practiced' (Schoub et al. 1988, p. 156).

Epidemiologists started to recognize that the AIDS epidemic was a serious and growing threat to South African women's health when the first anonymous antenatal clinic surveys were conducted in some parts of the country in 1988. By 1990, the first national, antenatal survey showed that infection rates remained below 1%, but as discussed in Chapter 1, some epidemiologists were clear that there was the potential for a more generalized epidemic to emerge. In the early 1990s, the national antenatal clinic surveys made epidemiologists more aware of the significant growth in the number of women who were becoming infected with HIV. But in the early 1990s, prostitution still remained at the centre of many of their explanations of how women were becoming infected with the virus. This dominant theory of migrant-labour-related prostitution as driving new infections was evident in an article by Anthony Zwi and Deborah Bachmayer that was published in the journal *Health Policy and Planning* which argued that the migrant labour system caused 'disruption to family life' and, thereby, facilitated 'the spread of STDs through casual sex, prostitution and "situational" homosexuality' (1990, p. 318). Figure 3.2 shows pie charts by Zwi and Bachmayer, representing data gathered by the AIDS Advisory Group (discussed in Chapter 2).

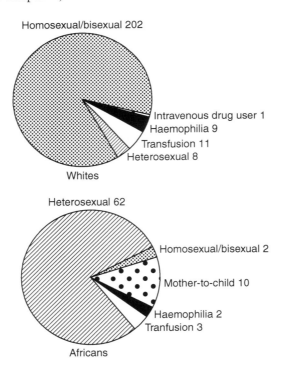

Figure 3.2   'Routes of transmission' in whites and Africans
Source: © Oxford University Press; Zwi and Bachmayer (1990).

Zwi and Bachmayer's pie charts obliquely referred to women's risk of infection using the androgynous categories of 'Heterosexual', 'Intra-venous drug user', 'Haemophilia' and 'Transfusion'. Indeed, in their pie-charts, women's risk of infection was only explicitly mentioned in relation to 'Mother-to-child' transmission, perpetuating the notion that HIV's threat to women mattered principally insofar as their children could become infected with the virus.

In the early 1990s, women epidemiologists also began publishing studies showing some of the socio-economic and cultural factors behind the growth in HIV infections in women. These studies demonstrated that while commercial sex workers certainly had an elevated risk of infection with the virus, they were far from the only group of women becoming infected with HIV. Moreover, they showed that like all women, sex workers' vulnerability to infection stemmed from their marginalization *as women* and the prevailing cultural ideas that men should exercise a greater degree of control in sexual relationships, even if they frequently exercised this to veto condom use. From the early-to-mid-1990s, epidemiologist Quarraisha Abdool Karim conducted and published a series of population-based HIV prevalence and socio-behavioural studies in collaboration with her colleagues. Abdool Karim had studied under Zena Stein at Columbia. When she started her research, the best available data on HIV prevalence among women in the country had emerged from the national antenatal clinic surveys. But these national surveys were entirely anonymous, and they did not measure the relationships between age, migration and gender-related factors and the spread of the epidemic in women: these were gaps which Abdool Karim aimed to address with her population-based surveys. Her studies showed that while sex workers had an extraordinarily high risk of infection (demonstrated in a study published in 1995), there were also other groups of women who were also at risk of infection (as highlighted by a study published in 1992): for instance, women in serious relationships or who were being faithful to their husbands were increasingly among the ranks of the newly infected (Abdool Karim et al. 1992; Abdool Karim et al. 1995).

The 1992 study – published in the journal *AIDS* – was especially notable, because it was the first which pointed to women's greater vulnerability to HIV infection. This study piggybacked onto ongoing malaria surveillance by the provincial and national health departments in areas of Natal where the disease was endemic. Approximately every six weeks, agents of this programme would visit almost all houses in malaria-endemic areas and take their inhabitants' blood to test it for the mosquito-borne disease. In addition, agents asked participants their age, gender, duration of residence, malaria sector code and whether they had had a fever in the previous fortnight. Abdool Karim's study involved also anonymously testing these blood samples for HIV. Her study showed that women had a 3.2-fold higher HIV prevalence than men. A graph reproduced from her doctoral dissertation

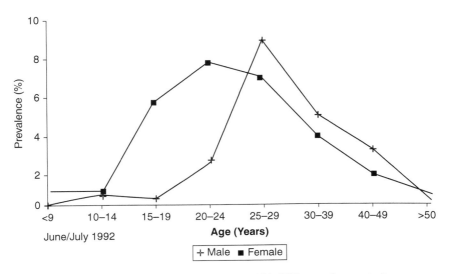

Figure 3.3   Data from Abdool Karim et al.'s 1992 HIV prevalence study: women generally became infected at an earlier age than men
Source: © Quarraisha Abdool Karim (doctoral thesis, p. 61).

(Figure 3.3) shows that infections peaked at an earlier age in females compared to males – most alarmingly, a 12-year-old girl who had participated in the study was diagnosed as infected with the virus (1992). The study also found a strong correlation between HIV infection and migration – that is, having changed place of residence recently. Those who had changed residence in the last year had a 3.1 times greater rate of HIV infection (Abdool Karim et al. 1992, p. 1538). This was particularly pronounced among the men studied, who had a 7.3 fold higher risk of HIV infection if they were recent migrants, compared to women's 2.4-fold higher risk of infection (Abdool Karim et al. 1992, p. 1538).

Abdool Karim described the body of research of which the 1992 study was a part in her 2000 doctoral thesis. She argued that her work showed that most South African women knew about HIV and were aware of how it was transmitted. Her community-based surveys also demonstrated that marriage was rare, but serial, monogamous relationships were common and the 'majority of women interviewed were sexually active' (Abdool Karim 2000, p. xxi). Young women in urban and rural communities were often undergoing early sexual debuts and engaging in unprotected sex which placed them 'at a high risk of acquiring HIV infection' (Abdool Karim 2000, p. xxi).

Catherine Campbell's social psychology research demonstrated some of the reasons why prostitutes' clients were often reluctant to use condoms. In her 1997 study based on in-depth interviews with miners, she pointed to the men's self-perceived need to 'compensate for reduced opportunities for assertion of masculine identities' in the difficult and dangerous workplace context of the gold mines (1997, p. 19). Even in the new South Africa, many miners were still migrant labourers who lived in crowded accommodation on the mines. While the miners Campbell studied were aware of the dangers of unprotected sex with multiple partners, they found that it relieved the stress associated with their living and working environment.

In the 1990s, such women public health researchers showed that prostitution needed to be situated among a mosaic of factors which placed females at risk of infection. Moreover, commercial sex only mattered in the growth of the epidemic, because the identities and practices associated with it were shaped by women's wider social marginalization. In this regard, Mark Hunter has fruitfully suggested that while 'prostitution may well have propelled HIV quickly through the major migrancy and transportation routes in its early stages', when taken alone, it cannot explain 'the tremendous speed and the persistence with which HIV has spread in South Africa' (2002, p. 100).

Peter Doyle, an actuarial scientist at the Metropolitan Life insurance company, issued further warnings that a massive HIV epidemic was developing in South Africa, which would heavily affect the country's women. Doyle developed an actuarial model to predict the future demographic impact of AIDS, based upon the assumptions that HIV would be spread 'mainly heterosexually' and that prostitution alone could not be blamed for the spread of the epidemic: future infection rates would be shaped by a wider range of risk-related behaviours such as mobility, whether people had other STDs, and whether they had more than one stable partner (1993). Doyle's model predicted that with no behaviour-change, HIV infection rates would peak at 27% of the 15–45-year-old population segment by 2010 (1993, p. 104).

The prostitute-as-vector epidemiological theory of infection is relevant to the history of AIDS activism because found its way into the mainstream media and, thereby, influenced public perceptions in ways which politically disempowered women. Those who were living with HIV were stigmatized as being prostitutes, a characterization which led many to believe that they were not at risk of infection prior to their own diagnosis. It also meant that the disease was accorded insufficient priority by many women's organizations. Even after evidence-based studies emerged predicting a generalized epidemic and showing how women's lesser social status placed them at risk of infection, these were inadequately amplified by the mainstream media for much of the 1990s, as the next section will show.

Mainstream print media coverage of women and AIDS

Like many women in the 1990s, prior to her own diagnosis as being HIV-positive, Promise Mthembu (who later became an AIDS activist) had little sense of her own risk of contracting the disease. Speaking of the early 1990s she told me that 'At the time, the way it was presented to me it wasn't a black [African] man's disease at all .... They were saying it affected sex workers and I believed that not many sex workers were black because [when they were pictured] you would see white women in magazines or coloured women, pretty women so it was not you, you know' (Interview 29 August 2003). Mthembu's story points to the ways in which mainstream newspaper and magazines' reporting on the issue made a substantial contribution to many South African women's false sense that their own risk of contracting HIV was low. The country's print-media began to report that the heterosexual population was primarily being infected through prostitution from 1988 onwards. But even though this implied for the first time that women were at risk of infection their *collective* risk of infection *as a gender* was seldom mentioned in early media reports on AIDS.

This problem was not unique to South Africa. Paula Treichler has commented, for instance, that the reporting of 'heterosexual' AIDS in the United States in the 1980s and early 1990s was contradictory and confusing and seldom identified women as being at risk of infection *as women* (Treichler 1999). Some American epidemiologists also grouped female sex workers, women with multiple partners, and promiscuous women together under the category of 'prostitutes'. According to Treichler, this confusing and contradictory early reporting on AIDS in the American medical and mainstream media 'made it difficult to conceptualize communities or cohorts of "women at risk" and discouraged the formation ... of a collective female identity a "we" around the issue of AIDS' (1999, p. 257). As we shall see, in South Africa, as in the United States, this confusing early reporting was almost certainly a factor which pushed AIDS further down the women's movement's political agenda.

Much early South African reporting on women's risk of infection either implied that AIDS chiefly affected prostitutes or discussed women's vulnerability to the virus using the euphemism of 'heterosexual' AIDS. While there was a long history of women mobilizing for their rights as 'women' in South Africa, stretching back to the suffragette movement and anti-pass demonstrations in the early twentieth century, there was no history of them organizing self-consciously as 'heterosexuals'. Similarly, while 'homosexual' was a category South Africans had organized around politically from the 1960s onward, 'heterosexual' was a broad, abstract category which only really made sense as the opposite of 'homosexual'. Furthermore, as philosopher Judith Butler noted, the category of the 'heterosexual' was created along with the modern, medically framed one of the homosexual – which only solidified in the nineteenth century (1999, p. 184).

For example, a 1988 article in *The Sunday Tribune* headlined 'Don't believe Aids is only a "gay" or "black" disease, warn experts' addressed the issue of 'heterosexual' AIDS (2 June 1988). The article warned readers not to become complacent by thinking that AIDS only affected gay men or black people; instead, it informed them that 'heterosexual' and white people were also at risk of infection. But it avoided any mention of the words 'woman' or 'women'. It also dealt with a symposium on 'how companies would cope with this growing problem' and on 'individual responses to the disease' and cautioned that if AIDS continued 'to be plugged as a gay disease, educational programmes' would become 'totally meaningless and a "waste of time and money" '. This was the feeling of 'AIDS experts' who wanted 'the gay and black tags to be thrown out of the window'. But the article contained no information on the number of HIV infections, or the epidemic's doubling time, or how 'heterosexuals' might prevent themselves from contracting the disease.

By the early 1990s newspaper coverage of 'heterosexual' AIDS had become more specific. An August 1990 article in *The Star* announced that most new 'AIDS sufferers' were 'heterosexuals' (20 August 1990). It opened by mentioning that of the 25 new AIDS cases (that is cases with progressive opportunistic infections) reported in the previous eight weeks more than two thirds were 'involving heterosexuals'. The article offered specific advice to 'heterosexuals': it quoted a health department statement which said that HIV had entered 'the heterosexual community' and that 'anyone with more than one sexual partner' was potentially at risk; therefore, the government urged the public to introduce 'safer sex practices' into all casual liaisons and relationships 'including marriage' where more than one partner was involved.

In the late 1980s and early 1990s, coverage of the new menace of 'heterosexual' AIDS in South African newspapers was also entangled with debates about the legalization of prostitution (*Cape Times* 22 October 1988). In 1991, there appears to have been a debate within the national health department about whether to legalize prostitution and homosexuality to combat the growth of the epidemic. A *Sunday Times* article of 26 May 1991, headed 'Legalise prostitution call to control AIDS', reported that the government was 'considering' legalizing prostitution and homosexuality 'to help curb the spread' of the disease. But the government's contemplation of the legalization of prostitution was short-lived and this is probably attributable to differences of opinion within the national health department. Just three days later an article in *The Citizen* countered that 'Legal prostitution [was] "not considered" '. The department hid behind a standard shield in instances of bad press: it stated that it had been misquoted and 'noted with regret the sensationalism of the Aids issue and the "deliberate" misinterpretation of a departmental response to a press inquiry' (*The Citizen* 28 May 1991). This back-pedalling by the Department needs be understood against the reality that South Africa was a country where public opinion veered towards social conservatism on issues of gender and sexuality.

Two years later, a similar article headed 'Heterosexual AIDS cases on the increase' appeared in The Natal Witness. The article reported that the national health department had warned that two-thirds of the 345 AIDS cases reported in 1991 were heterosexually transmitted (26 March 1992).

Paediatric cases accounted for one sixth of this figure. But the article failed to explicitly name 'women' *as women* being diagnosed with AIDS: a remarkable omission given that it was in no insignificant way indirectly pointing to the fact that women were being diagnosed with AIDS.

The widespread social opprobrium attached to prostitution and same-sex sexuality, which were generally understood to be the dominant modes of transmission, was shown in a November 1993 *Sunday Times* article (reproduced in Figure 3.4) which reported that in a survey of black South

Not much comfort on social issues

THE politically "correct" can hardly take much comfort from the poll.

In the week that black communities in Natal's Dukuduku Forest were being moved because they were threatening the flora, the poll showed two-thirds of blacks support the chopping down of trees to create more jobs.

The same percentage supported the mining of sand dunes if it meant creating jobs. A third of blacks also believe game reserves should be opened to farming.

Only six out of the 2 200 people interviewed thought spending on improving human rights should be a major priority.

Less than a quarter of black South Africans thought women should be allowed legal abortions and fewer than 10 percent thought prostitution should be legalised.

Forty percent thought

that people who caught AIDS deserved it. The same number thought a waiter with the disease should be fired.

Less than a fifth approved lesbian or gay relations.

But not all was lost to the cause. Seventy percent thought it was wrong to deny women top jobs and most believed in animal rights.

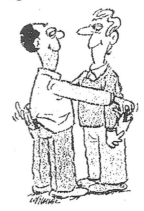

Figure 3.4   Report on a study showing that black South Africans lacked 'political correctness'

Source: © Avusa Media Ltd.; *Sunday Times* (4 November 1993).

Africans, of 2,200 interviewed, less than a quarter supported legalization of abortion and less than 10% legalization of prostitution; less than a fifth 'approved [of] lesbian or gay relations' (4 November 1993). Similarly, 'Forty percent thought that people who caught Aids deserved it. The same number thought a waiter with the disease should be fired.'

Just under a year later, The *Cape Times* reported that 794 new HIV cases had been identified in the Western Cape in the first six months of 1994 (21 October 1994). According to the report, 60% of these were 'infected by heterosexuals'. Yet again, the report used the euphemism 'heterosexuals' to sidestep referring to the fact that *women* were becoming infected. But it shied away from blaming prostitutes, reporting that of the cases 'none were found to have been at risk [of infection] from blood transfusions, female prostitution or drug use'. Reading between the lines, it was clear that heterosexual, non-prostitute women were also becoming infected with the virus.

As we have seen, over the period, any efforts to promote decriminalization of same-sex sexuality or prostitution had to contend with widespread social conservatism on these issues. A 1996 article in *City Press* – a publication with a mainly African readership – quoted Rev. Muzi Kunene, Secretary-General of the 'controversial' organization 'Christians for Truth', as calling for the government to wage 'chastity campaigns' because 'the only safe sex' was supposedly 'no sex' (07 August 1996). And, the reverend argued, it was contradictory that the Health Department went to ' "such lengths to fight Aids" ', while the same government supported ' "the homosexual lifestyle" ' and was ' "even considering decriminalizing prostitution" '.

While the risk AIDS posed to women *as women* was seldom stated unambiguously in the mainstream media, there were significant exceptions, especially towards the end of the decade. A 1996 article in *The Star* headed 'Women bear the brunt of Aids in SA' reported on a seminar on the epidemic's impact on the economy which was hosted by Business Report and Southern Life insurance company (22 November 1996). It quoted Clem Sunter, head of corporate affairs at Anglo American – one of South Africa's largest companies – as having predicted that 26% of the female population would be HIV-positive by the year 2010. He also apparently 'attacked women of influence' for not pressing for more 'political attention' to be paid to the 'high incidence of sexual attacks on young girls'. But this article was an exception to mainstream media coverage at the time which generally failed to address the link between violence against women and AIDS.

Women AIDS activists thus had to overcome journalists' common replication of the earlier prostitute-as-vector epidemiological model and their frequent use of confusing euphemisms such as 'heterosexual AIDS', which masked women's real risks of infection. Reporters' deployment of such confusing terms needs to be viewed in the context of the popularity of socially conservative views on prostitution and same-sex sexuality. In addition, in the early 1990s, activists in the women's movement often initially accepted the dominant prostitute-as-vector model and only researched and organized around the links between violence against women and AIDS in a later period, as the next section will demonstrate.

The women's movement and its activists' writings on AIDS

The lack of social support women initially experienced *as a woman* living with HIV (discussed in the final section of this chapter) paradoxically occurred at a time when the South African women's movement was at its apogee. Indeed, the transition-era advocacy of the Women's National Coalition (WNC) resulted in unprecedented numbers of females entering government and some important pieces of gender-equality-promoting law reform in the post-1994 period. While AIDS was not a central concern for the women's movement as a whole, the disease was a growing area of interest for some sexual and reproductive health activists within it. These women's health activists wrote on the issue in women's rights-promoting publications such as *Agenda* journal and *SPEAK* magazine; unsurprisingly, their writings did not obscure the risk AIDS posed to ordinary women in the same manner as the mainstream media. But there was no consensus among them on which groups of women were being exposed to infection and also the set of factors that lay behind their vulnerability.

Women's organizations' limited involvement with the issue was observed by concerned public health experts at the time. In 1990 Zwi and Bachmayer noted that 'women organizations and youth groups' needed 'to be sensitized to the issues concerning HIV infection and other STDs' (1990). This was because their 'involvement' would have done much to 'facilitate grassroots understanding of the nature of STDs and how to combat them' (Zwi and Bachmayer 1990, p. 324).

On the rare occasions when feminist academics and women ANC activists did mention AIDS in the early 1990s, they deployed the dominant prostitute-as-vector epidemiological model. For instance, in a statement to the 1990 Maputo Conference, Liz Floyd argued that it was 'natural' for men who were migrant labourers to seek out relationships which provided 'the comforts of home' and for the women they were involved with to 'accept compromises, with their partners having a wife at home and a girlfriend at work'.[3] Floyd went on to argue in the same speech that women who were impoverished by the migrant labour system became prostitutes and were often involved in financially dependent relationships with multiple boyfriends. Manto Tshabalala (who later became the second post-apartheid Minister of Health) also pointed to prostitution as the main reason for the spread of AIDS.[4] Similarly, Anna Strebel wrote in *Agenda* feminist journal that migrant labour had 'forced on women and men sexual practices which can only increase the risk of HIV infection' (1992, p. 50).

The problematic idea that AIDS mainly affected prostitutes was also a common view among South African women, more generally in the early 1990s.

Montsho Matlala published an article in *SPEAK* magazine in 1993 which described her embarrassment at accidentally removing a condom from her back pocket in front of three young women while taking a taxi from Jane Furse to Pietersburg. Her mortification at this mistake was based on experience: she knew women who would get 'angry' when the use of condoms came up and would tell her that if it came up in a relationship they would say 'Do you think I'm a prostitute infected with STD's? Never use that rubber in my body.' (Matlala 1993, p. 33). The stereotype that AIDS primarily affected prostitutes generated an artificially low sense of risk among uninfected women and in the minds of many it connoted that all women living with HIV were sex workers.

Moreover, some women still adhered to the older stereotype that AIDS was a 'gay plague'. One woman living with HIV – who chose to remain anonymous – told *SPEAK* magazine that prior to her own diagnosis she had not believed that she was at risk of infection because when she had first heard about the disease in the 1980s, it had been described to her as one which only affected gay men in San Francisco (SPEAK 1993, p. 14).

The limitations of the South African women's movement's response to AIDS did not stem from its lack of power: it was far from weak or disorganized in the 1990s. While the Women's National Coalition (WNC) was made up of several ideologically and socially diverse organizations, it managed to generate a consensus on its goals and a unified strategy that led to a series of women's rights-focused law reforms (Hassim 2006). The two main self-defined 'feminist' publications in the country were *SPEAK* magazine and *Agenda* journal. *SPEAK* (founded in 1982) was a newsletter published in English and isiZulu which profiled the activities of community-based women's organizations in Durban. It later became national in distribution and in terms of the issues it covered. *Agenda* journal, established in 1986, aimed to provide a forum for feminist academics and activists to publish theoretical discussions about women and gender.

SPEAK and *Agenda* were among the few outlets which published pieces by self-described 'feminists'. But not all participants in South African women's organizations in the 1980s and 1990s referred to themselves as 'feminist', and some women's organizations were not even founded with the aim of promoting women's rights. SPEAK founders Shamim Meer and Karen Hunt told me that in some cases, their genesis can be traced back to male activists having urged for women to 'organize' other members of their gender in order to strengthen the overall 'struggle' for national liberation (Interview 10 February 2006).[5] Even in cases where women's organizations and activists did promote gender equality, they did not necessarily describe themselves as feminists. This reluctance to use the term 'feminist' to describe projects promoting women's rights related to the fact that the ideology was widely stigmatized in anti-apartheid circles in the 1980s and early 1990s as a 'separatist' strategy promoted by Rape Crisis activists (some of whom were lesbians) at white universities. In this context, many anti-apartheid women who were actually articulating and organizing around gender-equality-promoting positions did not refer to themselves as feminists, for strategic reasons (Hassim 2004).

But these complexities of organizing for gender equality did not seriously hinder the women's movement's march. Its limited response to AIDS came at a time when it was engaging in effective campaigning on other issues: its relative inaction on the issue chiefly related to the fact that it did not prioritize the epidemic. Indeed, the movement, as embodied in the creation of the multi-party, multi-sectoral WNC, was instrumental in the inclusion of females in negotiating teams at the Congress for a Democratic South Africa (CODESA) and of the incorporation of the gender equality clause into the post-apartheid Final Constitution's Bill of Rights (Hassim 2006). By contrast the movement lacked a coherent strategic response to AIDS: its main manifesto, the WNC's 'Women's Charter for Effective Equality' produced in February 1994, included only one minor mention of AIDS under the health article (11) which called for women to have access to 'information pertaining to reproductive health services'.[6]

This focus on providing women with information on how to prevent HIV transmission was certainly necessary, but it was not sufficient: as a lone strategy, its success rested on the assumption that they exercised full control over their sexual decision making. It was only towards the end of the decade that women's health activists came to recognize that coercion and violence played a significant role in the spread of HIV: factors which could not be altered merely by giving women the relevant information about how the virus was transmitted. Yet at the close of the 1990s, neither feminist academics nor women's NGOs had developed effective and sustained programmes aimed at illuminating and addressing this nexus.

But the movement did not neglect gender-based violence, per se: its participants were active on the issue alongside other women's health issues such as cervical cancer and the need for abortion law reform. One activist who campaigned on sexual and reproductive health in the period was Helen Rees, an anti-apartheid physician who co-chaired the ANC Women's Health Policy committee with Manto Tshabalala in the transition era. With hindsight, Rees could see that 'ANC policy was not really getting its head around the enormity of the impact of the epidemic,' and the party's women's health policy committee which she was part of 'didn't really touch on it' (Interview 7 February 2007). Instead, they focused on 'sexually transmitted infections, cancer of the cervix... [and] a woman's right to choose [to have an abortion]'. In the early 1990s, Barbara Klugman led the Women's Health Project (WHP), an anti-apartheid NGO which advocated abortion law reform and reproductive rights in a new South Africa. Looking back on the WHP's work in the period, Klugman told me that 'I don't think we got what its [the AIDS epidemic's] impact would be. We had a feminist analysis before many others but we dealt with it as one of many issues' (Interview 24 October 2007).

Feminist publications contained sporadic assertions of the links between violence against women and HIV transmission, but these had yet to be systematically demonstrated through epidemiological research. For instance, women attending a 1991 meeting of the Township AIDS Project told reporters at *SPEAK* that it was 'men who control[led] women's sex lives'. Indeed, it was seen as 'a man's right to have sex whenever he wants to, and with who[m]ever he wants' (SPEAK 1991, p. 11). Another report on AIDS education highlighted the fact that women's requests to use condoms could result in men being violent or ending relationships (SPEAK 1992, p. 25).

In 1992, Shireen Hassim – a political scientist – stated in a paper she wrote for Oxfam Canada that there was a dearth of research on phenomena which prevented 'women from making choices about sexual practices'.[7] As we have seen, a small, local body of research on the gendered social factors which placed women at greater risk of infection developed from the mid-1990s, but it seems as if this research did not readily translate into effective feminist activism until the next decade.

When the ANC swept to power with an overwhelming majority in 1994, the new parliamentary system of proportional representation enabled it to handily implement a gender quota system where 30% of its members were women. Several women also joined the cabinet, including Nkosasana Zuma, the Minister of Health. The new government adopted a 'gender mainstreaming' approach to advancing women's rights. Gender mainstreaming refers to the principle that all government policies should entrench women's rights to equality with men. As political scientist Amanda Gouws has pointed out, since 1994, an elaborate matrix of South African state institutions has also evolved to promote gender mainstreaming, including the following:

- The Office for the Status of Women
- Gender focal points in each state department
- A Women's Empowerment Unit
- A multi-party women's caucus in parliament
- The Joint Standing Committee on the Quality of Life and Status of Women
- The Commission for Gender Equality (Gouws 2005a, p. 10).

But some feminists have also been critical of gender mainstreaming. Gouws has contended that it has replaced state engagement with women's concrete, lived experiences of oppression *as women* with technocratic, abstract readings of gender (2005b). She has also persuasively made the case that because mainstreaming has placed gender policy everywhere in the South African state, it has become no one's responsibility (2005b, p. 78).

In the post-1994 period, South African women also attended the Fourth World Conference on Women in Beijing, China in 1995. The Beijing Platform for Action committed governments – including South Africa's – to develop policies to promote gender equality and women's empowerment. South African women's participation at the Beijing conference was an important badge of honour in their home country. But such activists' participation in prominent international meetings was reflective of hierarchies within the country's women's movement. Deborah Mindy avers that 'Politically savvy women ... knew that Beijing was the place to be, to network, and to credential oneself as a leader in the South African local and national arenas' (2001, p. 1191). While some women activists engaged in power-brokering in Beijing, 'young women were left out of women's organizing [back in South Africa] or, at best, were marginal and silent (and silenced) in women's organizations' (Mindy 2001, p. 1206). Moreover, young women living with HIV were among the ranks of the young women who were excluded from such global networking opportunities.

In assessing the post-apartheid accomplishments of the women's movement, it is also worth noting that two important pieces of gender legislation were passed: the Termination of Pregnancy Act of 1996 and the Domestic Violence Act of 1998. The drafting and passage of these two laws must be viewed in the context of the women's movement's reconfiguration into a set of sector, or issue-based, networks. In the 1990s, the most influential of these networks were the National Network on Violence Against Women (NNVAW) and the Reproductive Rights Alliance (RRA) (Hassim 2006). Unsurprisingly, these two important pieces of women's legislation (listed above) passed in the 1990s addressed these networks' demands.

But powerful women in government and influential NGOs did not always represent *all women* – especially poor women. In this respect, those living with HIV were by far the only group of females who had a limited voice within the women's movement. The economic empowerment of poor women – which Hassim has referred to as 'substantive gender equality' – has, therefore, proved to be elusive in post-apartheid South Africa (2006). Hassim was not alone in her assertion of the interwoven nature of women's economic marginalization and their low social status. Indeed, feminist philosopher Nancy Fraser has argued that gender is a 'hybrid category simultaneously rooted in the economic structure and status order of society' (2003, p. 19). For Fraser, 'redressing gender injustice, therefore, requires attending to both distribution and recognition' (2003, p. 19).

South African feminists, concerned about what Fraser has referred to as the 'class-like dimension of gender' (2003, p. 21), have critiqued the government's 1996 adoption of neoliberal policies under the rubric of the Growth Employment and Redistribution (GEAR) strategy. In particular, they have criticized policies such as the privatization of essential services, associated aggressive cost recovery, and reductions in social spending.[8] They have also characterized these policies as having rested on the sexist assumption that poor women would (and should) have 'naturally' undertaken additional, unpaid reproductive labour such as wood/paraffin/water collection and care of children and sick/disabled relatives (including those who were AIDS-ill) (Gouws 2005b; Benjamin 2007). Such critiques were pronounced at the time when the policy was passed: for instance, the Women's Budget Initiative argued that 'the [GEAR] policy contained elements which had been detrimental to women in other countries' (Budlender 2001, pp. 337–8). Debbie Budlender positioned women's unpaid labour at the centre of their economic disadvantage because it constrained the work that women could take; indeed, she equated such labour to a tax which women paid before entering the job market.

Another feminist critic of the GEAR policy at the time it was adopted was ANC Member of Parliament (MP) Pregs Govender (2007). Govender cut a lonely figure in parliament in her feminist opposition to the macroeconomic policy and she was also the only ANC parliamentarian to vote against the multi-billion rand arms deal. Her singular feminist opposition to both policies showed that party loyalty and the disciplinary procedures associated with the proportional representation system hindered many ANC women MPs from taking independent, feminist positions. She opposed the ambitious rearmament plan on the grounds that she found it morally indefensible that funds which could have been used to improve the plight of poor women were instead spent on arms (Govender 2007).

South African women's subordinate economic status was multifaceted. They were more likely than men to be unemployed or employed in the informal sector and, therefore, to be the first to lose their jobs when economic conditions worsened (Budlender 1996; Gouws 2005b). Women also faced a gendered disadvantage in education – a major route out of poverty – as the schooling of girl children and young women was disproportionately harmed by teenage pregnancy, their additional share of domestic labour and their greater victimization through sexual violence in schools (Gouws 2005b). Likewise, rural women's access to land often depended upon their intimate and familial relationships with men (Cross and Friedman 1997). Many women's economic subordination prevented them from leaving abusive relationships with wealthier male partners (Abdool Karim 2000).

A further relevant feminist critique of the women's movement in this period is that NGOs that focused on intimate partner violence and sexual assault seldom engaged with how the issue interlocked with HIV transmission and, when they did, such efforts were not prolonged. For instance, in 1995, the National Conference Against Violence Against Women, NGOs called the compulsory testing of rape suspects and for district surgeons to be trained to offer counselling to women who had been raped both before and after they were tested for HIV. There is little evidence, however, of sustained campaigning subsequent to this call (*The Citizen* 27 November 1995).

A further crucial, if isolated, initiative was an AIDS-related special edition of *Agenda* journal which was published in late 1998. The overall idea behind the edition – compiled by feminist AIDS activist Vicci Tallis – was to showcase the small, but growing, number of studies demonstrating how gender was shaping the AIDS epidemic. As was customary for the journal, the edition included articles which were both academic and activist in tone and content. Abdool Karim published a research-based article showing that the root of women's greater vulnerability to infection lay 'in the imbalance in power between men and women' (1998, p. 18). By contrast, Mthembu offered personal testimony of her experiences of intimate partner violence as a consequence of her involvement in AIDS activism (1998). The special edition of the feminist journal also included a report on a seminar on violence against women and HIV transmission, attended by representatives from 30 NGOs, held at the offices of the Commission for Gender Equality in Johannesburg on 12 August 1998 (Pendry 1998). According to the report, Helen Rees discussed her view that violence against women was likely a significant factor in the spread of HIV because of the high prevalence of both in the country. Both doctors who presented at the seminar – Rees and Des Martin – also discussed the efficacy and feasibility of HIV prevention through the provision of ARVs to rape survivors for use as post-exposure prophylaxis (PEP).

But as late as 2001, researchers concluded that 'current responses to HIV/AIDS and violence against women remain split from one another and typically exist as parallel rather than complimentary initiatives' (Vetten and Bhana 2001). The researchers argued that the link was eventually brought to the public's attention in 1999 when journalist Charlene Smith wrote about her experiences as a rape survivor. Smith used her articles about her ordeal to lament rape survivors' limited access to counselling and PEP with ARVs (Smith 2001). There was, however, limited epidemiological research and information available at the time, which made it harder for women's organizations to develop 'comprehensive responses' to address the connections between rape, intimate-partner violence and HIV (Vetten and Bhana 2001, p. 1).

Feminist writers did, on occasion, publish articles on AIDS, and a few activists affiliated to the progressive health and women's movements sometimes spoke out on the issue at conferences, but they lacked a common understanding of the problem AIDS posed for the country's women – a critical first step to developing effective policy advocacy around the issue. The collective inability of the women's movement to develop a shared vision of the problem meant that it was relatively inactive on the sexism behind AIDS, especially compared to its work on other sexual and reproductive health issues or the gay rights movement's response to the epidemic (discussed in Chapter 2).

Activism by women living openly with HIV

Women living with HIV often felt that mixed-gender AIDS NGOs did not provide adequate social support for them *as women* living with HIV. So they began to found their own non-governmental networks and to develop feminist critiques of sexism within mixed-gender AIDS NGOs. The most trenchant of these critiques argued that the mixed-gender NGOs had sometimes failed to foresee the unbearable consequences some women AIDS activists faced following public disclosure of their HIV status – assault and murder. While activist Gugu Dlamini's murder received the most media coverage, it was hardly singular.

Prudence Mabele was pivotal in founding the Positive Women's Network (PWN), one of the first South African organizations run by and for women living with HIV. Mabele was born in Watville Township outside Benoni on the East Rand. In the late 1980s, she started studying analytic chemistry at Witwatersrand Technikon, but her studies were interrupted, and so she moved to Cape Town and started studying at a similar institution there. During that time she began a relationship with a male, and her main concern was avoiding an unwanted pregnancy, especially as that had been the fate of some of her female friends. She noted that her partner had a packet of 'Rough Rider' condoms in his drawer, but when she asked him to wear one he said 'No' (Interview 22 November 2006).

In 1990, she went to a hospital in Cape Town because she had started having migraines. The doctors took her blood and did several tests. Mabele told me that she remembered being told that she had 'full-blown AIDS'. They apparently kept coming 'in and out' and asked whether she was a sex worker and how many boyfriends she had. At the time of her diagnosis, she found that the only existing AIDS support organizations – Body Positive and GASA 6010 – were run by white gay men. She only discovered these organizations by seeking out the company of other AIDS patients while visiting Somerset Hospital. Women like Mabele who were diagnosed with HIV in the early 1990s found that there were few social spaces where they felt comfortable discussing their experiences of living with HIV *as women*. Mabele found that many early AIDS organizations were dominated by white gay men who had homes with Jacuzzis, while she had gone to a school that had no water. She was there to deal with her HIV status and was going to 'different places' and meeting new kinds of people.

Though male dominated, the existing mixed-gender AIDS support organizations offered Mabele the opportunity to meet some other women who were living with HIV. For instance, at the Triangle Project (a successor organization to GASA 6010 and ASET) she met a female sex worker who was HIV-positive. This sex worker had a six-year old child and was pregnant because her clients refused to use condoms. Later, Mabele met Mercy

Makhalamele and two other women living with HIV through her membership of NAPWA (founded in 1993, as discussed in Chapter 4). She also
decided to be proactive in seeking out other HIV-positive women and
began writing to hospitals and clinics informing them that she was living with the virus and expressed her desire to connect with others in her
position because she needed 'someone to talk to with the same condition' (Interview 22 November 2006). But it was extremely difficult because
healthworkers would tell her that the names and contact details of patients
living with HIV were confidential. Around the same time, Mabele began
getting small contract-based jobs translating for the Red Cross Children's
Hospital. Through this work, she started informally meeting women whose
children had been diagnosed with HIV at that hospital to express solidarity,
seek solace and provide advice.

Mabele formed the PWN in 1995. During this period, she also visited
hospitals and clinics across the country giving talks on her HIV-status as a
participant in the Department of Health's FACES of AIDS project: an opportunity she used to further consolidate PWN. As she described it to me, this
work remained informal and was done on a shoestring budget: 'I'm funding the network [PWN] and I'm earning and I'm using their [Department of
Health] resources. It's so crazy! But it worked, women were there [at different
clinics], they were meeting ... things were happening.'

Promise Mthembu was another woman AIDS activist who lived openly
with HIV in the 1990s. Mthembu was diagnosed as HIV-positive at the age
of 20 in 1995. She hailed from Umlazi township in Durban and like many
black South African young people had received her primary politicization
about the apartheid system at high school in the 1980s. Mthembu told
me that 'we started to challenge the government you know and I sort of
developed an interest in community action, you know boycotting things,
or staying away ... so I started to get involved' (Interview 29 August 2003).
Her involvement in student politics was interrupted when she became pregnant at the age of 16. Mthembu's child was born disabled which took her
'back to politics' because her daughter 'was not treated like other children'.
In her last two years of high school she was the president of the Students'
Representative Council (SRC) which was 'not very usual, I mean being a
female' but she was nevertheless elected because 'I was quite vocal ... and
my mates believed in me.' The SRC to which she belonged was affiliated
with the ANC's Youth League which, from 1990, could legally operate in the
country.

Mthembu did participate in some AIDS awareness workshops in the early
1990s, none of which 'personalized the risk' that she could become infected.
In the summer of 1992, she recalled having attended a Catholic youth camp
where she was shown a film about AIDS which featured 'sick and dying
people ... from Africa'. The film apparently denounced condom use, in line
with Catholic doctrine. In this period, she also remembered having seen the

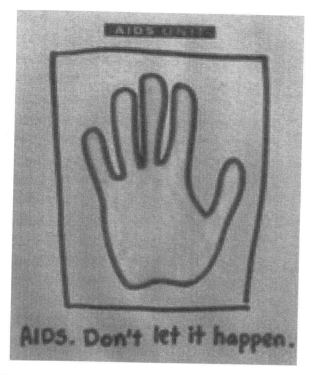

Figure 3.5 The 'yellow hand' campaign
Source: © Department of Health; Personal collection of Bridget Schutz.

Department of Health's vague 'Yellow Hand' campaign (shown in Figure 3.5), which urged people to 'Stop AIDS.'

Around the same time, an NGO called Drama in AIDS Education (DramAidE) held 'train-the-trainer' workshops at her school. These workshops offered useful information such as what the acronym AIDS stood for, the various stages of HIV infection and how to use a condom. Mthembu could pass this information on to other young people, but she did not leave the meetings feeling that she, herself, was vulnerable to infection. Nor did she think about AIDS as a political issue prior to her own diagnosis; indeed, to her 'the most important thing' at the time was 'for Nelson Mandela to be released and for the first democratic elections [to be held] on April the 27th'.

In her first year at university, Mthembu became pregnant again. She went to a clinic and tested positive for tuberculosis, a result which meant that she was also encouraged to give a blood sample to be tested for HIV. As a woman in a 'committed relationship' with a man, Mthembu did not expect to be diagnosed as HIV-positive. And she felt very angry 'with myself' and 'with the system'. She had participated in AIDS projects at school, but they did not help her to think of herself as a person at risk and so post-diagnosis her whole outlook on life changed and 'this whole new world suddenly opened up to me like, oh my goodness. Now I had HIV and I mean surely there are loads of other people that have HIV. Where are they? Why are the issues not on the agenda?'

After her diagnosis, she received counselling which helped her adjust to living with HIV. She also began attending NAPWA's meetings where she talked about living with HIV five months after her diagnosis. In 1996, she started volunteering with the National AIDS Convention of South Africa (discussed in Chapter 4). But this work had adverse consequences for her relationship, experiences which informed her gender-based critique of NAPWA. Like many South African women, she was the first partner in her relationship to be diagnosed as HIV-positive by virtue of having been tested for the virus while pregnant. Her HIV-infection resulted in her second child being stillborn. This tragedy compounded the problems her HIV-diagnosis had caused, and her partner began assaulting her. Despite this she decided to marry him because he had paid *ilobolo* (bride-price) for her, but

> Marriage changed nothing. He became more and more angry with me for attending AIDS meetings and giving talks about my personal story. He was jealous of my meeting other people who were HIV-positive, saying that I cared for and supported other people at his expense. My life became an endless circle of beatings and unprotected sex, especially if he was drunk. I could not take it any longer and I left him, despite the cultural disgrace and shame that it caused.[9]

In 1996, Mthembu was hired by Vicci Tallis, a committed feminist, to work at Durban's AIDS Testing, Training and Information Centre (ATTIC). Mthembu's interactions with Tallis helped her frame her personal experiences as related to societal sexism and were also influential on her later decision to leave NAPWA and join TAC.

Both Mthembu and Mabele's stories of being diagnosed with HIV and getting involved in political work around the issue share many similarities. They both demonstrate early male-dominated, mixed-gender AIDS organizations' neglect of the needs of women living with and vulnerable to HIV infection. Similarly, neither story contains an established women's NGO (such as those in the violence against women sector) or political organizations (such as the ANC Women's League) offering social support to either female living with HIV or conducting advocacy on her behalf.

As Mthembu's story showed, women activists who were living with HIV could also be violently attacked as a consequence of disclosing their diagnosis. Dlamini's murder brought the issue to the public's attention, and AIDS activists were unified in their outrage about it, but they had diverging political reactions to it. While some wanted to continue focusing on providing counselling and safe spaces for people living with HIV to discuss their experiences living with the disease, others developed a feminist critique of NAPWA's approach and felt more radical demands and tactics were required. Mthembu told me that she left NAPWA because 'I credited Gugu's death to the campaign. Because I just felt that she was not ready to reveal her HIV status, she had not communicated with her family or her community.'

Jo Manchester – an AIDS activist and gender and development researcher – has expressed scepticism as to whether people living with HIV who disclose their diagnosis are always, thereby, automatically empowered. Ugandan, South African and Zimbabwean AIDS activists revealed to her in interviews that their disclosure sometimes enabled them to see AIDS though a more external, political lens. But Manchester has pointed out that if activists living with HIV are to move beyond personal testimony and towards policy-focused analyses of the epidemic, they need to be 'educated around issues and trained as effective speakers' (2004, p. 91). As late as the mid-2000s, Manchester asserted that while women made up the majority of members of networks of people living with HIV in Southern Africa, 'the paid or elected positions are filled mostly by men' and this gendered glass ceiling was related to their 'lack of professional experience or educational qualifications' (2004, p. 100). Dlamini's murder needs to be interpreted in this context, against a range of shortcomings of public personal testimony as a lone strategy to empower women living with HIV in South Africa – a society in which they were marginalized in many ways.

Radicalized South African AIDS activists like Mthembu increasingly started making policy-related demands and developed campaigns based upon strategic analyses of how to obtain and wield political power. Durban-based activists who shared Mthembu's sentiments organized themselves into a Gugu Dlamini Action Committee which demanded access to AZT to prevent mother-to-child transmission. Around the same time, the Treatment Action Campaign (TAC) was formed (discussed in Chapter 4). TAC activists who were involved in the movement at an early stage told me that it was Zackie Achmat – the new movement's head – who designed defiant new t-shirts bearing Dlamini's image on the front and the words 'H.I.V. POSITIVE' on the back (depicted in Figure 3.6).[10] The next flipped-around edition of these t-shirts, which had 'H.I.V. POSITIVE' on the front, would go through multiple versions. By March 1999, the Durban-based Gugu Dlamini Action Committee had started collaborating with the TAC, which became a formidable adversary of the two Mbeki administrations on AIDS, as Chapter 4 outlines.

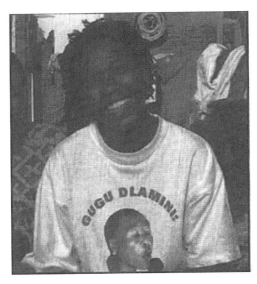

Figure 3.6 An unnamed activist wearing an early TAC t-shirt depicting slain activist
Gugu Dlamini
Source: © TAC (TAC 2008 diary, p. 6).

Conclusion

There were limited sources of social support in the 1990s for women AIDS
activists who were living openly with HIV such as Dlamini, Mabele and
Mthembu. They had to contend with sexism in AIDS-related science, the
media and mixed-gender AIDS NGOs and the women's movement's relatively low prioritization of the epidemic. In this chapter, I have pointed
to the intellectual, sociocultural and organizational factors behind their
isolation and political disempowerment in the period.

In the epidemic's early years, epidemiologists hypothesized that prostitution was driving new infections in women. This framing of AIDS was
taken up by journalists writing for the mainstream print media, reports
which made many women relatively unconcerned about their own risk of
contracting HIV. It was also taken up by sexual and reproductive health
activists in the women's movement, which was hardly surprising as it was
in keeping with the best thinking on the issue in the early part of the
1990s. Indeed, women public health academics only published evidence-
based studies showing a wider array of factors which placed women at risk of
infection from 1992. As these scholars showed women's vulnerability to HIV
infection extended far beyond sex work and was also shaped by their age,
mobility and male resistance to condom use. But this more sociologically

informed gender-focused research remained in its infancy, and the links between violence against women and AIDS were merely anecdotally alluded to in feminist publications, which did not provide an intellectual basis for sustained, effective advocacy dealing with the nexus between the two issues.

The marginalization of activists living with HIV within the women's movement cannot, however, merely be chalked down to the timing of the development of epidemiological research, especially given that more sociologically accurate research on AIDS and gender was emerging by the end of the decade. In the 1990s, the women's movement was very effective in empowering certain groups of women – NGO leaders and politicians and civil servants who moved in government – and obtaining significant legal reform. But certain groups of women were also marginalized within the movement – young women, poor women, women living with HIV – which meant that it did not represent their interests in either domestic or international policy forums. For similar reasons, neither the South African women's movement nor its international allies came to play a role in the founding and consolidation of the TAC.

Poor, HIV-positive and young women's lack of representation in the women's movement partially accounts for women in government's immobility around the 'class-like' aspects of gender oppression, discrimination which certainly shaped female vulnerability to HIV infection. Moreover, after 1994, the women's movement slowly lost its former unity of purpose, and a disconnect developed between women NGO leaders, those in government and those living with HIV. While some women in government such as Govender took independent feminist positions on issues affecting women who were poor and/or living with HIV, this was very rare given the reality of strict party discipline within the ANC. Indeed, two female health ministers (Zuma and Tshabalala-Msimang) who had participated in the women's movement in the early 1990s refused to widen access to ARVs, despite the fact that by the end of the decade AIDS had become a leading killer of young women.

Of course, this 'broken telephone' in the women's movement was far from the only dimension of the political marginalization of those living with HIV. Mixed-gender AIDS NGOs must also feature in a fair account of the social isolation and political marginalization of women AIDS activists living with HIV. While NAPWA encouraged women to speak out about living with the virus, it did not fully prepare for the fact that this could result in intimate partner violence, the termination of their relationships and even their deaths via homicide, as illustrated by the tragic demise of Gugu Dlamini. Following her murder some women AIDS activists such as Mthembu developed feminist critiques of mixed-gender groups such as NAPWA. In the process, they created a new model of AIDS activism which yoked HIV disclosure to strategic-policy-focused activism, a phenomenon the next chapter (Chapter 4) describes.

Part II

The TAC and Global Health Politics

4
Science and Sexuality in the Formation of the TAC, 1994–2001

In August 1998, Zackie Achmat wrote a letter to individual members of the National Coalition for Gay and Lesbian Equality (hereafter, the gay and lesbian coalition) informing them that he was living with HIV.[1] The letter was an important precursor to his call to form a Treatment Action Campaign (TAC), and included many of the movement's later demands. Achmat said that up to that point only his 'closest friends, family, past lovers and colleagues' had known about his HIV status.[2] New therapies and drugs with 'a proven track record for improving the quality of life' of many people living with HIV and 'previously sceptical' health professionals were suggesting that the new treatment could suppress the virus to low levels, thereby prolonging the lives of those who could access them.[3] But few could access the novel therapy, and Achmat held that the majority of people living with HIV could not 'afford the new drugs because of the profiteering and waste by the drug companies' and governments' lack of 'political will to deal with this crisis'.[4] He spelt out the implications of this lack of access to HIV treatment for sexual orientation equality – at the same time that gay right activists had obtained a constitutional guarantee of equality, their lives were becoming 'more expendable'.[5] By World AIDS Day, South Africa had lost one of its most effective gay rights activists Simon Tseko Nkoli to the disease and Achmat founded the TAC, partly, in his memory. In the late 1990s, South African AIDS activism became more radical: a development that this chapter traces. This radicalization can be linked to the greater immediate rewards that the new drug therapies offered to people living with HIV, developments which the South African activists learnt about from their counterparts who were based in the global North. People living with HIV/AIDS (PWAs) could now fight for life-extending treatment, which they learned about through correspondence, phone conversations and interactions with Northern AIDS activists at international AIDS conferences: as a consequence they began to educate themselves and members of their communities about the new treatments and to investigate ways of reducing their costs in South Africa.

This chapter maps the role of sexuality- and science-based treatment advocacy networks in the formation of the TAC, a radical new social movement. It discusses how the TAC can be viewed as having been partially, but significantly, generated by elements of the country's gay rights movement. It also demonstrates that the TAC can be seen as a newly transnational manifestation South African AIDS activism because the activists in the movement began to work extensively with AIDS, gay rights and medical humanitarian activist allies abroad to create novel treatment literacy and efficacy-demonstration programmes (also called treatment 'pilot' programmes).

The creation of such programmes to explain and demonstrate advances in HIV medicine was necessitated by the Mandela and Mbeki administrations' resistance to the development and implementation of ARV treatment programmes in line with the best science. In the initial post-apartheid period AIDS activists experienced warm relationships with progressive health activists who had gone into the government's Department of Health, which meant that the emergence of conflict over the development of an HIV treatment plan was entirely unexpected. Indeed, in the immediate post-apartheid period, there was every reason for those activists who did not go into government to be optimistic, after all former anti-apartheid activists were now running the country and the state had been fundamentally reshaped by the political negotiations and first democratic elections. Furthermore, the right to access to health care was also among the social democratic values that were enshrined in the country's final Constitution (1996). But these activist–government relationships quickly soured over four scandals, namely: *Sarafina II* (a controversial AIDS play); Virodene (an untested AIDS remedy); notification (compulsory case reporting) and AIDS denialism. In this period, the government also started to demonstrate resistance to providing a short course of AZT for prevention of mother-to-child transmission (PMTCT) of HIV. A group of activists linked to the gay and lesbian coalition, the ALP and the AIDS Consortium coalesced around Achmat to collectively found the TAC as a campaign of the National Association of People Living With HIV/AIDS (NAPWA). As the TAC's advocacy became more radical, the two organizations (the TAC and NAPWA) rapidly parted company owing to disagreements over political strategies and tactics.

This chapter also discusses how TAC activists collaborated with American and European AIDS activists to fashion programmes to popularize the science around HIV and AIDS. Achmat initially came into contact with American allies in groups such as the Treatment Action Group (TAG) and Gay Men's Health Crisis (GMHC) via his gay-related arts-based and activist social networks in New York City, which he had developed through his work as a film maker. The new South African AIDS movement also worked in tandem with MSF to establish a pilot programme in Khayalitsha township in Cape Town, one which was also critical to demonstrating the safety and efficacy of ARV drugs. Doctors in the medical humanitarian NGO reached out to the TAC after having heard about it via international HIV treatment access advocacy e-mail list-serves. These treatment literacy and efficacy-demonstration programmes contributed to the growth of the South African movement which was increasingly peopled by informed activists from heavily affected communities. They also laid the basis for it to become a mass movement with the political muscle to tackle both the pharmaceutical industry's excessively high drug prices and the government's scientifically irrational AIDS policies – campaigns which are discussed in subsequent chapters.

Gay rights and AIDS activism in the 'New South Africa'

Achmat addressed his 1998 call for action on HIV treatment to the gay and lesbian coalition. Gay rights organizers such as Achmat, Phumzile Mthethwa and Edwin Cameron formed the coalition at a 1994 conference, which brought together 40 gay and lesbian activists and 32 organizations. Its goal was to ensure that the Interim Constitution's sexual orientation equality clause be retained in the Final Constitution which was still under negotiation. Activists such as Jack Lewis were well aware that it was by no means guaranteed that the clause would remain in the Final Constitution, not least because many South Africans continued to hold conservative views on same-sex sexuality (*The New York Times* 28 December 1994).

Despite its interim nature, the new Constitution (of 1993) led to the unbanning of sexually explicit films and magazines and the flowering of sex clubs and cabarets in the country (*The New York Times* 28 December 1994). The government no longer placed images of stars over women's nipples in photographs in 'girlie' magazines: these magazines were instead placed in plastic wrappers and their sale was age restricted. It was in this context that activists such as Lewis and Achmat arranged the first national 'Out in Africa' gay and lesbian film festival in 1994. The festival was made possible because film companies felt empowered for the first time to show cinema with gay and lesbian themes in South Africa. As a consequence of the gay and lesbian coalition's very effective advocacy, the right to sexual orientation equality remained in the 1996 Final Constitution's Bill of Rights (Croucher 2002).

In the early 1990s, activists had formed multiracial organizations for gay and lesbian equality which were black-led and which rejected racism. Their activism went beyond a narrow understanding of gay and lesbian equality: they saw it as part of a tapestry of struggles for human dignity and frequently also described themselves as activists who were committed to human rights, in general. As we shall see, many had multiple political commitments and participated in networks which spanned the work of the AIDS Law Project, the AIDS Consortium, the gay and lesbian coalition and the Communist Party. In addition to their commitments to lesbian and gay equality, there was also a great deal of ideological diversity along the left spectrum among members of this group: some described themselves as also being socialist, others communist, Trotskyite and feminist. Achmat, like several other lesbian and gay activists, was also very cosmopolitan: his transnational links to American AIDS activists and the Europeans in MSF certainly influenced how the movement's treatment literacy programmes developed.

AIDS policy, science and the New South African state

The formation and political direction of the TAC was far from inevitable, especially when viewed in terms of AIDS policy making in the immediate post-1994 period. South Africa held its first democratic elections in April 1994. The new government faced the challenge of trying to implement the new National AIDS Plan while transforming the state from being a white-run enforcer of racial segregation to being a 'non-racial', human rights-respecting, development-orientated entity. As we have seen, anti-apartheid activists concerned about AIDS had begun to meet and form social networks around the epidemic from the late 1980s. These meetings culminated in the development of the first National AIDS Plan through the National AIDS Convention of South Africa (NACOSA) process. The new government doubled the AIDS budget to R75 million and announced its intention to adopt the Plan, and so in the immediate post-election period, relations were cordial between progressive health activists who had entered government and those who had remained in civil society (*The Dallas Morning News* 25 September 1994). Activists also had every reason to be optimistic because the Plan was adopted at a time when the government was radically overhauling its health care system as part of its Reconstruction and Development Programme (RDP).

South Africa's Final Constitution of 1996, reflected the developmental nature of the new state, and its socio-economic rights also later provided a basis for AIDS activists' litigation. Whether socio-economic rights should have been included in a new South African Constitution was a matter of much debate in progressive legal circles from the late 1980s, when they arose within the ranks of the ANC-in-exile. These debates then migrated to the transition-era Constitutional deliberations at CODESA. Much of the disagreement hinged on whether such rights were *justiciable* – whether their content could be correctly determined and enforced by courts of law. Opponents of their inclusion mounted many arguments, such as that they would undermine judicial deference to the executive in policy making and so upset the balance of powers in the new democracy (Dugard 2004; Pieterse 2004). However, judicial deference had a problematic history in South Africa. It had been interpreted by liberal and left-wing legal scholars and lawyers as having dovetailed with narrow, positivist interpretations of the law (the idea that the law should be literally interpreted) and parliamentary sovereignty (the idea parliament should be supreme in making the law), which had been cornerstones of apartheid jurisprudence (Davis 2006). The proponents of socio-economic rights won the argument, and they were included in the Final Constitution's Bill of Rights. As we shall see in chapters 5 and 6, within a few years of the Constitution's coming into effect, AIDS activists started making legal and political arguments based on one of these rights – the right to access to health care services.

NACOSA itself became an umbrella organization, which aimed to bring together civil society, business and government to plan a collective response to AIDS. From 1994 to 1996 Edwin Cameron and Clarence Mini were co-chairs of the organization. Cameron was appointed as an Acting Judge of the High Court by President Mandela in 1994, a position which was made permanent in 1995. The AIDS Consortium (whose formation was discussed in Chapter 2) continued to grow and also provided a basis for the emergence of a new activist NGO called the AIDS Law Project (ALP), which took on increasingly influential cases as the decade wore on.

The AIDS Consortium grew from having 18 initial affiliates to being a human rights umbrella organization with 225 member organisations in 1998.[6] This growth reflected a rise in the number of AIDS NGOs in the country.[7] The coalition provided a key networking space for activists and a sociopolitical basis for the emergence of the TAC. In late 1994, Achmat started working at the newly formed AIDS Law Project (ALP). He also invited his old friend Heywood to join the organization. Hence, when Cameron became a judge in late 1994, Heywood and Achmat took over the running of the ALP.

Initially, AIDS activists who had remained in civil society expressed their satisfaction with the new government's approach to addressing the country's epidemic. Shortly after her appointment, the new Health Minister expressed her desire to implement the National AIDS Plan (*Weekly Mail & Guardian* 28 July 1994). While there were some initial disagreements in the immediate post-election period, AIDS activists had relatively ready access to senior members of government. What soured relations between the Mandela administration and AIDS activists was a series of scandals, the first of which concerned tendering procedures for an AIDS play.

Sarafina II

The *Sarafina II* controversy demonstrates the challenges which activists-turned-bureaucrats faced in familiarizing themselves with state mechanisms. According to the Public Protector's report, prominent playwright Mbongeni Ngema was approached by the minister to give his views on producing an AIDS play. He put in a tender for R14.2 million to produce a play called *Sarafina II*.[8] Owing to the proposed project's obvious extravagance, the department's tender committee did not issue its approval for it. Nevertheless, an official in the department signed a contract with Ngema for the R14.2 million play and immediately wrote a R3 million cheque for its development.[9]

Judy Seidman, an activist aligned to the AIDS consortium who saw the play, recalled that it reinforced existing, harmful social prejudices, which encouraged risky sexual behaviour and generated HIV-related stigma (Interview 4 December 2006). Morna Cornell, of the AIDS Consortium, told me that she came away from the play upset that it fed into gender stereotypes driving the epidemic: it featured a character Crocodile who was lionized for having multiple partners while female characters wore very short skirts (Interview 28 March 2007).

In early 1996, the allegations that the government had flouted tendering procedures in commissioning the play hit AIDS activists when they were contacted by the media for comment. In particular, the media reported claims that the Department of Health had ' "relaxed" ' tender procedures because donor funds from the European Union (EU) were involved, as opposed to taxpayers' money (*Eastern Province Herald* 14 February 1996).

As a result of the media storm, and following calls from NACOSA, the Parliamentary Portfolio Committee on Health held a hearing on the controversy. After this, Mike Ellis a Member of Parliament (MP) for the Democratic Party, asked the Public Protector to look into the tendering procedures around the play. Staff at the AIDS Consortium found that making a submission to the Public Protector involved a great deal of work. According to Consortium staff member Morna Cornell, this included gathering information and fact checking and then the submission itself, which took two and a half hours (Interview 28 March 2007).

The media glare surrounding the scandal only grew when the Public Protector's report was presented in parliament in early June 1996. His report found that the 'awarding of *Sarafina II* contract ... *was an unauthorized expenditure.*'[10] *Sarafina II* brought serious embarrassment to the government – Quarraisha Abdool Karim who led the Department of Health's AIDS programme from 1995–6 told me that the government 'closed ranks' (Interview 18 October 2006). The fall out from the affair in terms of activist–government relations was shown by the AIDS Consortium's widely publicized statement on the Public Protector's report, which blamed the Minister and Director General of Health for the debacle and argued that it had 'put further donor funding of AIDS activities into question ... [and] demoralized countless organizations and activists'.[11]

In this context, according to Hein Marais, NACOSA began to malfunction from 1996 onwards, because in the wake of the *Sarafina II* scandal, it found it increasingly difficult to fulfil its mandate to coordinate the formulation and implementation of AIDS policy by bringing together people across sectors (including business and unions, who ceased attending its meetings) (Marais 2000). From 2000 it ceased to exist as a national organization and pursued its goals simply as an NGO in the Western Cape.[12] Therefore, from

1996 to 2000, the AIDS Consortium became the main, national AIDS NGO policy-advocacy-focused umbrella body.

Virodene

The dust had barely settled on the *Sarafina II* affair, when allegations emerged that the government was offering inappropriate support for Virodene – a largely untested substance which, its promoters claimed, could treat HIV. Virodene matters in the history of AIDS in South Africa for two reasons. Firstly, as political scientist James Myburgh has argued, two of Virodene's key protagonists, Zigi and Olga Visser, were important in introducing Mbeki to AIDS dissidence (2007). Secondly, as economist Nicoli Nattrass pointed out, it set a dangerous precedent of the government meddling with the independence of the national drug regulatory authority, the Medicines Control Council (MCC), a South African equivalent of the US Food and Drug Administration (FDA) (2007).

The story of Virodene began in the mid-1990s with the experiments of Olga Visser, a cardiovascular perfusionist at Pretoria's H F Verwoerd Hospital. Visser was investigating the heart-freezing properties of N Dimethylformamide (DMF). In December 1995, her husband Zigi Visser registered a company called Cryopreservation Technologies to patent and develop DMF. Through the press coverage of their experiments they met the Minister of Health in July 1996 and told her that their compound had antiviral properties (Myburgh 2007). Myburgh alleges that unofficial clinical trials of the drugs were conducted on patients living with HIV and that the product's investigators discussed these with the Minister at this stage (2007). The Vissers had not gone through the MCC, as they were obliged to in accordance with the law, before commencing this trial. In mid-January 1997, they contacted Zuma again, reporting the glowing results of their clinical trials (Myburgh 2007). The Vissers were then invited to address the cabinet on their claims that they had found effective, affordable HIV treatment at a time when the widespread provision of combination ARV treatment was prohibitively expensive (Lawson 2008). At the heart of the controversy lay the fact that the Vissers had conducted an illegal and unethical clinical trial without first obtaining approval from the MCC – the country's drug regulatory authority.

In this period, the MCC was led by Professor Peter Folb a specialist in Internal Medicine and Pharmacology at the University of Cape Town. On 23 January 1997, the day after the announcement of the supposedly miraculous results obtained in trials of the AIDS drug was made to the press, the University of Pretoria announced that it would launch an urgent investigation into the researchers' 'deviation from established research practice' (*Business Day* 24 January 1997). The MCC rapidly swung into action and the following day halted the trial which also meant that patients had to stop taking the drug (*Pretoria News* 25 January 1997). By this stage, there was 'widespread criticism from scientists of the unorthodox way in which the researchers released the initial results' which lacked scientific credibility (*Pretoria News* 25 January 1997). Barry Schoub of the National Institute of Virology said that the drug did not enjoy scientific credibility, because scientists did not know much about it (*Pretoria News* 25 January 1997).

Folb was contacted by AIDS activists such as Mark Heywood, Fatima Hassan and Mary Crewe (Interview 17 January 2006). The AIDS Consortium used the information Folb and other doctors gave them casting doubt on Virodene to run a letter-writing campaign by member-organizations. At that stage, claims were published in the *Weekly Mail & Guardian* that the government aimed to own the unproven drug so that it could distribute it more cheaply to state hospitals (31 January 1997).

In late February 1997, the findings of a joint committee of inquiry into Virodene, constituted by the University of Pretoria and the Gauteng Health Department, were announced. It found that the Virodene researchers had failed to present evidence that the drug could inhibit HIV, contravened 'accepted scientific procedures' and conducted trials on patients 'without sufficient evidence' (*The Sowetan* 27 February 1997). AIDS activists announced to the media that they felt 'betrayed' by the Minister because of her 'ill-considered and premature support' for Virodene (*Weekly Mail & Guardian* 28 February 1997). It was a 'cruel trick', which had raised 'the hopes of millions of South Africans infected with HIV only to see them dashed' (*Weekly Mail & Guardian* 28 February 1997).

In late 1997, Folb met twice with both Zuma and Deputy President Mbeki to discuss the MCC's reasons for not granting approval for the continuation of the Virodene clinical trials. Folb was placed in a very unusual position for a scientist at a regulatory authority – he was being asked to meet with senior politicians to *lobby* them to accept the body's rulings (Interview 27 January 2006).

But the Minister continued making statements in favour of Virodene and by December publicly urged the MCC to 'work with researchers to resolve the status of Virodene P058' (*Weekend Saturday Argus* 7 December 1997). The scientists at the MCC refused to give way to the pressure and declined repeated applications for the drug to continue to be tested in humans, because there was insufficient evidence that it would be safe to do so or that the product would work in treating HIV (*The Citizen* 3 February 1998). DA MP Mike Ellis released a memo from the manufacturers of the drug, Cyropreservation Technologies, which appeared to state that the ANC had shares in the drug manufacturing company, allegations which would be subsequently reiterated (*Weekly Mail & Guardian* 13 March 1998). In late March, it emerged that a recent study had found that Virodene may have actually activated the HI Virus by 'stimulating the part of HIV that controls how much of the virus is made ... [and it] also caused other HIV activators to replicate the virus more efficiently' (*Weekly Mail & Guardian* 20 March 1998). Despite further revelations of the harm the drug could cause, Peter Folb and two of his colleagues were unceremoniously axed from the MCC, which as a consequence briefly ceased to function (Interview 27 January 2006).

At the end of April, Helen Rees, a former anti-apartheid health activist took over Folb's post, and the MCC became active again. She took the same hard line as Folb, and the drug was finally rejected once and for all by the MCC. Under her leadership, she said, the council's position was that 'Virodene was an unsafe product for which there was no proof' (Interview 7 February 2007).

Notification

The tensions between the government and civil society over AIDS also grew when, in a speech to a national meeting reviewing the country's AIDS policies, the Minister called for notification – compulsory reporting – of AIDS cases to the health authorities (Schneider 2001). In September 1997, Zuma again expressed in parliament her ministry's desire to make AIDS notifiable.[13]

The controversy around notification hinged on the fact that it involved breaching doctor–patient confidentiality. This had been a key preoccupation for AIDS activists since at least the early 1990s (as discussed in Chapter 2). In January 1998, the Minister of Health argued, in correspondence with Morna Cornell of the AIDS Consortium, that her 'responsibility as Minister of Health' was to 'obtain sufficient information to plan appropriately for the health service needs of persons diagnosed with AIDS'.[14] At this stage, the regulations were still merely 'under consideration' by her Ministry and the aim of the proposals would be to 'implement an efficient reporting system' that would safeguard 'the patient's confidentiality'.[15] This was also a view which was held by her Director-General Olive Shisana who told me that she did not believe in people living with HIV being 'paraded' but was in favour of notification 'for planning purposes' (Interview 27 March 2007). Cornell said that the AIDS Consortium's opposition to the measure was based on the fact that 'the risks to an individual were so huge' that they 'could not support the change' (Interview 28 March 2007).

In February 1999, Mark Colvin, an epidemiologist at the MRC, used an editorial in the *South African Medical Journal* to batter notification as an inefficient method of collecting scientific data. Colvin argued that 'Our experience [as epidemiologists] of using notification data for surveillance purposes of other diseases is dismal owing to substantial under-reporting' (1999, p. 147). To keep AIDS cases confidential while reporting them would require 'a coded number system', which would produce 'substantial numbers of incomplete and difficult to match records because of the relatively high infection rates' (Colvin 1999, p. 147). He queried the merits of monitoring AIDS cases, when it would have only provided an historical snapshot of who had become infected with HIV ten years before – hardly the most effective way of preventing new HIV infections. Instead, he suggested that government efforts to track the epidemic should have focused on the collection of high quality data from sentinel sites such as Hlabisa in KwaZulu-Natal and more detailed enumeration of cases of HIV-related illnesses at health facilities.

Meanwhile, the Department of Health announced more far-reaching notification plans, which were supported by their regional counterparts at a meeting of the Southern African Development Community (SADC) in April 1999. According to a media report, the regional body adopted several policy guidelines at the meeting, including those that HIV-positive people ought be have been obliged to tell their close family and partners about their HIV status, doctors and hospitals needed to keep records of their patients' HIV statuses and authorities were urged to document all HIV-related deaths (*The Daily News* 21 April 1999). According to health department spokesperson Vincent Hlongwane, the resolution would be taken to the SADC council of ministers for ratification before each head of state would implement policies in line with the regional body's recommendations.

The proposals appeared to enjoy support at a high level. Deputy President Mbeki and his spokesperson indicated he was in agreement with Zuma's proposals as they were 'for the good of the country' (*The Star* 22 April 1999). Cornell shot back that that Mbeki's suggestion was ' "appalling" ', as she feared that it could have caused more attacks on people living with HIV such as that on Gugu Dlamini who, as we have seen (in Chapter 3), was murdered for publicly revealing her HIV status (*The Star* 22 April 1999).

On 23 April 1999, proposals to make AIDS notifiable were published in the *Government Gazette*. Activists from the Consortium and NACOSA were 'outraged' by this step, because they feared that the adoption of the measure would drive the epidemic underground and increase the 'spiralling' infection rate (*Sunday Tribune* 25 April 1999). They also alleged that it violated the principles of confidentiality and non-discrimination, which were included in the 1994 national AIDS plan.

Mbeki's inter-ministerial committee on AIDS endorsed the SADC resolution making it seem as if it were 'only a matter of time' before the government adopted the measure (*Financial Times* 30 April 1999). AIDS activists ratcheted up the rhetoric in the media by arguing that notification of AIDS could create a ' "new style apartheid" ' (*The Sowetan* 3 May 1999).

Activists also had a legitimate fear that notification could lead to a slippery slope to the criminalization of HIV transmission. In early 1998, the South African Law Reform Commission (hereafter, referred to as the Law Commission) had been asked by the parliamentary Justice Portfolio Committee to investigate whether such legislation was required, a request which was conveyed via the Department of Justice.[16] For much of 1999, the Law Commission was considering the need for a separate statutory offence prohibiting the 'deliberate transmission of HIV'.[17]

Activists such as Achmat feared that notification could be used to identify people suspected of committing the 'crime' of 'deliberate infection', who would then be arrested.[18] The proposed notification of HIV and AIDS cases was a policy that was never implemented, and it appears to have dropped off the public radar after the June 1999 elections. There are a number of factors that may have influenced this outcome. Nkosazana Zuma became Minister of Foreign Affairs and Manto Tshabalala-Msimang was appointed Minister of Health by the new president, Thabo Mbeki. Also, it is likely that the bureaucratic problems posed by notification – suggested by Colvin – were also recognized to be immense. Lastly, from October 1999, it became utterly eclipsed by a conflict over the merits of AZT, a controversy which would take the government's policy to the very heart of AIDS dissidence.

In late October 1999, the Law Commission advised against passing a new law specifically aimed at criminalizing 'deliberate infection' (*Mail & Guardian* 28 September 1999). The Law Commission argued that rather than protecting women vulnerable to infection, they would be more likely to be prosecuted and imprisoned under the putative law. Rather, the Commission urged the state to use existing laws, especially those dealing with sexual assault, to prosecute partners in such circumstances. As the government failed to capitalize on new advances in HIV treatment, AIDS activism became more radical, developments which led to the formation of the TAC.

Formation of the TAC: A radical South African AIDS movement

Achmat was one of several gay rights activists who were central in founding the TAC. The new movement was based upon social networks formed between activists based at AIDS NGOs such as the ALP, NAPWA, the gay and lesbian coalition and the Positive Women's Network, all of which were closely linked to the AIDS Consortium. The TAC's formation must also be viewed in the context of scientific developments and the ways in which the epidemic itself was progressing.

NAPWA was formed in 1993 at the first national conference for people living with HIV held in Durban.[19] By 1994, it had a national committee with members such as John Pegge, Rick Stephens, Prudence Mabele and Mercy Makhalemele. It was initially a very small organization, as few people were prepared to be open about living with HIV in the mid-1990s.[20] AIDS activists who were living with HIV commonly self-identified with the acronym People living with HIV/AIDS (PWAs). NAPWA was certainly successful in providing the only real nationwide 'space' for PWAs to meet each other and to obtain social and psychological support in this period.

In 1996, startling breakthroughs were announced in the United States that triple combination ARV therapy was effective in treating HIV. While their PWA colleagues in the North were living longer because of these new therapies, every day South Africans were dying *en masse* from the disease. AIDS activists such as Promise Mthembu and Zackie Achmat were well aware of these developments in HIV medicine.

The increasing radicalism of the TAC's advocacy for treatment access compared to earlier AIDS activism may have related to the greater immediate rewards the new drug therapies offered to people living with HIV. PWAs could now literally fight for their lives, as they learned through emails, phone conversations and interactions with Northern AIDS activists at international AIDS conferences: as a consequence activists like Judy Seidman began to investigate ways of reducing the costs of the drugs in South Africa (Interview 4 December 2006).

A group of South African AIDS activists formed the TAC in December 1998. The movement's first chairperson Mazibuko Jara told me that its formation followed months of informal discussions between activists about the need for a treatment access movement, following AIDS Consortium meetings (Interview 26 March 2007). Morna Cornell and Mazibuko Jara both said that the TAC came into existence at a meeting where the following activists were present, amongst others: Zackie Achmat (NCGLE), Mark Heywood (ALP), Edwin Cameron, Mazibuko Jara (NCGLE), Prudence Mabele (Positive Women's Network), Mercy Makhalemele (NAPWA), Morna Cornell (AIDS Consortium) and Phumzile Mthethwa (NCGLE) (Interview 26 March 2007; Interview 28 March 2007). This group of founding members helped to write the TAC's Constitution and unofficially managed it for the first two or three months of its existence.

At the time of the TAC's formation there were numerous links between these founder organizations. Firstly, members of staff rotated between the organizations: for instance, the AIDS Law Project hosted Mthethwa as a full-time organizer of the 1994 conference, which had led to the formation of the gay and lesbian coalition. Similarly, Achmat worked for both organizations (the ALP and gay and lesbian coalition) across the period. Secondly, as we have seen, the AIDS Consortium was closely associated with the formation of the ALP. Thirdly, all the organizations to which the activists who co-founded the TAC belonged were members of the AIDS Consortium. Lastly, there were also close personal friendships between some of the activists, such as those between Cameron, Achmat and Heywood.

The epidemic was also taking an increasingly grim toll. By the late 1990s, rising HIV prevalence, as measured by antenatal clinic statistics, was widely reported in South Africa's media: by 1998, there were an estimated 3.2 million people living with HIV in the country (*Business Day* 10 December 1998). AIDS-related sickness and deaths were on the rise, as suggested by the fact that medical wards were becoming inundated by seriously ill adult and paediatric patients living with HIV (*The Star* 26 June 1998; *Sunday Tribune* 29 March 1998). However, most people living with the disease did not know their HIV status (*Business Day* 10 December 1998). But the majority of those with 'full-blown' AIDS had been infected with HIV five to eight years before, so the full social impact of rising infections in the 1990s had yet to be felt and so many people were still not yet seeing the 'evidence' that AIDS was a serious socio-economic and political issue. AIDS-related mortality continued to rise: a trend which would continue into the next decade. Indeed, a 2001 Medical Research Council (MRC) Study showed that 'about 40% of the adult deaths [of people] aged 15–49 that occurred in the year 2000 were due to HIV/AIDS' (Dorrington et al. 2001). From the few hundred AIDS deaths in the late 1980s, AIDS had become South Africa's leading cause of death by the early 2000s (Dorrington et al. 2001).

By the late 1990s, AIDS activists faced the daily reality of losing colleagues to the disease. Simon Nkoli's death in December 1998 came as a big blow to many activists. Mthethwa remembered Nkoli's last hours as follows: 'That Sunday all of us running to hospital and hearing the horrible machine that goes "Beep, Beep".' When the activists returned during a lunch break on Monday, 'two minutes after we arrived, he basically passed away. We came back to this office and we say "Hey! What shall we do?" There's all of our sadness, but something needs to be done' (Interview 15 April 2008).

In a 2000 TAC newsletter, Achmat recalled the rationale behind his decision to publicly call for the movement's formation at Nkoli's funeral. He took a new approach of discussing normally private aspects of living with HIV to reveal the wider social injustices which were expressed in the epidemic. Achmat wanted to campaign for access to the drugs,

> But whoever I spoke to said it was impossible; the drugs were way out of reach. Around that time I became very sick myself and I thought I was going to die. I had terrible thrush in my mouth and throat and I couldn't swallow anything. Eventually I was prescribed fluconazole, a very expensive drug. My friends helped me pay for it and still it nearly bankrupted me. I knew that if I hadn't been able to afford the treatment I would have died, like so many other people. On top of Simon [Nkoli]'s death it was just the last straw.[21]

The new movement's first event was a fast and protest on the steps of St George's Cathedral in Cape Town on 10 December 1998.

Cameron was not a member of the TAC since he felt it was more appropriate for him to maintain a judicial posture of formal political non-alignment. But he remained a close friend of Achmat's and took action in his personal capacity which advanced the movement's goals. In 1997 his health began to deteriorate. As a judge, his medical aid (health insurance) covered the expensive new combination ARV therapy. The judge's immune system recovered and he returned to full health. He told me that he decided to speak out about living with HIV because a black woman secretly living with the disease in a township or a suburb experienced 'feelings which in all respects are comparable to what I experienced 15 years ago when I was diagnosed – a sense of ostracism, a sense of fear, a sense of terror, a sense of no connection, a sense of no help being available' (Interview 4 October 2004). There were also practical reasons for him to reveal his HIV status when he was interviewed for a Constitutional Court post – he wished to counteract rumours that he had been unwell (*The Daily News* 20 April 1999).

While he knew NAPWA activists such as Mercy Makhalemele and Sean Mellors through his prior work at the ALP and AIDS Consortium, Cameron wanted his disclosure to move beyond the older model of telling a moving personal story about living with HIV at conferences, in the manner of Mellors and Busse. He told me in an interview that 'When I made my own statement, I said "My statement is relevant only insofar as it points to what social action should be taken" ' (Interview 4 October 2004). His thinking in this regard was also influenced by that of Achmat.

In this period, the two organizations were often referred to in a hyphenated way as NAPWA-TAC.[22] But conflict soon developed between them, for reasons which Mary Crewe described to me (Interview 18 October 2006). The TAC grew rapidly and began using a greater proportion of NAPWA's resources. At a NAPWA board meeting in 2000, Zackie Achmat levelled accusations that Peter Busse had been mismanaging the organization. NAPWA moved out of its offices in the same building as the AIDS Consortium and up to the University of Pretoria. Busse experienced a period of severe AIDS-related illness, recovered and reinvented himself as an AIDS consultant who mostly worked internationally. A new Director, Nkuleleko Nxesi, was appointed to the leadership of NAPWA, which ceased to have any sort of working relationship with the TAC.

Responses to Mbeki's AIDS denialism and early advocacy for AZT for PMTCT

From late 1998, Achmat and the movement he led advocated for all patients to be able to benefit from important advances in HIV medicine. At the Vancouver conference in 1996, David Ho, a Taiwanese-American clinician, announced that combination ARV therapy could durably suppress HIV from copying itself in the bodies of people living with the disease. People living with HIV who could afford to purchase the new protease inhibitors or who were lucky enough to live in countries where the state provided them for free were given a new lease on life. But in one of the worst affected countries on earth – South Africa – AIDS mortality continued its steep climb in these years.

In 1998, a study in Thailand showed that a short course of AZT could be effectively used for PMTCT, and South African AIDS activists and scientists increasingly called for the measure to be universally implemented in the country. The South African activists started out by calling for AZT to be provided for PMTCT, and only later shifted to full-throated advocacy for the combination ARV drug therapy.

Initially, the cost of AZT appeared to be the main barrier to wider access to the drug. So the TAC's advocacy on the issue began by pressuring the pharmaceutical industry to halt its legal efforts to block parallel importation of branded medicines from countries where they were cheaper and prevent the manufacture and importation of generic medicines. But from October 1999 onwards, activists had one more challenge to contend with – President Mbeki's adoption of dissident views on AIDS. Despite the renewed public controversy between scientists and senior government leaders that now centred on the president's views, the TAC's advocacy in this period focused on the pricing issue.

James McIntyre and Glenda Gray, doctors at Baragwanath Hospital in Soweto, were also important in advocating universal access to AZT for PMTCT in the late 1990s. At a meeting of the Department of Health's National AIDS Programme in Pretoria from 21–22 April 1998, Glenda Gray gave a presentation on PMTCT which noted that the Thai study had proved that a shorter course of AZT could be effectively used to prevent infants from contracting HIV.[23] In particular, the study showed a 50% reduction in transmission when a much shorter course of AZT was administered during the last month of pregnancy and during labour (Shaffer et al. 1999). The regimen in this study was, therefore, much more suited to implementation in developing countries like South Africa. According to the minutes of the meeting, Gray's presentation was well received and those at the meeting expressed their support for the measure to be piloted provided 'implementation issues' could be addressed.[24] 'Pilot sites' were clinics and hospitals where new health services were tested prior to their wider provision. It was agreed that the policy implications of Gray's presentation would be debated by a meeting of the national Minister of Health and the nine members of the Provincial Executive Councils for Health (hereafter referred to as provincial Health MECs).[25] This government forum was usually referred to as the Health MINMEC. Information, education and counselling of HIV-positive expectant mothers were also to be addressed by the putative pilot sites, which would be aimed at operational research and training.[26]

Rose Smart who was then the head of the Department of Health's AIDS Directorate recounted in an interview with me that at this stage PMTCT was 'an issue' but not yet a source of 'conflict' (Interview 6 May 2007). A few months later, in July 1998, the decision was taken by Smart at the Department of Health to introduce the Thai regimen for PMTCT at pilot sites in Gauteng and the Western Cape to research the feasibility of the intervention (Myburgh 2007, p. 268). This programme was extremely short-lived, because in early October 1998, Health Minister Nkosazana Zuma 'announced that an AZT programme for HIV-positive pregnant women would not be implemented because the country couldn't afford it' (*Cape Argus* 16 January 1998). Doctors and AIDS researchers expressed 'disbelief' at the decision. Glenda Gray was quoted in the *Cape Argus* as having said ' "I'm surprised at this decision. I'm also sad. We've evaluated the economic side and it's quite clearly of benefit" ' (16 January 1998). Medical researchers like Gray argued that the cost of caring for HIV-positive babies was twice that of caring for those who were HIV-negative. Robin Wood, head of the HIV Unit at Somerset Hospital in Cape Town concurred with Gray that PMTCT using AZT was a cost-effective intervention because preventing infection meant a lifelong benefit was offered to children (*Cape Argus* 16 January 1998).

Zuma hit back by arguing that making AZT available to all who needed it was too expensive and that it was not the best use of resources to combat the disease. The Minister argued that it would merely halve the transmission rate: from 30% without the intervention to 15% with it (*Mail & Guardian* 16 October 1998). Instead, Zuma told the *Mail & Guardian* that she wanted to encourage vaccine research efforts which were underway at the MRC (16 October 1998). According to the same report, Glaxo Wellcome had reportedly already reduced the price of AZT 'by more than 70% of the world average' which would have enabled 'mothers to be treated for under R400 over a period of weeks'. The drug firm was also quoted in the piece as having announced that it was willing to consider further cuts to the prices of AZT and 3TC.

Government provision of AZT for PMTCT was one of the TAC's core early demands from its inception on 10 December 1998. The first report of NAPWA activists' plans to pursue legal action to force the government to provide greater access to ARVs for PMTCT emerged in December 1998, in an article in the *Sunday Tribune* (06 December 1998). According to the article, lawyers acting for NAPWA had written to the Minister of Health demanding 'exact reasons for the cancellation of the programme'. If reasons were not forthcoming by the end of the following week, NAPWA's lawyers had planned to 'go to the High Court to compel the Government to disclose the details of its decision'.

Demands for the government to reinstate funding for PMTCT pilot programmes were central to the newly formed TAC's first public event on International Human Rights Day in December 1998. On this day, 20 activists held a one-day fast at St George's Cathedral in Cape Town in support of provision of treatment (TAC 2008, p. 149). Passers-by were apparently largely unaware that HIV was now a treatable illness or that the medications which could be used to treat it were readily available in Western countries.[27] By the end of the day of action, the TAC activists had collected over a thousand signatures calling for the government to develop a national treatment plan.[28]

The conflict dragged on in 1999, as media articles continued to ratchet up the rhetoric on the subject. In an article in the *Sunday Independent*, AIDS activist Mark Heywood opened a new line of legal argument which would be extremely significant in the TAC's later campaigns. Heywood said that the government had ' "a legal obligation to at least proceed with the pilot projects" ' given the constitutional right to access to health care services

(*Sunday Independent* 24 January 1999). Moreover, he announced that the AIDS Law Project (ALP) planned legal action along these lines.

The dispute grew more vituperative as the year wore on. In late January 1999, it emerged that some international AIDS activists planned to boycott the International AIDS Conference which was to be held in Durban in July 2000, because of the government's refusal to provide AZT for PMTCT (*Sunday Times* 31 January 1999). In mid-February the results of the Perinatal Transmission (PETRA) multi-country study were released, which pointed to the fact that when AZT and 3TC were administered to an HIV-positive mother a week before labour and to both her and her baby for another week thereafter, there was a 63% reduction in early mother-to-child transmission (MTCT) and a 61% reduction in HIV transmission to infants at six weeks (Hudson et al. 2002). This was also superior to the Thai regimen because it involved a shorter course of drugs. The findings of this study were reported on in the *Daily News* under the headline 'Hope for Aids babies' (17 February 1999).

South Africa's new Constitution gave the provinces a high degree of autonomy in health policy making and spending. While the ANC had won a hefty majority in South Africa's national parliament in the 1994 elections, two of the country's provinces were controlled by other political parties. The Western Cape was controlled by the rebranded 'New National Party' (NNP) and KwaZulu-Natal by the Inkatha Freedom Party (IFP). The NNP government in the Western Cape announced that it would go ahead with supplying AZT to HIV-positive pregnant women at two sites in Khayalitsha township, contravening the Minister's decision not to adopt such measures (*The Citizen* 20 February 1999).

Another entirely new line of argument entered the debate about AZT for PMTCT in South Africa when Anthony Brink, a lawyer from Pietermaritzburg, attacked the drug as a toxic 'medicine from hell' in an article in *The Citizen* on 17 March 1999. Brink declared that people living with HIV were being 'killed by the cure' of ARVs and that AZT headed 'like a heat-seeking missile for one's immune and energy transporting cells', and he questioned whether the presence of anti-bodies to HIV was evidence of an 'active infection'.

In an international context, Brink's article presented nothing new and was based upon the work of AIDS dissidents. Since the late 1980s, Peter Duesberg, an American molecular biologist, had consistently questioned the link between HIV and AIDS, arguing that the former was an entirely harmless retrovirus (Epstein 2996). Another group of scientists in Perth also asserted that HIV was entirely harmless. Nattrass has observed that 'What unites them [the dissidents] all is the unshakable belief that the existing canon on AIDS science is wrong and that AIDS deaths are caused by malnutrition, narcotics and ARV drugs themselves' (Nattrass 2007, p. 23). At this stage, Brink's arguments were not significant in the national political dialogue around AIDS. Myburgh claims that Zigi Visser, the husband of Virodene researcher Olga Visser, wrote to Mbeki in April 1999 bringing Brink's article to the President's attention, along with a dissident journal article on which it was based (2007, p. 273). As we shall see, Mbeki did not publicly articulate these views until October 1999.

Brink's article did not go unchallenged. A fortnight later, Des Martin of the Southern African HIV/AIDS Clinicians' Society tore into Brink's assertions in an article in the Johannesburg-based *Citizen* headed 'AZT: a medicine from heaven' (31 March 1999). Contrary to Brink's view that AZT caused AIDS deaths, Martin argued that it was HIV infection itself that had led to a massive increase in AIDS-related mortality in infants and children. He also refuted Brink's position that AZT was inherently unsafe; instead, Martin said, when it had been used as a component of combination therapy it had allowed patients to 'maintain or, more importantly, improve their quality of life'. Where combination ARV therapy was available AIDS had been changed to being a 'chronic manageable disease'. Addressing Brink's statements on AZT's toxicity, Martin pointed out that it was only a problem in patients with 'advanced HIV disease' whose 'bone marrow function' was already possibly impaired by HIV disease. Toxicity was not a problem during the drug's short-term use for PMTCT.

Meanwhile, the TAC's mobilization around PMTCT began to take on a more radical tone. The new movement held its first major protest at Baragwanath Hospital on 21 March 1999. This day was chosen because it was Human Rights Day, a new post-apartheid national public holiday which commemorated the Sharpeville massacre of 1960. Mazibuko Jara told me that the Johannesburg Central Branch of the South African Communist Party (SACP) was also involved in the demonstration and produced leaflets calling for lower drug prices (Interview 26 March 2007). According to a report in *The Star*, 'About 300 HIV/Aids sufferers, as well as their supporters, were at the main gate of the huge hospital to stage a six-hour fast, lie down in the entrance for a minute and listen to speeches reminiscent of the pre-1994 "struggle" days' (22 March 1999). This 'die-in' strategy of lying down to symbolically represent AIDS deaths had been pioneered by American AIDS activists in the AIDS Coalition to Unleash Power (ACT UP) in the late 1980s (Epstein 1996). According to the article, the TAC had three objectives at that time. Firstly, it wanted to get the Minister of Health and the Minister of Finance, Trevor Manuel, to meet with NAPWA (to which the TAC remained affiliated) and other NGOs to discuss implementation of free AZT and baby formula for PMTCT. Its second aim was to campaign for 'affordable and quality treatment to be made available for people with HIV and Aids'. Lastly, it called on drug companies to reduce the prices of AIDS medicines. The new movement had outlined a whole plan of action for the next two quarters. It had collected 50,000 signatures to be handed to President Mandela on 27 April, the Freedom Day holiday, commemorating South Africa's first democratic elections five years before. Marches were also planned on the

Union Buildings and Parliament on 16 June (a holiday commemorating the Soweto Uprising of 1976).

Jara was the movement's chairperson for the first year of its existence. He was chosen as the first chair of the TAC partly because he participated in many different activist networks, all of which could be used to recruit new members and allies. Not only had Jara coordinated the gay and lesbian equality coalition's legislative reform-focused Equal Rights Project since 1996, he was also a member of the AIDS consortium, the ANC and the SACP. Jara recounted that the TAC initially allied with the minister in her 'anti-imperialist' fight (court case) with the pharmaceutical companies (Interview 26 March 2007), a development which is discussed in Chapter 5.

Accordingly, while many early TAC actions called on the government to provide AZT for PMTCT, they were also aimed at pressuring pharmaceutical companies to reduce the prices of AIDS drugs. Indeed, on two occasions in this period (the first in April 1999), the TAC's leadership met with Zuma to discuss AZT for PMTCT and the pending court case on the Medicines Act, once in Cape Town and once in Pretoria. Phumzile Mthethwa then of the ALP, NCGLE and the TAC remembered that these meetings were 'very productive', and they 'were good, at least in the way of collaborating and a large part [of the agenda] around that time was also around the court case, you know, that the PMA had' (Interview 15 April 2005).

In June, Thabo Mbeki became South Africa's second democratically elected president when the ANC won the 1999 national elections. The new Minister of Health Manto Tshabalala-Msimang initially appeared to be open-minded about state provision of AZT for PMTCT. Indeed, at a parliamentary media briefing in early June, she announced that she wanted to review the government's decision not to provide AZT to pregnant women. After the briefing she told the *Star* that ' "I cannot say what it will take to convince me that we should provide the treatment...but I need to listen to all the arguments" ' (*The Star* 30 June 1999). In July 1999, the results of the HIVNET 012 trial which had been conducted in Uganda were released. The study demonstrated the efficacy of an even cheaper, simpler, effective ARV regimen for PMTCT: a single dose of the ARV drug Nevirapine could cut mother-to-child transmission by half when it was given to mothers as they went into labour and to infants, shortly after birth, in the form of paediatric syrup (Guay et al. 1999).

The TAC continued its energetic advocacy for cheaper drugs, which was still its major focus. But the movement's campaign for access to AZT for PMTCT simultaneously came up against an entirely unexpected challenge, when President Mbeki gave an address to the National Council of the Provinces (NCOP) on 28 October 1999, which questioned the safety of AZT. Mbeki said it had been brought to his attention that there were 'legal cases pending' in South Africa, the United Kingdom and the United States 'against AZT on the basis that this drug is harmful to health' (Mbeki 1999). He also noted that there was 'a large volume of scientific literature alleging that, among other things, the toxicity of this drug is such that it is in fact a danger to health'. Mbeki argued that it would be 'irresponsible' for the government 'not to head the dire warnings' which 'medical researchers' had made. Accordingly, the president announced that the Minister of Health had been tasked with investigating AZT so that the government and the country's medical authorities could know where the truth lay. The drug's manufacturer, Glaxo Wellcome, claimed that no such court cases in respect of AZT had been brought to its attention (SAPA 28 October 1999).

This was an entirely unexpected development for the TAC, because, as Heywood has mentioned, until that point 'it looked as if TAC's [P]MTCT campaign would be one primarily targeting the manufacturers of antiretroviral medicine to reduce their prices' (2003, p. 281). Indeed, the TAC found Mbeki's intellectual embrace of AIDS dissidence 'an unanticipated and unfortunate diversion' from its campaign on the price of drugs (Heywood 2003, p. 281).

Mbeki had been sent more dissident material by AIDS-dissident journalist Anita Allen in July and again by the Vissers on 21 October 1999 (Gevisser 2007; Myburgh 2007; Nattrass 2007). Nattrass makes the point that irrespective of whether it was Brink, the Vissers or Allen who first alerted Mbeki to dissident ideas, several of his speeches from October 1999 onwards indicate that he took the scientifically refuted set of arguments 'very seriously indeed' (2007, p. 48). The exact timing and reasons behind the president's adoption of AIDS-dissident views have been documented extensively elsewhere. Mbeki's adoption of AIDS dissidence certainly needs to be seen in the context of the high prices of the drugs and the conflict with the pharmaceutical industry over the intellectual property law surrounding them (Bond 2001; Lawson 2008). It was also motivated by his belief that those holding mainstream views on AIDS were racist, which related to Mbeki's reassertion of African nationalism as part of his vision of generating an 'African Renaissance' (Mbali 2004; Posel 2005; Gevisser 2007; Myburgh 2007).

The TAC reiterated its threat of legal action in January 2000, when its lawyers wrote to Manto Tshabalala-Msimang asking whether the government intended to develop a PMTCT programme using ARVs.[29] Tensions between the government and activists and scientists were also heightened in January 2000, when the President appointed no doctors, scientists or representatives of the AIDS Consortium or the TAC to the newly formed South African National AIDS Council (Nattrass 2007, p. 65). From 2000 to 2005, South Africa's main AIDS policy was the HIV/AIDS/STD Strategic Plan for South Africa 2000–2005 (hereafter referred to as the 2000–2005 Strategic Plan). The Council was created in accordance with the Plan to bring together different sectors to oversee its implementation.[30] In the same period, the TAC continued to step up its protest actions: on 4 February 2000, the movement protested at the opening of Parliament (TAC 2008, p. 27).

But the government's AIDS policy continued to be mired in AIDS dissidence. In May 2000, the Ministry of Health announced that a Presidential Panel would be held to investigate the science behind AIDS (*The Star* 5 May 2000). From then until the July 2000 International AIDS Conference – which was the largest bi-annual global gathering of AIDS-related scientists – the debate, as it played out in the media, revolved around Mbeki's questioning of the link between HIV and AIDS, which was emerging as a major barrier to the government's adoption of a PMTCT programme. Mbeki sent a letter outlining his views on AIDS to US President Bill Clinton in a diplomatic pouch. This letter was leaked to the Washington Post and according to a report in *The Star*, it denounced his critics as part of a ' "campaign of intellectual intimidation and terrorism . . . born by a degree of fanaticism, which is truly terrifying" ' (20 April 2000). He also apparently defended his interactions with AIDS dissidents who denied the link between HIV and AIDS, saying that the West could not dictate Africa's response to the epidemic. One of South Africa's top scientists, Salim Abdool Karim of the MRC, countered that the debate had been resolved in the 1980s.

The first meeting of the Presidential Panel was held in May 2000. One of the main reasons why it failed to reach a consensus was that it included an equal number of scientists holding dissident and mainstream views, which meant that its members were fundamentally at odds on AIDS-related science (Nattrass 2007, p. 54). So while the 33-member group included Luc Montagnier, the co-discoverer of HIV, it also included Peter Duesberg who argued that the idea that HIV caused AIDS was ' "inconsistent, paradoxical and absurd" ' (*The Star* 5 May 2000). At the opening of the panel's first meeting the President said he had convened the panel to ' "understand this matter [of AIDS] better" ' and expressed surprise at the divisions that his questioning of scientific orthodoxy had generated, insisting that ' "It must surely be because people are exceedingly worried about the large numbers of people who are dying, and therefore any suggestion that dealing with that is being postponed because somebody is busy looking at abstruse scientific theories, it becomes a betrayal" ' (*Sunday Times* 7 May 2000).

Zena Stein had played an important role in alerting the ANC to the threat that AIDS would pose while it was still in exile in 1990. By the early 2000s, Stein was a professor of Epidemiology at Columbia University in New York. She was one of the scientists invited to attend one of the panel's meetings, and she found that it was 'terrible and a waste of time because they [the government] did not listen. They invited an equal number of scientists from each side. They did not invite Jerry [Coovadia] to the first one. Manto [Tshabalala-Msimang] was there and it was dreadful' (Interview 18 October 2007).

In 2000, Malegapuru William Makgoba was the President of the MRC. Like Stein, Makgoba found participating in the Presidential Panel an unpleasant experience: 'it was a shambles' (Interview 7 September 2007). He told me that he attended because 'we had to honour the President, but actually the Presidential Advisory [Panel] didn't achieve anything' (Interview 7 September 2007). Makgoba was one of the country's top African scientists. He knew Mbeki, who had written the foreword to a book that Makgoba had published in 1997 offering his reflections on the academic's experiences in the racial controversy surrounding his credentials and conduct during his time at Wits University (1997). In January 2000, Mbeki contacted Makgoba requesting his advice on some of the dissident literature that he had been sent by Allen and Brink (Gevisser 2007, p. 742). Makgoba quickly read through the 2000 pages over seven days and wrote to Mbeki telling him that the dissident literature was 'rubbish'. The arguments were not based on scientific facts, but on 'wishful thinking'. In correspondence addressed to Mbeki, the then President of the MRC made the point that unlike the dissident theories, the theory that HIV caused AIDS 'came out of a scientific process of reiteration, review, challenging, discarding, improving upon. You could see why this hypothesis was robust that HIV causes AIDS, because in every AIDS patient you could identify the virus and there was nobody who had ever been described as having AIDS in whom the virus did not exist' (Interview 7 September 2007).

By contrast, as he argued in his correspondence with the President, the dissident critique was merely a critique, not backed up by any experimental data.[31] Over and above the sheer irrationality of AIDS dissidence, Makgoba was concerned about the impact Mbeki's adoption of such views would have on the country's reputation because it could make South Africa 'the laughing stock, if not pariah, of the world again'.[32] Makgoba's advice was not followed.

South African and international scientists continued to lean on Mbeki to unequivocally state his support for proven scientific theories about AIDS in the lead-up to the 2000 Durban International AIDS Conference. In a move redolent of activism, 5000 of the world's top scientists signed a declaration in support of mainstream scientific views on AIDS which was published in *Nature*, one of the world's top scientific journals. Presidential spokesperson Parks Mankahlana told the media that the document belonged in the dustbin (*Business Day* 5 July 2000).[33] Meanwhile, the Presidential Panel met again in July and was tasked with re-evaluating the reliability of HIV tests (*Sunday Times* 19 July 2000). This was despite the fact that mainstream scientists such as Helene Gayle of the United States Centers for Disease Control (CDC) and Makgoba were in no doubt as to the accuracy of such tests.

On 9 July 2000, the TAC held a march from the Durban City Hall to Kings Park Stadium where the opening of the International AIDS Conference was held. At the beginning of the march Winnie Mandela addressed the crowd from the steps of the City Hall wearing a white TAC t-shirt with 'H.I.V. POSITIVE' emblazoned on it in purple.[34] Holding the microphone, she made an unequivocal statement directly opposing Mbeki's stance. To roars of approval from assembled demonstrators, she said 'Let me state what appears to have become less than obvious in South Africa in the last few months: AIDS exists! HIV causes AIDS!'[35] Her vocal expression of support for the TAC's PMTCT campaign was important as it demonstrated that the movement was multi-racial and that its demands could be framed in a popular manner. At the end of the 3000-person demonstration, Mark Heywood, a founder member and leader of the movement, renewed its call for 'the South African government to immediately implement a countrywide program to reduce the risk of mother-to-child transmission'.[36] Accepting the marchers' memorandum, Tshabalala-Msimang gave a warm response: she accepted the petition with 'a great sense of humility'.[37] She reminded those assembled that 'Only six years ago I myself was a political activist and, therefore, I admire and support what you are doing.'[38]

After a spectacular theatrical light display and acrobatics which represented the conference's theme of 'breaking the silence', Mbeki gave his speech. With the undivided attention of the world's media and its top AIDS researchers and activists, it was the perfect opportunity for him to lay the AIDS dissident controversy to rest by endorsing the evidence-based position of the country's top scientists. This opportunity was squandered when Mbeki gave one of his most dissident-aligned speeches up to that point. After referring to AIDS as a 'health crisis of enormous proportions' he said that 'One of the consequences of this crisis is the deeply disturbing phenomenon of the *collapse of the immune system* [my emphasis]', and it 'seemed' to Mbeki that *"we could not blame everything on a single virus* [my emphasis]."[39]

He omitted to mention that HIV was the cause of both the syndrome of AIDS and the local and global epidemics of the disease. Instead, he implied that poverty was the cause of AIDS. Indeed, he said, 'The world's biggest killer and the greatest cause of ill-health and suffering across the globe, including South Africa, is extreme poverty.'[40] This assertion was not necessarily entirely incorrect in relation to socio-economic aspects of the epidemic, but was inaccurate in describing the disease's causation at a microbiological level. The speech bore the discursive hallmarks of AIDS dissidence in its refusal to describe HIV as the cause of a syndrome which stemmed from immune-system collapse, an epidemic of which was killing hundreds of thousands of South Africans and millions worldwide annually.

Edwin Cameron used his Jonathan Mann Memorial Lecture on Health and Human Rights at the conference to attack Mbeki's speech. He told the delegates that he wished the president had 'unequivocally' stated that HIV is 'a virally specific condition ... that is sexually transmitted ... [and] if uncontained precipitates, on its own, debility and death' for which 'antiretroviral treatments exist that can be affordably and effectively applied.'[41] To his 'grief and consternation,' Mbeki's speech was 'bereft of any of this.'[42]

Nelson Mandela seldom mentioned HIV/AIDS while he was in office, but after he stepped down from the Presidency he came to recognize the seriousness of the issue and began to speak out on it more frequently. Mandela closed the conference calling for an end to the debate between scientists and President Mbeki, pointing out that experience from other countries had shown that 'introducing measures to reduce mother-to-child transmission has been proven to be essential in the fight against AIDS'.[43]

The image evolved in the media of Mbeki as a president who made AIDS policies based upon his late-night Internet-surfing – as depicted in a cartoon in *The Star* of 20 July 2000, shortly after the Durban International AIDS Conference (Figure 4.1). In his October 1999 NCOP address, Mbeki had urged MPs to consult the Internet on AIDS, which created the myth that it was the chief source of his views.[44]

Following the Durban conference and into September, Mbeki reiterated dissident positions on AIDS in correspondence with Tony Leon, the leader of the Democratic Alliance (DA), the country's main opposition (Myburgh 2007; Nattrass 2007). In mid-October 2000 the President reportedly told the ANC's National Executive Committee (NEC) that he was 'withdrawing' from the debate (Myburgh 2007). However, he did not repudiate his views and continued to make dissident statements on HIV over the period. In April 2001, the findings of the presidential AIDS panel were released. Given the panel's even split between dissidents and mainstream scientists, it failed to reach a unanimous agreement on the cause, prevention and treatment of

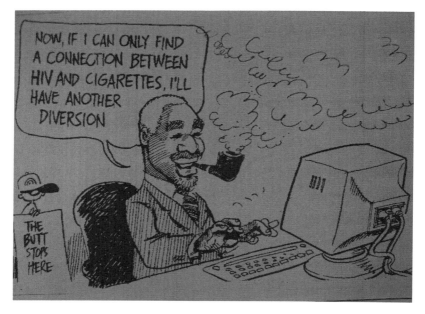

Figure 4.1   Cartoon of President Mbeki on the internet
Source: © Independent Newspapers; *The Star* (20/07/2000).

AIDS and on the use of ARVs; after much expenditure of scientists' time and energy, the report recommended that the government should not change its AIDS policy (*Natal Witness* 5 April 2001). Prior to April 2001, the TAC spoke out against the president's adoption of AIDS dissidence, but much of its actual campaigning was around the medicines' pricing issue, which is discussed in the next chapter. Meanwhile, it developed its influential treatment-efficacy demonstration and literacy programmes in tandem with its international allies.

The TAC and the founding of the Khayalitsha MSF clinic

TAC activists continued to die because they were too poor to afford AIDS drugs. In order for its organizing to be strengthened, the TAC also needed a project providing HIV treatment, thereby, demonstrating that to do so was both feasible and effective in a poor community. For these reasons, the TAC collaborated with MSF to create a clinic to provide ARVs to patients in Khayalitsha in Cape Town on 4 January 1999. Central to this effort was Eric Goemaere, an MSF physician. Goemaere was a Belgian doctor who had joined MSF because he wanted to apply his skills in resource-limited settings and enjoyed travel and intercultural exchange. He had been seeing cases of AIDS in patients in the developing countries where he worked from the 1980s onwards. The introduction of the simplified AZT PMTCT regimen in Thailand in 1998 gave Goemaere a great deal of hope: finally a regimen had been identified which could affordably reduce the number of infants living with HIV in developing countries.

The Belgian doctor first got in touch with the TAC and Zackie Achmat in 1999 via a transnational AIDS activist e-mail listserve. He had sent e-mails to the listserve looking for NGO-allies who could assist the medical humanitarian charity in starting a project providing ARVs in an African country. He had originally wanted to start the project in Kenya, but re-routed it to South Africa, because he realized that it had stronger traditions of civil society advocacy. Other activists on the listserve recommended Achmat as a potential collaborator. Originally Goemaere had thought about doing the project in Alexandra township in Johannesburg, but decided against it following a meeting with Nono Simelela who was then the Director of the HIV/STI and TB programme at the Department of Health. Semelela apparently told Goemaere that it would not be possible to use ARVs in the public sector, which the Belgian later came to attribute to the Mbeki administration's AIDS denialism (Interview 20 December 2010).

Achmat and Goemaere met in person in the days when the TAC was still small. In response to Goemaere's question about how MSF could assist the TAC, Achmat apparently told the Belgian doctor that ' "We need activist doctors who will treat the patients that nobody's treating in the public ser-vice. You treat the patients and we'll do the advocacy part" ' (Interview

20 December 2010). MSF faced less political barriers to providing ARV drugs at its clinic in Khayalitsha because the Western Cape province, where it was situated, was ruled by an opposition party and its government had already started a pilot PMTCT programme, as we have seen. Also the ANC-aligned MEC (provincial cabinet member) for health, Ebrahim Rassool, was broadly supportive of providing ARVs for PMTCT. Rassool and Fareed Abdullah the head of the Western Cape province's HIV programme signed agreements with MSF which enabled it to start operating. Hermann Reuter, an early member of the TAC was one of the first doctors to work with Goemaere to start the programme in June 2001.

Goemaere found that the MSF doctors had to rapidly 'learn by doing'. In addition to the high prices of the drugs, one of the greatest early challenges was that many of the local nurses were fearful of being around people living with HIV. Very few of Khayalitsha's residents had tested for HIV in the late 1990s: in 1999, only 450 had taken an HIV test. By contrast, by 2010, MSF was testing 45,000 of the township's residents per year. As we shall see in the next chapter, this fledgling programme soon began to develop impressive results in patients. But in the late 1990s, few community members knew about the disease or how it was transmitted. Meanwhile, the TAC and MSF also had a great deal of work to do to design an effective treatment literacy programme, which they did with some help from their American allies.

American allies' collaboration on the TAC's treatment literacy programme

TAC leaders such as Achmat also recognized that it was important to educate the public about how HIV treatment worked, both to combat government leaders' confusing statements about combination drug therapy and to generate greater demand for it in wider society. Yet again, international collaboration was vital in countering public mistrust of ARVs. In an interview, American AIDS activist Gregg Gonsalves described to me how he came to work with Zackie Achmat and the TAC on designing their treatment literacy programme.

Gonsalves and Zackie Achmat met in early 2000 through their mutual friend Loring McAlpin who, like the South African activist and his friend and former partner Jack Lewis, made films which dealt with gay themes. McAlpin apparently rang Gonsalves and told him that 'I have a friend from South Africa who would like to meet you guys to talk about how TAG could help this new group TAC to learn about HIV treatment' (Interview 19 May 2011). By this stage, Gonsalves was GMHC's director of treatment literacy and advocacy and McAlpin had previously been a member of Gran Fury, ACT UP's art collective. Achmat was visiting Manhattan and so Gonsalves showed him around GMHC's library: the American activist recounted that 'The treatment literacy program was run out of it and he [Achmat] was overjoyed, he said "Look at all this treatment information and all this stuff." ' Gonsalves described how his and Achmat's social networks meshed, noting that 'an LGBT arts threat that tied Zackie into America' in that McAlpin was both an AIDS activist and 'an artist and supportive of artists' (Interview 19 May 2011).

During that same trip to New York, Achmat invited Gonsalves to South Africa to conduct treatment literacy trainings for the TAC. This was some-thing that Gonsalves was well placed to assist with both because of his extensive experience as a treatment activist-expert and his participation in the North American Treatment Access Forum, which gathered annually to conduct training workshops on relevant developments in HIV medicine for AIDS activists. While in New York, Achmat also met Mark Harrington of TAG, who worked with Gonsalves to arrange the treatment literacy workshops that the TAC planned to hold in South Africa. Gonsalves then contacted activists from Project Inform, a San Francisco-based ally, and TAG and requested their assistance with the designing the workshops.

This group of American AIDS activists' relationships with the TAC was further consolidated when they visited South Africa to attend the Durban International AIDS Conference in July 2000. Mark Harrington recalled in an interview with me that the Durban conference was a turning point for 'the global AIDS research establishment' who 'discovered that the activist movement was really huge ... and that Africans were real and that you could really do things there' (20 May 2011). He added that 'for a lot of people it was a big eye-opener that just deconstructed the idea that you couldn't do treatment, that Africa was this giant wasteland and humanized the epi-demic'. The South African activists arranged a march for universal access to treatment which Gonsalves referred to as the movement's 'international coming-out party,' and a moment which permanently altered many visiting academics and activists' approach to the world's pandemic, particularly in the global South (Interview 19 May 2011).

After the Durban conference, the small cluster of American AIDS activists – including Gonsalves – continued their preparations for the South African treatment trainings. In New York, TAG raised funds from the NIH and the Aaron Diamond Foundation for the trainings. The workshop plan-ning also continued via international teleconferences between August and November 2000.

The American AIDS activists returned to South Africa in November 2000, to co-conduct the three to four day workshops with their South African counterparts in the country's three major cities of Johannesburg, Durban and Cape Town. They decided to cover a variety of topics including how HIV adversely affected the immune system in people living with the virus, the opportunistic infections which they could then contract and how the combination ARV therapy worked, including specific information about HIV treatment in women and children. The audiences for these trainings largely consisted of the TAC's township-based members. TAC activist Sipho Mthathi later developed these trainings into a nationwide treatment literacy programme, which Gonsalves characterized as having been 'much more sophisticated and elaborate and widespread than anybody else, I think, had ever done' (Interview 19 May 2011).

Both the Americans and the South Africans were very conscious of the fact that, given their target audience, it wouldn't be enough to simply show PowerPoint slides or handout copies of scientific articles or extracts from relevant textbooks. According to Gonsalves a lot of the TAC's early treatment literacy work involved putting information about HIV treatment 'into language and formats people could relate to' (Interview 19 May 2011). And so, for instance, the South African activists put words describing how to prevent mother-to-child transmission to the melodies of popular 'struggle' songs. They made posters with striking artwork about how to diagnose and treat opportunistic infections, and they enacted dramas showing how HIV treatment worked.

But, perhaps the most powerful element of the trainings was the personal testimony that the American activists openly living with HIV on combination ARV therapy could offer to their South African counterparts. In a 'digital age' where activists in different countries communicated via e-mails and the Internet, the American activists' physical presence was still necessary to demonstrate the effect of the drugs to most TAC's members. In this regard, it is worth noting that over 80% of South Africans had never had an Internet experience in this period, so such digital communication was only accessible to the movement's leaders and middle-class supporters.[45]

Harrington recalled that at the training in Durban 'there were just a lot of women at the conference that never spoke up, all sat together and just looked totally petrified' (20 May 2011). This was because information was both 'very technical' and 'very scary'. But, Harrington recalled that in each of the workshops 'there was always this great dramatic moment where you would be taking out your pills and saying "You know, I've been HIV positive since 1985 and I started therapy in 1996, my CD4 count went from 150 to 900" and people would gasp.' Harrington noticed that the TAC members in the audience 'knew enough about AIDS to know about CD4 counts and that it was bad to have low CD4 counts' but few knew people whose CD4 count had dramatically rebounded. Some of the American activists themselves were living, 'concrete examples' of how treatment worked, its success and they could discuss the side effects and how to manage them in an accessible way.

Conclusion

The TAC was formed by a group of former anti-apartheid activists, including gay rights activists. Its early treatment literacy and demonstration programmes' design benefitted from the South African activists' leveraging of expertise contained by people in their transnational sexuality and science-based treatment-advocacy networks. The South Africans used their networks effectively to obtain the assistance of American and European activist-experts in generating greater domestic public understanding of the science behind HIV treatment and, hence, support for their demands steadily grew. Achmat, a key moving force behind the TAC's formation, was also a leader in the post-apartheid, black-led, multiracial gay rights movement. Through his simultaneous involvement in the gay arts world as a filmmaker, he came into contact with American HIV treatment activist-experts who were pivotal in the design of the South African movement's early treatment literacy campaigns. In this period, MSF connected with the TAC via an HIV treatment activist e-mail list-serve, contact which culminated in the two groups co-founding a clinic in Khayalitsha, Cape Town.

Such programmes were especially necessary given the Mandela and Mbeki administrations' intransigence in the face of the South African activists' demands that the government provide ARVs in the public sector of the health system. This conflict was not inevitable: initially the activists enjoyed an amicable relationship with the government, especially as some former progressive health activists who had worked on AIDS joined its ranks. While the controversy of *Sarafina II* largely focused on allegations of tendering irregularities, the latter two controversies – over notification and Virodene – involved the worrying trend of government-imperviousness to independent scientific advice and, in this way, they ominously foreshadowed Mbeki's adoption of AIDS dissidence. Mbeki's position rendered HIV treatment literacy and demonstration projects all the more necessary both to counter growing public mistrust of ARVs and to save activists' lives, and, hence, sustain the movement itself.

While years of humming conflict over post-apartheid AIDS policy came to a crescendo over what Edwin Cameron has aptly referred to as 'the dead hand' of Mbeki's AIDS denialism, it was far from the only barrier to universal access to HIV treatment in the country (2003). The TAC's first major campaign used anti-apartheid symbolism and socio-economic rights-based rhetoric to urge multinational pharmaceutical companies to cease blocking the implementation of an act aimed at widening access to generic medicines – a campaign to which this book now turns.

5
'Pharma' v Mandela: South African Moral Capital in a Global Movement, 1998–2001

Introduction

On 19 April 2001, cheers, song and dance erupted in a packed room in the Pretoria High Court. The world had just witnessed a dramatic turn in the latest legal challenge faced by Nelson Mandela and his government. Just moments before, lawyers acting for South Africa's Pharmaceutical Manufacturers' Association (PMA), which represented 40 multinational pharmaceutical companies, had informed Judge Ngoepe that it was unconditionally withdrawing its case against the country's government and that it would bear all costs in the matter. The Mandela administration was now free to pass the Medicines and Related Substances Amendment Act (hereafter, the Medicines Act) to enable wider access to cheaper generic and imported patented drugs. Civil society activism had forced one of the most powerful industries in the world to retreat in a high-profile legal dispute with the government of a middle-income developing country. Moreover, this successful campaign against the court case had meaningful impacts for poor patients in developing countries. This favourable outcome permanently altered the politics of HIV drug pricing and, in a broader sense, global health in developing countries. The pharmaceutical industry – which was also sometimes informally referred to as 'pharma'[1] – introduced substantial reductions to the prices of certain branded ARV drugs, which facilitated a significant widening of global access to this treatment, especially in sub-Saharan Africa. Similarly, as discussed in Chapter 7, it also altered global health governance in terms of the World Trade Organization's (WTO's) Doha Declaration of 2001: a development which was inconceivable without the activism surrounding the court case, especially as it clarified states' public health-promoting rights to take the very same measures contained in South Africa's Medicines Act that had been challenged by the industry Association's litigation.

This chapter describes how the transnational activists in the TAC contributed a specifically South African type of moral capital to the international

HIV treatment access movement's challenge to the industry association's case. This chapter uses the term 'moral capital' in the sense suggested by Christopher Brown to describe how a civil society campaign can frame a policy as unethical in a politically impactful manner (2007, p. 29). It argues that the South African activists' moral capital had three main components: the effective use of anti-apartheid or 'struggle' symbolism to equate the actions of the pharmaceutical industry with those of the country's former racist regime; the presentation of legally convincing arguments based on the socio-economic right to access to health care; and the demonstration that there was a large, visible constituency of affected and aggrieved people.

The 'struggle' background of many of the TAC's leaders, such as Zackie Achmat, enabled the South African and international movements to convincingly deploy anti-apartheid-derived narratives to claim moral legitimacy for their cause. Achmat's leadership of the TAC provided powerful moral justifications for the American AIDS activists' solidarity actions which targeted Vice-President Al Gore during the early months of his election campaign because of his support for threats of US trade sanctions against South Africa for passing the Act. In South Africa, anti-apartheid narratives deployed by the TAC during its first civil disobedience campaign used the 'struggle symbolism' of the ANC's 1950s Defiance Campaign to generate domestic support for its advocacy on drug pricing. As we shall see, the South African and international movements had to challenge the dominant development consensus which was opposed to wider provision of combination ARV therapy in developing countries because of utilitarian arguments that it was not 'cost-effective' to do so and arguments that Africans lacked the 'cultural competency' to adhere to them. Locally, there were also suspicions and misunderstandings about the safety and efficacy of ARV therapy which the TAC overcame through careful treatment literacy programmes which explained how the drugs worked.

The TAC successfully argued to be admitted as an *amicus curiae* in the case. It deftly used legal arguments based upon the constitutionally enshrined socio-economic right to access to health care. This litigation strategy was an important legal factor in the industry association's decision to drop the case. International allies such as James Love of the Consumer Project on Technology (CPT) and Eric Goemaere of Médicines Sans Frontières (MSF) provided critical expert testimony on international trends in drug pricing. Litigation based upon the socio-economic right to access to health care was new in the history of South African AIDS activism. The movement invoked these rights to press for the state and pharmaceutical industry to play a more substantive role in fulfilling their positive obligations in law in terms of the right to access to health care. By contrast, earlier AIDS activism in the country had emphasized the right to privacy, a 'negative' right, which generally provided that the state should refrain from taking various actions in relation to individuals (described in Chapter 2).

The Medicines Act and global trade

The new South African government passed the Medicines Act to address racial and class disparities in access to health care services in the country. But it did so in a context where access to affordable medicines in developing countries was being increasingly threatened by 'free trade' agreements. In April 1994, 12 days before the country's first democratic elections, trade ministers from around the world, including South Africa, signed a new global free trade agreement in Marrakesh, Morocco. It brought into being the WTO, which was a new trade negotiation and arbitration body. Annexed to the main WTO agreement was one on Trade Related Aspects of Intellectual Property (hereafter, the TRIPS agreement) which came into effect in January 1995. The TRIPS agreement imposed 20-year pharmaceutical patents on WTO members and extended such 'intellectual property rights' to apply to both manufacturing processes and finished products (that is, to the drugs themselves). Middle-income developing countries had until 2005 to comply with this agreement.

A patent is an intellectual property right granted by a government to an inventor to exclusively manufacture, market and trade a product. Modern patents were first granted to engineers by the Republic of Venice in fifteenth-century Renaissance Italy. Since then, the thinking behind patents has been that inventors need incentives to innovate. But the scope and length of patents has changed over time and has only recently been made more globally uniform. For instance, prior to the TRIPS agreement, the Paris Convention for the Protection of Intellectual Property of 1883 (which was revised multiple times, up to 1967) allowed for countries to have diverse patent laws (Dutfield 2008; Adusei 2010). Most significantly, this earlier convention had enabled countries such as India to only grant patents to pharmaceutical manufacturing processes as opposed to the finished products (i.e. the drugs themselves). In this context, India, Brazil and Thailand had developed thriving generic drug industries, which, as we will see, would became critical in reducing the prices of ARV drugs in developing countries.

Critics of the granting of long and inflexible patents such as MSF and the TAC have charged that the market exclusivity they grant inflates the prices of drugs because it grants pharmaceutical companies a monopoly and, thereby, inhibits competition (Adusei 2010). Scholars of the impact of intellectual property on health in developing countries have also noted that 'patents only generate investment where profitable markets exist' (Hollis and Pogge 2008; Smith et al. 2009). This has created a dearth of new drugs for malaria, neglected tropical diseases and formulations of ARV drugs which are appropriate for children living with HIV. A dispute over the correct interpretation of the TRIPS agreement would lie at the heart of a monumental struggle over the Medicines Act, which was aimed at reducing the price of drugs. This conflict would prove all the more charged given that the country, led by Nelson

Mandela, had just emerged from apartheid to face one of the fastest growing HIV epidemics in the world. As discussed in Chapter 1, during the apartheid era, South Africa had a racially segregated public health system and a well-resourced private system, largely patronized by whites. Mark Heywood has argued that during this period, the 'absence of regulation of medicine prices' allowed the pharmaceutical industry to inflate their cost (2001). This was a factor behind general medical inflation which also hindered more people being able to access private health care (Heywood 2001).

To address some of these issues, the Mandela government developed a new National Drug Policy in 1996. Among its many goals were drug cost reduction and increased access to essential medicines (Zuma 1997; Heywood 2001). The concept of essential medicines can be traced back to 1977, when experts at the WHO decided to draft a list of drugs it regarded as truly 'essential' to improve access to health care for the greatest possible number of patients internationally. The thinking behind drawing up such an 'essential medicines' list was that it would enable ministries of health to focus upon the maximal provision of drugs which were necessary to improve patients' health in their respective countries.

In October 1997, South Africa's National Assembly had passed the Medicines Act with this aim in mind. The Act was signed into law by President Mandela on 25 November 1997. Section 15c of the Act included compulsory licensing and parallel importation. Compulsory licensing involves a government forcing a patent holder to allow another entity (either the state or a private company) to use its patented knowledge. In most instances, the company will be paid a royalty which is either negotiated with or legislatively enforced by the state. It is an effective tool to reduce the prices of medicines, because it enables generic competition. Parallel importation involves a government taking advantage of the fact that pharmaceutical companies frequently charge varying prices for patented drugs in different countries. When a government parallel imports a brand name drug, it has sourced it in another country where it is cheaper.

In February 1998, the entire multinational pharmaceutical industry in South Africa obtained an urgent high court interdict which prevented the 1997 Medicines Act from being signed into law by President Nelson Mandela. This was on the grounds that the association deemed section 15 (c) of the Act, which allowed for compulsory licensing and parallel importing, to be unconstitutional. At the time of the case, James Love, an activist at the Consumer Project on Technology (CPT), wrote that

The PMA not only threw everything at the Medicines Act, challenging virtually every aspect of the government's actions, but it went deep into the new South African constitutional protections, and used a number of human rights arguments against the Medicines Act, which the companies can exercise as a corporate persons. Generic drug substitution was the subject of a long line of attacks [based] on the right to [free] speech and conscience, as were other parts of the act.[2]

The association's motives in blocking the legislation were to stop generic competition and cheaper imports of their own products from reducing the prices they had set for their brand name drugs in South Africa. Because the WTO's TRIPS agreement contained clauses enabling compulsory licensing, the greater area of contention was parallel importation. Heywood has argued that '[i]n effect the legal action was an attempt by the PMA to use the Constitution to annex additional powers and safe-guards for intellectual property that are not part of TRIPS; to fill in some of the ambiguities in TRIPS, particularly its vagueness around parallel importation and to warn other developing countries off a similar path.'[3]

The progress of this litigation was slow moving for two reasons. It took a relatively long time, partly because the state requested numerous postponements.[4] Also, in September 1999, the industry announced its intention to voluntarily 'suspend' the lawsuit to enter into negotiations with the government.[5] This was a decision that was influenced by the withdrawal of the US government's diplomatic support for the litigation in response to American HIV treatment access activism at the time of Al Gore's presidential election campaign, which is discussed later in this chapter.

Meanwhile, the South African activists singled out individual companies for placing ARVs out of reach for most people living with HIV in the country. In 1999 and 2000, much of the TAC's early campaigning was focused on demands for Glaxo to reduce the price of AZT and for Pfizer to reduce the price of fluconazole. These campaigns had global dimensions. At a meeting on 19 April 1999, the TAC decided to write a memorandum to Glaxo Wellcome, the manufacturer of AZT, and to hold a picket outside its South African headquarters in Midrand, Johannesburg.[6] Three days later, the TAC sent a letter to Brian Collier Glaxo's Chief Executive. The letter stated that cost was a barrier to the government implementing a short course of AZT for PMTCT in the public sector of the health system.[7] It framed the issue in stark moral terms: the country and the continent faced 'a holocaust simply because we are poor and cannot afford the latest medications'.[8] The TAC had learnt through the media that Glaxo had committed itself to helping poor countries to access AZT. It asked Glaxo to reveal what it really cost to produce AZT, when the patent had expired on the drug, whether their offer of price reductions was unconditional and if they would make it available at cost price to all pregnant women living with HIV. The authors concluded that '[w]e believe this can be done and there is a *moral imperative* [my emphasis] for Glaxo to do this to realize its expressed commitment to assisting developing countries in fighting the epidemic'.[9]

By 1999, it was clear that the country was facing a devastating HIV epidemic. The 1998 annual national survey of pregnant women attending public antenatal clinics had found an HIV prevalence rate of 22.8%

(Department of Health 2009). In 1998, the Joint UN Programme on HIV/AIDS (UNAIDS) noted that 'South Africa, which trailed behind some of its neighbours in HIV infection levels at the start of the 1990s' was 'unfortunately catching up fast': one in seven new infections on the continent that year were 'believed to be in this one country' (1998, p. 3). The UNAIDS 'Epidemic Update' also projected that AIDS would knock 17 years off life expectancy in South Africa by 2005–10 (1998, p. 7). Children were far from exempt from this 'dismal decline' in life expectancy: South Africa was a prime example of the way in which HIV was 'contributing substantially to rising child mortality rates in sub-Saharan Africa' (UNAIDS 1998, p. 8). It was projected that by 2005–10, 61 out of every 1,000 infants born in South Africa would die before the age of one; by contrast, without AIDS, infant mortality in the country would have been as low as 38 per 1,000 (UNAIDS 1998, p. 8).

Silent or hostile: The international 'development' consensus on treatment access

Despite the unfolding demographic disaster being caused by AIDS in Sub-Saharan Africa, the newly formed TAC and its international allies faced an uphill battle advocating universal access to ARV drugs in developing countries in important global forums. This was chiefly because the dominant development discourses of the day were hostile to the HIV treatment activists' demands. Two main sets of arguments were put forward to oppose providing ARVs to poor patients in developing countries: utilitarian arguments that it was not 'cost effective' to provide ARVs in 'resource poor settings' and the view that Africans lacked the cultural sophistication to successfully adhere to ARV treatment regimens.

Peris Jones has argued that Western donor policy on HIV/AIDS remained largely silent on the provision of ARV drugs in developing countries in the early 2000s (2004). In an analysis of documents, reports and speeches by the UK's Department for International Development (DFID) and the Norwegian Agency for Development Co-operation (NORAD), he found that the overwhelming emphasis was on funding programmes for the prevention of new infections. Such donors also feared that widening access to ARV therapy would undermine prevention.

These aid agencies also viewed combination ARV therapy as 'too technical' and 'ultra-modern' for Africa's existing health capacity (Jones 2004, p. 396). Sweeping generalizations were frequently made about the limited capacity of health systems on the continent to provide access to ARVs. Instead, there was a focus on individuals' responsibilities to change their sexual behaviour, often divorced from a substantial analysis of the impact of structural factors such as gender inequality in the growth of the HIV epidemic.

Similarly, while the UNAIDS Epidemic Updates in the period under discussion were eloquent about the demographic and economic impacts of AIDS in sub-Saharan Africa, they failed to suggest that these could be ameliorated by universal access to HIV treatment or to indicate the pharmaceutical industry's role in constraining it. For instance, the UNAIDS 1999 epidemic update noted that sub-Saharan Africa bore the brunt of HIV and AIDS, as it contained close to 70% of the global total of people living with HIV and that most of them would die from the disease in the next decade (1999, p. 5). It went on to state that '[t]he challenge for the leaders of Africa and their partners in development' was to 'adapt and massively expand successful approaches' that made it 'harder for the virus to spread' and 'easier for those affected to live full and rewarding lives' (UNAIDS 1999, p. 5). But it did not mention that limited access to ARVs was a factor in Africa's elevated AIDS-related mortality compared with Europe or that this was partly caused by multinational drug companies' patent-induced monopolies on drug production and marketing.

The 2000 epidemic update stated that scaling up the response to Africa's epidemic was both 'imperative and affordable' (UNAIDS 2000). The update went on to state that '[s]etting ambitious but achievable targets' for HIV prevention measures would cost countries at least US$1.5 billion a year (UNAIDS 2000, p. 5). It added that '[f]or people with HIV and their families, the bill for palliative care for pain and discomfort, the treatment and prevention of opportunistic infections, and care for orphans would come to at least US$ 1.5 billion annually' (UNAIDS 2000, p. 5). By contrast, '[a]dding antiretroviral therapy would cost several billion dollars more a year' (UNAIDS 2000, p. 5). UNAIDS's failure to specify the cost beyond 'several billions' made it sound unfeasible.

The World Bank – a constituent part of UNAIDS by virtue of its membership of the UN 'family' – took a similar position. Its 1999 strategy for 'Intensifying Action Against HIV/AIDS in Africa' supported the procurement and provision of drugs for sexually transmitted diseases (STDs) and opportunistic infections such as TB, but it barely discussed the issue of the provision of ARVs on the continent. Indeed, it only mentioned the new drugs in an annexed case study describing a fictional country called 'Muzumbuka' which was supposedly based on an unnamed real African nation's response. Apparently, Muzumbuka did not include ARVs in its strategy, because they were 'simply not affordable' for reasons the report failed to specify (World Bank 1999, p. 49). The fictional country's government would, however, have been prepared to reconsider this 'based on new advances such as the development and accessibility of other affordable, low-cost drugs' (World Bank 1999, p. 49). But the strategy was silent on the role of generic competition in reducing the costs of ARVs and on the extant trade agreements which diminished their affordability and availability in developing countries.

The Bank's strategy document touched upon ARVs again in another appendix, where it recommended their wider usage for PMTCT. This support doubtless related to the fact that where 'basic services' were 'already in place and operating efficiently, the cost of providing counselling and testing, antiretroviral drugs and replacement feeding' was 'likely to be well distributed across the health system and relatively easy to absorb' (World Bank 1999, p. 70). A country with a 15% HIV prevalence rate and a birth rate of 40 per thousand would pay only US$0.8 per capita to roll out PMTCT (World Bank 1999, p. 73). The Bank argued that the cost of the intervention also compared well with other developing country health programmes: at HIV prevalence rates of 5% and above, the strategy cost around US$35 per Disability Adjusted Life Year (DALY); this was compared with US$20–40 per DALY for polio and diphtheria vaccination and US$200–400 per DALY for river blindness prevention (1999, p. 74).

A section of this annex entitled 'Questions of ethics' raised the issue of whether a mother being able to access ARV drugs only during her pregnancy and labour amounted 'to treating the mother for the sake of her baby alone' (World Bank 1999, p. 70). The Bank countered that this question was 'based on an erroneous perception', for an ARV drug used for the purpose of preventing MTCT was 'not really a treatment, but a "vaccine" for the infant' (1999, p. 70). Instead the issue of 'antiretroviral treatment for infected people' should have been 'considered separately from the issue of antiretroviral drugs used for the prevention of MTCT', because it required 'debate and policy decisions outside the scope of MTCT policy-making' (World Bank 1999, p. 70).

This type of development rhetoric and the policies it fostered had a devastating real-world humanitarian impact in South Africa and other heavily affected countries on the continent. For example, Dr. Peter Mugyenyi, a paediatrician and HIV/AIDS specialist who co-founded the Ugandan HIV/AIDS Joint Clinical Research Centre (JCRC), was deeply disheartened by the price tag of US$14,000 per patient per year for triple ARV drug therapy when it was first announced in 1996. He described his experiences as a physician working in Uganda in his 2008 book *Genocide by Denial: How Profiteering from HIV/AIDS Killed Millions*. In the book, he recounts that for much of the 1990s he faced a 'complex dilemma involving the huge numbers of poor and desperately ill AIDS patients, who swarmed my clinic and the JCRC, yet almost always left empty-handed'; this was 'simply because they were too poor' to pay for ARVs produced by multinational pharmaceutical companies (Mugyenyi 2008, p. 149). Another part of his 'predicament' was that 'no donor would fund antiretroviral therapy or even subsidise it, as this was then a no-go funding area often described as a "bottomless pit" ' (Mugyenyi 2008, p. 149). This meant that the only ARV drugs available in the country were those that his clinic had imported using the very limited funds raised from 'a small section of my patients who had the means to purchase their own drugs on a cost-recovery basis' (Mugyenyi 2008, p. 149).

Mugyenyi has pointed to the fact that there was not a total dearth of international initiatives to reduce HIV drug prices in this period (2008).

There were UN-led initiatives to reduce the prices of ARVs, but the problem was that these had proved ineffective. Indeed, from 1996, UNAIDS had held meetings in Geneva with major drug companies where interventions to increase access to HIV medicines were on the agenda: but these discussions seldom moved beyond the idea of pharmaceutical companies offering lower cost branded drugs, while their monopolies remained intact. This 'Accelerated Access Initiative', therefore, failed at significantly increasing access to the drugs. In 2001, absent decisive multilateral action on the issue, he was driven to import Indian generic medicines produced by CIPLA to Uganda, despite not being entirely clear about the legality of doing so; bold actions which enabled him to negotiate with the Ugandan government and other generic manufacturers for more of the cut-price drugs to be imported into the country (2008).

The Ugandan medical specialist's critique of the UN's role substantially overlapped with those of the transnational activists in the international HIV treatment access movement. As far as they were concerned, development as usual was insufficient to realize the rights of people living with HIV to access ARVs. One of the activists' rhetorical strategies at the Durban 2000 conference was to frame HIV treatment access as being crucial to development, more broadly (TAC and Health GAP 2000). The nascent international HIV treatment access movement's 2000 march memorandum made specific development policy demands of UNAIDS, the WHO and the US and EU governments at the Durban conference. These governments were urged to 'renounce' the use of trade sanctions as retaliation for parallel importation and compulsory licensing (steps facilitated by South Africa's Medicines Act). It also called for them to provide development financing to widen access to HIV treatment. The activists also pressed for UNAIDS and the WHO to move beyond gathering and publishing data on the epidemic. Like Mugyenyi, they concluded that their negotiated price reduction initiatives were 'showy but ineffective' and, further, alleged that the UN agencies had allowed themselves to be 'courted' by pharmaceutical companies with few results (TAC and Health GAP 2000).

They also visually projected their idea of universal treatment access as integral to, and enhancing, development. Activists at the demonstration held a banner showing these ideas which is reproduced in Figure 5.1. The banner's bold purple and red lettering proclaimed that 'Treatment Will Sustain Development', words which were placed against an orange background in the shape of the continent of Africa. The TAC's 'HIV POSITIVE' logo was right at the centre of the banner framed by red hands reaching out to each other, evoking the red ribbon which had come to symbolize AIDS.

But donor and UN arguments that the provision of ARVs was not 'cost-effective' were hardly unique in the health policy world. By the late 1990s, the dominant approach to health policy analysis had become a market-friendly consequentialist (consequence-focused) approach of assessing the

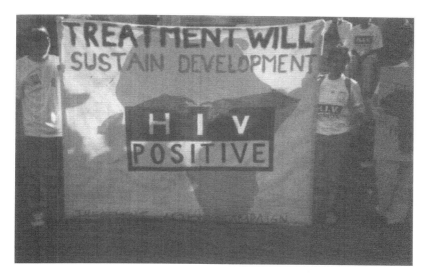

Figure 5.1   Activists hold TAC, Health GAP and ACT UP banner at Durban 2000 conference
Source: © Mark Harrington.

worth of health interventions in terms of their cost-effectiveness and reduction of disease burden as measured using DALYs (Ruger 2009). Measures which were deemed to not be 'cost-effective', such as the provision of patented ARV drugs for HIV treatment, were widely discounted within development circles, without ascertaining whether this was actually equitable, and despite the fact that the failure to provide these drugs was a violation of patients' human rights to access to health care.

Dan Brock has noted that cost/benefit or utilitarian approaches to health policy prioritize preventing or treating a prevalent but low-impact disease or condition if it produces greater overall benefits to society as a whole over treating or preventing a disease with a high impact on each individual affected (2004). Brock argues that part of the reason why this is controversial is that it runs counter to many people's sense of moral obligation to the sickest and neediest and also the manner in which a great deal of clinical decision making takes place in resource-constrained contexts – through triage. More precisely, when doctors are forced to prioritize, most are inclined to treat the patient who will suffer the most serious clinical consequences of non-intervention and obtain the most benefit first (Brock 2004, p. 216).

DALYs which are commonly used to measure 'disease-burden' and 'cost-effectiveness' have been critiqued as prioritizing the needs of working-age, relatively healthy adults at the expense of the disabled (Anand and Hansen

2004; Brock 2004). Critics have also charged that such metrics ignore the wider economic effects of ill-health and its disproportionate social impact on the poor (Anand and Hansen 2004).

In opposing this prevailing 'development consensus' on HIV and TB treatment in the early 2000s, Paul Farmer argued that '[t]he poor need access to the best clinical interventions available' and questioned a 'double standard' of clinical care, where the poor in developing countries were not seen as deserving access to the best available therapeutic technologies (2001, p. 15). He went on to argue that 'Many of the positions advanced in the development field are underpinned by a zero-sum approach: only exceedingly limited funds are available for "sustainable" projects, goes this logic, and so those who work for the poor must choose between, say, high-tech interventions and preventative services' (2001, pp. 21–2).

Perhaps the most egregious public enunciation of treatment-hostile rhetoric in the period was a speech given in June 2001 by Andrew Natsios, the administrator of USAID before the International Relations Committee of the US House of Representatives on AIDS in Africa. Natsios said that providing AIDS drugs to Africans was unrealistic because of limited infrastructure and capacity on the continent. He went on to argue that, even if the drugs were provided, a barrier to their efficacy would be Africans' supposed failure to understand 'Western time'.[10]

This is an example of what Farmer identified as a conflation of structural violence with cultural difference which was common both within the discipline of anthropology and among Western human rights and development practitioners, more generally (2001). He argued that this conflation led to the role of inequality in poor health outcomes being underplayed and exotic beliefs and practices of the Other being over-emphasized (2001).

Although the path to attaining foreign trade and aid policies to enable wider access to antiretrovirals was steep, it was not a route avoided by American AIDS activists. Indeed, as the next section will show, alliances between American and South African AIDS activists were critical in shifting US public policies in a direction aimed at widening access to HIV treatment in developing countries.

'Gore's Greed Kills': American AIDS activism in solidarity with South Africa

In January 1999, the Health Global Access Project (Health GAP) coalition was formed by American activists from HIV treatment, gay rights and consumer advocacy organizations. Health GAP quickly became one of the TAC's critical allies and a core component of the global HIV treatment access movement. The adverse humanitarian situation caused by growing AIDS-related sickness and death in South Africa provided a critical motivation for certain key American AIDS activists to begin advocacy around the global ARV treatment 'health gap'. Health GAP came to play an influential role in shifting US trade policy away from threatening South Africa with trade sanctions for passing the Medicines Act.

Raymond Smith and Patricia Siplon have provided a detailed account of the origins of Health GAP in their book *Drugs into Bodies*, a history which is worth briefly restating to shed light on their South Africa-focused solidarity actions. By 1999, Alan Berkman, a radical physician and former member of the Weather Underground, was a fellow in public health at Columbia University. He was stirred into action on the issue by a visit to South Africa. He told Raymond Smith and Patricia Siplon that, when attending the Geneva International AIDS Conference shortly after his stay in South Africa, he had the idea that the high price of HIV treatment was a ' "man-made obstacle" ' that could be changed (2006, p. 56). The example of Brazil's generic HIV drug industry – which produced ARVs costing less than a quarter of the patented versions – proved to Berkman that the drugs could be reduced in price (Smith and Siplon 2006, p. 57).

Activist John James of AIDS Treatment News had also begun to question the role of US trade policy in inflating the price of the drugs when he came into contact with James Love of the CPT (Smith and Siplon 2006). Love had acted as a consultant to the South African Department of Health. He shared with James his view that AIDS activists' demands for cheaper HIV drugs had a strong basis in international law and also informed him about the South African litigation.

Around the same time, Berkman called for the creation of a ' "multi-level strategy rooted in grassroots activism" ' to demand that the private sector, governments and civil society ' "dramatically expand access to life-sustaining medications, nutrients and nutritional supplements to HIV-infected individuals around the world" ' (Smith and Siplon 2006, p. 58). He also thought that activists should demand that pharmaceutical companies provide ' "drastic bulk discounts" ' of their drugs in the short term and relinquish their patents over the long term so that developing countries could produce their own generic ARVs (Smith and Siplon 2006, pp. 58–9). Health GAP was formed to implement Berkman's ideas.

Its first protest in support of South Africa's Medicines Act was held at one of Vice-President Al Gore's first presidential campaign appearances in June 1999. AIDS activist Mark Milano has described in an autobiographical article the ethical outrage which motivated him to participate in the demonstrations (2006, pp. 12–13). By June 1999, Milano had attended several demonstrations which had been held by AIDS Coalition to Unleash Power's New York City chapter (NYC) (2006, p. 12). He received a phone call one Sunday afternoon that he was being invited to a meeting that evening to plan a ' "party" ' – an ACT UP code word for a protest (2006, p. 12). Prior to attending that meeting, he had never advocated on global AIDS issues, as he had thought that there were plenty of domestic issues to address in relation to the epidemic and that 'the problem with AIDS around the world was too big for a simple activist to grapple with' (Milano 2006, p. 12).

According to Milano, the immediate impetus for the demonstration was provided by a leaked State Department memo detailing how the US government was preventing cheaper HIV drugs from being used in South Africa through blocking the implementation of the Medicines Act via trade negotiations (2006). Moreover, the office of the U.S. Trade Representative (USTR) had placed South Africa on its 'Special 301 Trade Watch', a warning that trade sanctions could follow. Milano noted that '[i]ronically, our [U.S.] government was threatening to restore the trade sanctions that had been lifted in 1993 when apartheid had ended' (2006, p. 12). He was outraged that the new South African government was being punished in a similar manner to the former apartheid government – merely for the 'crime' of trying to save its own citizens' lives. Gore was singled out both because of allegations that he had personally pushed the South African government to drop its Medicines Act at meetings of the Bi-national Commission held with Deputy President Thabo Mbeki and also because of the political opportunity presented by his campaign appearances (Behrman 2004; Smith and Siplon 2006). These American AIDS activists also noted that Anthony Podesta, one of Gore's closest campaign advisors, was a top lobbyist for the American industry body – Pharmaceutical Research and Manufacturers' of America (PhRMA) (Milano 2006).

On 16 June 1999, the first 'zap' occurred when Gore officially launched his campaign in Carthage, Tennessee. Health GAP activists arrived at the venue in Carthage after a 16-hour drive from New York City wearing fake ' "Columbia Students For Gore" ' t-shirts and as they were without tickets they 'sweet-talked' a ticket-taker into allowing them in and assumed a camera-friendly spot close to the stage. In the middle of Gore's speech Milano recounted that

> I got up on a fence, ripped off my t-shirt to reveal one that said 'GORE's GREED KILLS' and blew my whistle.
>
> All hell broke loose. We began chanting, 'Gore is killing Africans – AIDS drugs now!' . . . . The cameras focused on us immediately and I could see Gore was furious.
>
> (Milano 2006, p. 13)

The next day activists from the organization's Philadelphia chapter (ACT UP/Philly) raced to protest at one of the presidential candidate's campaign appearances in New Hampshire and held a banner reading 'AIDS Drugs for Africa' right behind where he spoke. On the third day of the protests, ACT UP/NY activists demonstrated at his appearance on Wall Street. For the rest of the summer of 1999, there were demonstrations as other fundraising events and activists came to dub Gore's election campaign, the 'Apartheid 2000' campaign (Smith and Siplon 2006, p. 66).

This equation of the PMA's case and the US government's actions in support of it with those of the apartheid government drew upon recent South African political history and the radical background of many Health GAP activists. South Africa had only emerged from apartheid four years before the industry association's challenge to the Act. As we have seen, the anti-apartheid movement had been global in scope, especially in the 1980s (Thorn 2006). It had also influenced a generation of liberal and left-wing young Americans, including AIDS activists and a future president, Barack Obama.[11] More directly, in the late 1980s and early 1990s there had been cross-pollination of ideas between American AIDS activists and their South African anti-apartheid colleagues. Eric Sawyer, an ACT UP activist and founding member of Health GAP, recounted that 'Some of ACT UP's most powerful actions – our political funerals – were copied from the South African anti-apartheid movement. During the 1990s, we carried the ashes of people who had died of AIDS, or the actual bodies of the dead, to the feet of those who had contributed to their deaths through inaction or inappropriate action' (2002, p. 92).

It is also important to note that – by definition – the industry association's decision to sue the Mandela administration to block the implementation of the Act invoked apartheid symbolism. The PMA's legal papers named Mandela as a First Respondent, and he had most famously been in the dock in 1963–1964 during his Rivonia Trial for 'sabotage and conspiracy'. That earlier trial had resulted in his conviction and notorious imprisonment for 27 years, a period when he became the world's most famous political prisoner and came to personify the global struggle for racial equality. Achmat, the leader of the TAC, had also been historically imprisoned for anti-apartheid activism, which lent further weight to the charge that the Clinton administration and pharmaceutical industry were enforcing a global medical 'apartheid'.

By the late 1990s and early 2000s, apartheid was part of the lexicon of terms used to describe invidious inequality around the world. For instance, some left-wing activists and 'movement intellectuals' used the term 'global apartheid' to describe globalization (Bond 2001). The sting of such apartheid metaphors lay in the accusation that the policies being criticized were as immoral as a racism-driven crime against humanity.

Gore's candidacy received a great deal of coverage in the US media, but his campaigning style had been deemed lacklustre by some commentators (Plotz 1999). Given his seeming lack of charisma, AIDS activists took over much of the story of his campaign for several months (Washington Post 18 June 1999). These protests, officially held under the ad hoc name 'AIDS Drugs for Africa', were also widely reported in South African newspapers

(*Business Day* 30 June 1999; *Sunday Times* 20 July 1999). The South African media reported that Gore was targeted because of allegations that he had personally threatened Mbeki with US trade sanctions against his country during a meeting of the Bi-National Commission between the two countries if his counterpart permitted 'the widespread sale of cheaper generic drugs that would cut into US companies' sales' (*Sunday Times* 20 July 1999). Perhaps most damning were the American AIDS activists' allegations that Gore had 'sold out' for 'drug-makers' cash contributions to his campaign' (*Pretoria News* 1 July 1999). According to the same media report, the industry tried to block the Medicines Act because it wanted to protect its profits and maintain the 'incentive to spend on costly research'.

In the fall of 1999, American AIDS activists redirected their energies to target the US Trade Representative (USTR), Charlene Barchefsky. On 17 September, the USTR released a statement that it had reached an agreement with the South African government that it would endorse that country's Medicines Act, if it agreed to adhere to all international trade agreements including the TRIPS agreement (Behrman 2004; Smith and Siplon 2006). According to Greg Behrman, that same press release claimed that the South African PMA had agreed to drop all litigation against the country's government (2004, p. 157). But AIDS activists wanted the US government to go further and pledge to refrain from sanctioning any African country for compulsory licensing and parallel importation. On 6 October, ACT UP organized a 750-person demonstration to the USTR's office in Washington, DC., and in November, activists occupied these offices. These wider goals were soon met: in December President Bill Clinton acceded to the activists' demands by pledging that no African country would face trade threats for compulsory licensing and parallel importation, and this was written into an executive agreement in May 2000 (Behrman 2004; Smith and Siplon 2006). While an important political victory had been won, it is important not to overstate its significance. The PMA's apparent offer to 'withdraw' from the case had no legal meaning on the ground in South Africa. The PMA had neither withdrawn its case from the Johannesburg High Court nor had it offered the South African government a fair settlement.

The fact that the case was still very much on was also not lost on certain members of the international media. Ed Vuillamy, writing in *The Observer* of London in December 1999, pointed out that 'The choice of "First Respondent" and principal defendant, at the top of the list was brazenly defiant: "The President of South Africa, the Honourable Mr N. R. Mandela N.O." It had been some years since Mandela was faced with a legal charge' (19 December 1999). This was not strictly accurate, as Louis Luyt, the former President of the South African Rugby Football Union, had taken Mandela to court in 1998, but it demonstrated that the pharmaceutical industry's case was eliciting unfavourable press, internationally, for the drug companies concerned.

Anti-apartheid symbolism in the TAC's domestic advocacy in South Africa

Meanwhile, in South Africa the TAC had started to pressure the PMA to withdraw its suit blocking the implementation of the new medicines law. While the case inherently invoked apartheid symbolism, in the domestic sphere the TAC used it even more explicitly than the international movement to organize large numbers of supporters in its campaign against the suit.

In September 1999, it demonstrated outside the PMA's offices in Midrand, Johannesburg.[12] The TAC wrote an open letter to Mirryena Deeb, the PMA's CEO, calling on the association's members (multinational pharmaceutical companies) to 'unconditionally' reduce the prices of three HIV medicines: fluconazole, gancyclovir and AZT.[13] It argued that the PMA's legal action against the Medicines Act was 'an unreasonable attempt to delay and deny South Africans' access to affordable treatment and care'.[14] Therefore, it called on the PMA to 'unconditionally withdraw' its legal action against the government.[15]

In May 2000, the dispute between South African AIDS activists and the pharmaceutical industry played out at the Parliamentary Portfolio Committee on Health's hearings on drug pricing. At a hearing on 9 May 2000, Deeb, the chief executive of the pharmaceutical industry body, reportedly placed the blame for AIDS squarely on the government by arguing that with its recent R30 billion arms deal, it was spending more on military hardware than on combating AIDS (*The Citizen*, 10 May 2000). By contrast, Deeb tried to paint the industry as caring about the epidemic because of its offers to donate ARVs and treatments for opportunistic infections for free or to sell them at reduced prices. She argued that although India did not respect intellectual property rights, the country was rife with disease. In a veiled reference to Mbeki's views on AIDS, Deeb apparently accused the government of making 'groundless excuses' for not treating poor, or pregnant, HIV-positive people (*The Citizen*, 10 May 2000).

A few days later, TAC activists Zackie Achmat and Chris Moraka used the hearings to 'lambaste' the drug companies (*The Sunday Independent* 14 May 2000). They told the committee that adults living with HIV had to pay more than R4,000 a month for combination ARV drug therapy. Achmat said that he had had to pay over R5,000 to treat a severe case of thrush, an HIV-related opportunistic infection. By contrast, the generic equivalent from Thailand cost roughly R400. Toby Jasper, the coordinator of MSF's 'access to essential medicines campaign', undercut the argument that the pharmaceutical companies would lose significant sales by allowing generic production and importation of cheaper drugs into South Africa by pointing out that Africa represented less than 1% of the industry's global market (*The Sunday Independent* 14 May 2000).

According to TAC activist Mandla Majola, Chris Moraka – one of the activists who testified in parliament – was a member of the South African Communist Party who had joined the HIV treatment movement in its early days (Interview 3 April 2008). He had been the chairperson of a street committee in Nyanga East township in Cape Town but then had given up the role owing to his ill-health. Majola recounted in an interview that Moraka decided to be open about that fact that he was living with HIV because of his concern about the disease being hidden and a fear that many others could become infected and die if more people did not publicly disclose that they were living with the virus. A frail, AIDS-ill Moraka spoke at the parliamentary hearing on drug pricing. He was suffering from severe thrush which could have been treated with the fluconazole produced by Pfizer.[16] Thrush was a debilitating, AIDS-related opportunistic infection which commonly manifested with symptoms in the mouth and throat which made it extremely painful for HIV-positive people to swallow and prevented them from eating comfortably. According to a 2001 TAC fact sheet, although no Pfizer representative was present, the dying activist made the following appeal to the company to save his life and those of people similarly afflicted: ' "Companies like Pfizer make a lot of profit. We ask them to lower prices of drugs because we HIV-positive people suffer most. Other people don't feel this pain; they want to make a profit you see".'[17] The TAC produced posters featuring the face of William Steere, the chief executive of Pfizer, labelling him as an 'AIDS Profiteer'.[18] Moraka died of AIDS-related illnesses later that month and was mourned at a funeral where his positive HIV-status was openly discussed. After the funeral TAC activists and Moraka's friends and family marched through Nyanga township to express their ire against Pfizer and call for universal access to HIV treatment.[19]

As we have seen, the first truly global march for universal access to HIV treatment was held at the opening of the Durban International AIDS Conference in July 2000. This march was jointly organized by the TAC and Health GAP, who co-produced a striking florescent yellow and black sticker stating that 'Cheap AIDS Drugs Save Lives' (see Figure 5.2). The marchers' memorandum symbolically linked global AIDS with apartheid. It was addressed to Deputy President Jacob Zuma and other senior government figures, among other targets. In it, they argued that the South African government had a 'unique potential to right the wrongs and inequalities' that existed around AIDS (TAC and Health GAP 2000). South Africa was both the 'worst affected in the world' and it also had 'the moral legitimacy' that had 'accrued to a nation' that had 'risen peacefully from apartheid under the leadership of Nelson Mandela'. As the government themselves had admitted, AIDS was a 'new struggle'. Several of the key South African activists and some of their international allies who organized the demonstration were former anti-apartheid activists which lent moral credibility to their framing of AIDS as a new form of apartheid. For instance, Action for Southern Africa

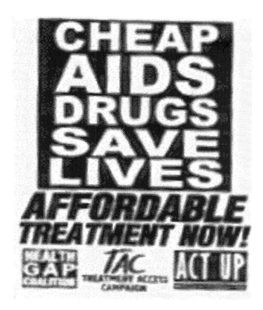

Figure 5.2 This sticker was distributed by Health GAP, TAC and ACT UP at the demonstration
Source: Author's own collection.

(ACTSA), which was established in 1994 as the successor organization to the British Anti-Apartheid Movement, had endorsed the 2000 Global March for HIV/AIDS Treatment Access (TAC 2001a).

The TAC's complex and changing political uses of the law were demonstrated by its decision in October 2000 to resort to civil disobedience for the first time, in the Chris Moraka Defiance Campaign. Sociologists who have studied social movements have noted that one of their characteristics is they use 'master frames' borrowed from past movements (Snow 2004). When the TAC chose to call their first civil disobedience campaign the Chris Moraka Defiance Campaign, they symbolically linked the master frame of the ANC's 1950s Defiance Campaign to the more recent memory and story of Chris Moraka: the TAC and SACP activist who had died because of being too poor to afford branded AIDS medicines.

Another documented characteristic of social movements is that their members take extraordinary steps to demonstrate their commitment to a cause and its moral and political legitimacy (Tilly 2004). In this sense, we can interpret Achmat and other TAC activists who broke the law in this civil disobedience campaign as having done so to demonstrate their dedication to what they viewed as being a morally worthy cause. The campaign began when Achmat illegally smuggled 3000 capsules of generic fluconazole (produced and sold under the trade name Biozole) from Thailand into South Africa and passed through customs without incident.[20] On 18 October 2000, the TAC held a press conference where Achmat revealed what he had done and used the opportunity to point out the dramatic difference between the price of the Thai generic and that of the branded versions sold in South Africa. Whereas Pfizer sold the patented version of the drug for R80.24 per capsule to the private sector and R28.57 per capsule to the public sector, the generic, Thai version cost a mere R1.78 per capsule (*The Sunday Independent* 29 October 2000). The next day, while the police began an investigation into Achmat's smuggling of generic AIDS drugs, the TAC simultaneously applied to the Medicines Control Council (MCC) – South Africa's drug regulatory agency – for an exemption from their registration.[21] On 20 October the drugs were confiscated from Achmat at the Narcotics Bureau and remained so even when the MCC later allowed the Brooklyn Medical Centre in Cape Town to prescribe them to patients.[22]

When Achmat adopted civil disobedience as a tactic, the South African media began to focus on him much more as an individual. Achmat had previously been quoted by the country's press over his support of Edwin Cameron's HIV-status revelation and in favour of people being open about living with HIV in 1999. But in October 2000, as he became the TAC's main media spokesperson and a recognizable figurehead, detailed 'human interest' stories began to be produced on him. An article in the *Cape Argus* of 1 November 2000 was based on a two-hour interview with Achmat. In line with the movement's evolving strategy of symbolically linking its campaigns to those against apartheid, the story emphasized Achmat's involvement in actions in solidarity with the 1976 Soweto student uprising. It related how

> Achmat, a schoolboy at Salt River High, and two friends decided to pledge their solidarity with the African children up north by burning down their school.

> 'I think it was the horror of what happened and how kids were shot down. It made me aware of the system of power, not simply the inequalities which are around all the time.'

The article went on to mention how his experience of being beaten and arrested for arranging a demonstration as a school student had taught him a lot about how the law could be used ' "to defend people even in the worst circumstances possible" ' (*Cape Argus*, 1 November 2000).

After describing the general steps he took to remain healthy while living with HIV, such as taking vitamins and eating well, Achmat made a striking pledge: ' "I know there's going to come a time when my body cannot carry me. I won't have the strength and then I want to have the right to go onto anti-retrovirals. But not if they are not available to the mass of people in our country" ' (*Cape Argus*, 1 November 2000). Achmat's drug-fast pledge was yet another extraordinary step he took to show his commitment to the goals of the TAC.

In the same period, the TAC stepped up its organizing efforts, especially in the townships surrounding Cape Town. Mandla Majola and Sipho Mthathi were central to these efforts. Concerned about how to expand the TAC's base, these two activists drew on their experiences of involvement in earlier struggles against apartheid. Majola was a young man from Gugulethu township in Cape Town who joined the TAC in April 1999 at the age of 29 (Interview 3 April 2008). He came from an anti-apartheid Pan-Africanist Congress (PAC) political background and was the chairperson of the Young Romans Football Club in the township. The activist had initially attended a TAC meeting on behalf of Imbizo, a Gugulethu-wide youth umbrella-body. He remembered that 'In those days we were very vocal in terms of "Settler, Settler, Bullet, Bullet, Settler, Settler."' We talked a lot about Pan-Africanism. We were taught a lot about Africa, that it should be united. 'Africa should unite. Africa must be independent. We must take back Africa from the imperialists and from the colonialists' (Interview 3 April 2008).

Because Majola came from this political background, he initially felt very suspicious of the TAC, particularly of the racial motives of Dr Hermann Reuter, a white doctor who played a leading role in the movement's treatment literacy workshops in Gugulethu.

As Majola became more involved in the TAC, he began to see that the drugs were safe and effective when correctly prescribed: he found that as he became more involved in the organization's work he got 'more information' and his 'understanding changed' (Interview 3 April 2008). Anthropologist Jonny Steinberg has noted that the racialized suspicions many Africans harboured in relation to HIV medicine was a barrier to the TAC's growth in the rural Eastern Cape, and Majola's experience illustrates how the same problems were present in urban areas (2008).

Majola's thinking about how to organize was informed by his earlier experiences as a PAC activist. In the same interview he recalled how 'My understanding of how to empower communities was lying with my time at the PAC, where you build branches, and you tell people about the aims of your organization.... Then we asked people in the communities to become members of the organization.'

When Majola had joined there was only one TAC branch, which Mthathi had established in Nyanga/Gugulethu. In conversations with TAC leaders like Nathan Geffen and Achmat, Majola began to advocate for changes to the movement's methods. They, in turn, gave him transport money to visit support groups for people living with HIV and tell them about the TAC's campaigns; on his urging, many of these support groups subsequently became branches, led by people living with HIV.

Majola wanted the movement to have its 'heart' in the communities and like other TAC activists, he knew that for the movement's base to grow, its activism had to be woven into the fabric of township life. He told me that Reuter spoke at a workshop about how pamphlet distribution had proved powerful in anti-apartheid township boycotts. When sharing ideas about how the TAC could mobilize more supporters, Majola recalled that activists who had come from a PAC background talked about how they had mobilized people while watching soccer: 'When we go to football matches, one of the ways of mobilizing people is when they are watching football. They are not watching football, we are talking about politics.' Similarly, from their days of opposing apartheid, such township activists had learnt the power of using the pulpit to mobilize people around social issues:

> Where people are waiting to hear more about the bible, you talk about what's going on today through the bible .... We would take advantage of, sometimes, unfortunate incidents where one of our comrades has fallen and use it [the political AIDS funeral] to educate people about HIV and the use of ARVs and all that stuff. That we have learnt from [the] liberation [struggle] in the days of apartheid.
>
> (Interview 3 April 2008)

Majola also successfully argued that, for the movement to grow, the way that marches were run had to change. In particular, the movement's initial adherence to the perceived Western tradition of merely chanting and giving speeches at marches did not excite many new African activists in the movement.

As a PAC activist he had seen

> the importance of using a song to mobilize a community. We, as Africans, we like to sing, we sometimes get comfort by just singing. A poet amongst you, that person motivates you in the face of fear, and then you have strength to move on. Because with AIDS people were dying, we have lost friends, we have lost comrades, we have lost many people. But still we are determined to move ahead. So there's a lot that we learnt from the liberation movement.
>
> (Interview 3 April 2008)

These painstaking efforts at branch establishment and awareness raising began to bear fruit in late 2000. By then, the TAC could mobilize large numbers of supporters to attend protests and meetings, even when there were not international conferences with many activist delegates, such as those which had been held in Durban some months before. In November 2000, 500 people attended a march at Groote Schuur hospital in Cape Town to demand that the illegally imported generic fluconazole ('Biozole') smuggled in by Achmat be released for use by AIDS patients (SAPA 1 September 2010). Majola was credited with playing an instrumental role in the high turn-out and was promoted from being a volunteer to the paid position of Western Cape provincial co-ordinator of the movement. The Chris Moraka Defiance Campaign continued into 2001 when Morne Visser, a South African soap opera star, smuggled a second batch of Biozole into the country in January 2001.[23] Shortly afterwards, and doubtless as a consequence of the TAC's activism, Pfizer and the government finalized an agreement in March 2001 for the donation of Diflucan (the multinational company's brand name for fluconazole) to be distributed in the public sector. Achmat's smuggled Biozole was never returned to the TAC by the narcotics' bureau, but Pfizer's free, donated, branded version arrived that same month.[24] With the PMA case looming on the horizon, the TAC's activities moved back to pressuring the pharmaceutical industry to drop the case.

Given the drug pricing issue's 'anti-imperialist' elements, the Congress of South African Trade Unions (COSATU) and the SACP joined the TAC's protests against the PMA's action to block the Medicines Act. What seems to have cemented these links is the fact that some of the TAC's founder members were also SACP members, such as Mazibuko Jara and Mark Heywood. Jara told me that in late 1999, he was recruited by Blade Nzimande to become the SACP's Media and Publicity Officer (Interview 26 March 2007). The movement also had ties to the union confederation because the TAC's first office space was rented from the COSATU-affiliated National Education Health and Allied Workers Union (NEHAWU). When the TAC decided to apply to be an *amicus curiae* in the case, they selected Theodora Steele – the Campaigns Coordinator for COSATU – as their founding affidavit's deponent (Heywood 2001). This alliance grew stronger when hearings in the PMA's case against the government commenced in March 2001. In media statements, both the SACP and COSATU framed the issue in anti-imperialist terms. The SACP told reporters at City Press – a South African newspaper with a largely African readership – that the PMA was trying to block the legislation so that ' "big capitalist drug companies would protect their huge profits at the expense of the health and lives of poor people around the world" ' (4 March 2001).

But one should not overstate the strength of the TAC's alliances with COSATU and the SACP, both of whom were part of the governing 'Tripartite Alliance' with the ruling party. After the TAC's march at Baragwanath Hospital in Johannesburg to call upon the government to provide AZT for PMTCT in March 1999, Jara perceived that the movement was seen by some powerful members of the Tripartite Alliance as 'anti-government' (Interview 16 March 2007). This perception restricted the extent to which COSATU and the SACP were prepared to support the TAC's activities – for fear of jeopardizing their primary political alliance with the ANC. As shall be shown, in

2003, for instance, COSATU was unwilling to support the TAC's strategy of renewed civil disobedience.

In the case of the SACP, support offered to the TAC was fleeting, and the movement was viewed with some ambivalence by the party. For instance, while Jara and other members of the Johannesburg Central Branch of the SACP had been supportive of the March 1999 Baragwanath demonstration, the party did not adopt a national position in favour of wider HIV treatment access in 1999–2000. Eventually, according to Jara, Nzimande (the Communist Party's leader) urged him to leave the TAC, on the grounds that an SACP spokesperson could not speak for both entities because the movement was seen by the ANC as anti-government (Interview 16 March 2007). In a similar vein, Jeremy Cronin pointed out in an interview with the author that the SACP was 'never directly aligned' with the TAC in the late 1990s and early 2000s (Interview 30 March 2007). He told me that this was because COSATU and the SACP were already under attack by the ANC for adopting what the ruling party termed 'ultra-leftist' (Trotskyite) positions and the Communist Party 'didn't want to open up too many fronts. We weren't sure if we could help as we were being attacked on so many fronts'. In particular, the SACP was being heavily criticized inside the ANC for attacking the ANC government's Growth Employment and Redistribution (GEAR) strategy (a strategy described in Chapter 3).

South African student groups were also organized in support of the case, for instance, in March 2001, AIDS Action from the University of Durban-Westville and ActivAID from the University of Natal organized a march on Merck, one of the litigants in the case. A pamphlet advertising the demonstration is depicted in Figure 5.3. The pamphlet emphasized that Achmat was a 'hero of the liberation struggle' and an 'internationally celebrated leader of the Treatment Action Campaign'.[25] Citing the example of Brazil, the pamphlet suggested that South Africa break the monopoly of big pharmaceutical companies through generic production and parallel importation.[26] It also asserted that the campaign for access to AIDS treatment was one to 'put human life before the profits of the big pharmaceutical companies'.[27]

As the court case drew near, the TAC and international HIV treatment access movement's demonstrations grew in global reach and radicalism. The night before the case commenced, the TAC held a vigil in Church Square near the Pretoria High Court.[28] According to Mark Heywood, in, the course of its social mobilization around the case the TAC had also significantly increased the number and strength of its international alliances: ACT UP, Health GAP, Consumer Project on Technology (CPT), MSF and Oxfam all supported the South African movement's campaign (Interview 14 April 2008). On the first day of the case, the TAC called for a 'global day of action' where the TAC's international allies organized demonstrations in Australia, Brazil, Britain, Canada, Denmark, France, Germany, Italy, the Philippines, Thailand and the United States.[29]

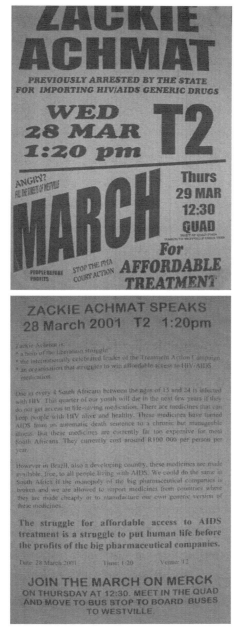

Figure 5.3   The front cover and reverse of a pamphlet advertising the march on Merck
Source: Author's own collection.

The right to access to health care in the TAC's court papers

Another key ingredient of the TAC's 'moral capital' was its successful deployment of legal arguments around the socio-economic right to access to health care as an *amicus curiae*. Mark Heywood has argued that 'The TAC's appropriation of the PMA case illustrates how legal action can be used to catalyze both national and international political mobilization' (2001, p. 3). He has gone on to argue that the case was an example of multinational pharmaceutical companies 'dressing [human] rights-incursions in the language of [intellectual property] rights-protection and using unlimited economic power to pursue legal strategies to consolidate this' (2001, p. 3).

According to Heywood, in January 2001 the TAC decided to apply for leave to intervene as an *amicus curiae* after being informed of the dates of the hearing by Maureen Kirkman, the PMA's Head of Scientific and Regulatory Affairs (Heywood 2001, p. 7). The TAC decided to present arguments in defence of three sections of the act (15C, 22F AND 22G) dealing with parallel importation, generic substitution and the establishment of a pricing committee. It argued that each of these measures was 'necessary and justifiable' given the need for HIV medicines in the context of South Africa's epidemic (Heywood 2001, p. 9). The movement said that epidemic 'created urgency and justification for legal measures to make medicines more affordable' (Heywood 2001, p. 12). Both the safety and efficacy of the medicines and the scale of the epidemic were beyond dispute, which meant that the TAC's argument could focus on the issue of the price of the medicines.

The TAC's legal argument was that none of the Act's three clauses was unconstitutional. Instead they were dictated by the government's '*positive duty* [my emphasis]' to ' "progressively realize" rights to access to health care services and to protect rights such as dignity, life, equality and the duty to act in the best interests of the child' (Heywood 2001, p. 12). Furthermore, the activists argued, the poor relied on the state's ability to progressively realize these rights. They also pointed out that under South African constitutional law (section 36 of the Bill of Rights), the state could limit certain rights (such as that to private property, including patents) as long as the infringements were 'reasonable and justifiable in an open and democratic society based on human dignity, equality and freedom' (Heywood 2001, p. 13).[30] It also pointed to the fact that in the new South Africa the legal rights of 'corporate persons' to intellectual property could be subordinated to individuals' human rights to dignity and access to health care. The movement further undermined the industry association's case by pointing to the fact that the research and development costs for several AIDS drugs had already been recouped and that, in any event, companies such as Pfizer and Glaxo had failed to provide these costs to the TAC.

Ronen Shamir has averred that '[t]he ultimate purpose of the [TAC's] brief...was to re-frame the dispute as a "right to health" case and, within this context, to establish a direct link between South Africa's AIDS crisis and the high cost of drugs incurred on the needy due to the pharmaceutical industry's economic leverage' (2005, p. 46).

This 'right to health' line of legal argument was very significant in the history of South African AIDS activism. Prior AIDS-related human rights litigation had centred on defending the right to privacy (as discussed in Chapter 2). South Africa's new Constitution and the medical innovation of combination ARV therapy had caused a shift in the role activists saw for the state in combating AIDS. Previously activists had conceived of the state's human rights obligations in relation to people living with HIV in classically liberal terms, emphasizing what Isaiah Berlin termed 'negative' freedom – freedom from unwelcome governmental intrusion into their privacy (2002, p. 169). Activists were now also supporting state intervention in drug pricing to enable it to provide medicines to millions of its citizens. By making their case through socio-economic rights, they were asserting a new vision for South African AIDS activism which was grounded in what can be termed 'substantive freedom' (Sen 1999; Ruger 2009). Differently put, they were advancing a view of social justice as enmeshing both personal freedom (in terms of the rights to privacy and bodily autonomy) and society-wide poverty reduction, and used the right to health in the manner suggested by political philosopher Jennifer Prah Ruger to 'make an ethical demand for equity in health' (2009, p. 125).

The PMA opposed the TAC's *amicus* application partly on the grounds that whether or not medicines were cheap or expensive was irrelevant to the main application (Heywood 2001, p. 13). It also argued that the TAC's *amicus* application had not mentioned the role of the state in addressing the AIDS epidemic.[31] Deeb complained to *The Guardian* of London that ' "This law is arbitrary and gives the health minister too many powers .... There is a lack of due process. The minister can make a decision that a drug is too expensive and the drug companies have no right to defend themselves" ' (5 March 2001). The industry's claim that many [unnamed] African countries received drugs 'at a large discount price' was repeated in the article. Deeb also said that the state had never asked the pharmaceutical companies what it cost to treat HIV. The TAC had indeed repeatedly requested this information from the industry and never been provided with it, as we have seen. The South African Director General of Health Ayanda Ntsaluba shot back that even with steep price reductions, the government could not afford to buy many 'brand-name' drugs.

On 6 March, Judge President Bernard Ngoepe ruled in favour of the TAC's application to be admitted as an *amicus* for the duration of the case. This meant that, even though the TAC was not a party to the case, they could submit arguments to the court in relation to it (*The Daily News*, 7 March 2001). Achmat told *The Daily News* that this ruling had restored the movement's ' "faith in the system" ' and showed that judges were ' "prepared to fulfil their constitutional duties in this country" ' (1 March 2001). The case was then adjourned to 18 April.

According to Heywood, the PMA tried to refute some of the TAC's *amicus* arguments in its 28 March Replying Affidavit (2001). It argued that the extent of poverty meant that any price was too expensive for many South Africans. The PMA also claimed that the high revenues the companies' acquired from their patent monopolies were required to finance innovation. According to the industry association, its members (multinational pharmaceutical companies) had already offered price reductions. In its view, the Medicines Act made South Africa a 'pariah state', because it alleged that no other co-signatories of the WTO's TRIPS agreement had legislation providing for parallel importation or generic substitution.

The TAC used the next month to obtain expert supporting affidavits which would also form a basis for its final affidavit. The TAC's international allies provided critical evidence. For instance, James Love from the Consumer Project on Technology (CPT) provided an affidavit dealing with the profitability of the pharmaceutical industry, the real costs of the research into new medicines and the critical role of the American National Institutes of Health (NIH) in co-financing medical innovation. As discussed above, Love had acted as a consultant to the Ministry of Health when it was led by Nkosasana Zuma.

Love claimed that the pharmaceutical industry had overstated its research and development costs and downplayed the extent to which the American government had financed such costs. He argued that the US Orphan Drug Act of 1983 provided a tax credit of 50% of the costs of conducting clinical trials in America.[32] The AIDS drug AZT, which was critical in preventing mother-to-child transmission of HIV, had received such a designation and so its manufacturer Glaxo-SmithKline had enjoyed this tax credit.[33] Love said the FDA had granted the orphan designation to 74 drugs used to treat HIV, which meant that the pharmaceutical companies that manufactured them had also enjoyed substantial tax credits in producing them.[34]

He also claimed that the pharmaceutical industry had overstated its drug development costs in its affidavits. In particular, he said, its papers had relied on a 1991 study by Joseph DiMasi and his colleagues which had put the cost of developing a new drug at US$231–500 million, but these figures were 'estimates of the costs of doing both the early discovery and preclinical work, the clinical trials and for obtaining the FDA's regulatory approval'.[35] For many drugs, the US government paid for either the preclinical or clinical work. In those cases, the companies' costs were lower.[36] In addition, there were huge differences between the costs of developing different products.[37] HIV drugs were typically fast-tracked for FDA approval.[38] In general, since DiMasi et al.'s study had been published, Love stated that there had also been a substantial reduction in the time between a patent being filed and the FDA offering marketing approval, and this reduced costs.[39]

The American activist countered the pharmaceutical industry's assertion that it needed to charge high prices to fund innovation by pointing out that the American government had played a significant role in the development of drugs. This was illustrated by the fact that the federal government was directly involved in the pre-clinical development of 18 of the 37 cancer drugs developed between 1955 and 1989, and it had also played a more limited role in pre-clinical research for ten other cancer drugs.[40] In the case of AZT, Love pointed out that it was synthesized by a scientist using a government grant, that its ARV potential was discovered by a publicly funded German scientist and that the first clinical pharmacology, immunological and virological studies from which it could be inferred that the drug might work were also state funded.[41]

The TAC's international supporters argued in their affidavits that Brazilian and Indian generic producers indicated the type of price reductions which were possible and had also played a critical role in reducing the cost of ARV drugs. For instance, Eric Goemaere of MSF argued in his affidavit that the prices of drugs produced by Indian and Brazilian generic manufacturers were 'the best estimates available of what commercial producers can achieve in terms of price as pharmaceutical manufacturers typically refuse to disclose publicly a breakdown of their drugs' price structures and specifically the marginal costs of these drugs'.[42] Love used competitive industry price data to show that Brazil's purchase of generic AIDS drugs had reduced their prices internationally over the preceding three years: 3TC had gone from US$ 10,000 per kilo to US$ 750; d4T, a drug invented at Yale University on a government grant had gone from US$10,000 per kilo to US$1,000.[43]

Achmat and the TAC also began winning the media war in South Africa and internationally. In April 2001, wearing a striking yellow t-shirt with 'H.I.V. POSITIVE' printed in purple across the front, Achmat confronted Deeb, who was wearing a plain black suit, in a debate on South African channel e-TV's current affairs show '3rd Degree' which was hosted by investigative journalist Deborah Patta. Achmat tore straight into the industry's argument that it needed to charge high prices for the AIDS drugs to recoup high research costs and create incentives for further innovation. On the contrary, argued Achmat, many AIDS drugs were developed using public funding, so public revenues had mainly contributed to companies' profits. A key part of the debate went as follows:

Achmat: AZT, dDI and d4T – were the drugs discovered by the pharmaceutical companies, or were they developed as, in fact I can prove, we can prove, they were researched with public funding?

Deeb: If one looks at the bulk of medicines . . .

Achmat: [Cuts her off] We are not talking about the bulk of medicines, let's talk about these three, specifics.

Deeb: I don't know the history of each specific one...

Achmat: [Cuts her off again] Why not? You're the CEO![44]

Achmat's superior debating skills and the TAC's meticulous research on the relevant issues, which was aided by their international activist allies, were clearly conveyed by the television programme.

On 18 April 2001, at the first hearing of the matter after its adjournment, the PMA dramatically reversed its strategy with its counsel requesting a day's adjournment to allow their clients to hold discussions aimed at achieving a settlement (*The Sowetan* 19 April 2001). The next day the PMA withdrew its lawsuit. It conceded that the Medicines Act complied with the WTO's TRIPS agreement, that the law could be enforced as it was written and agreed to pay the government's legal costs (*The New York Times* 20 April 2001). This was only part of what the TAC activists and their global supporters had achieved; they had also forced several companies, in March 2001, to make dramatic cuts in the prices of ARVs in developing countries. South African AIDS activists and their allies abroad had created a global public relations crisis for one of the most powerful industries in the world.

The TAC's growing global moral and political legitimacy on the issue of HIV treatment access was indicated when Achmat was chosen as *TIME* magazine's person of the week. So began Achmat's status as a globally recognized activist-celebrity. The article began by addressing the reader stating that 'You've probably never heard of Zackie Achmat. Not unless you're a South African AIDS patient demanding your government's help to stay alive, or a global pharmaceutical corporation' (*TIME* 19April 2001). The magazine had given Achmat the award 'For leading the campaign that shamed the corporations into backing down, raising hope for millions of AIDS sufferers throughout the developing world'. It also mentioned that Achmat's work against 'perpetrators of injustice' dated back to his 'tireless' anti-apartheid activism as a high school student. The power of the TAC's 'international networking' had become clear when ACT UP protestors had began 'dogging' Al Gore, a campaign that had been effective in pushing for the Clinton administration to change its stance on threats of trade sanctions. The TAC's 'politics of shame' had generated a 'public relations nightmare' for the industry, which had influenced some companies to make steep price reductions and even waive their patents.

Achmat's refusal to take ARVs until the government agreed to provide them involved his moral inability to 'take advantage of the privileges' that attached to 'a middle-class position in a society where almost all AIDS sufferers' were 'doomed' by poverty (*TIME* 19 April 2001). It also gave him a 'deeply personal stake in winning his campaign' and it was a 'noble stand'.

The affected companies began major public relations exercises to mend their damaged reputations (*TIME* 19 April 2001). J. P. Garnier, Chief

Executive of GlaxoSmithKlein, told the *New York Times* in a telephone interview from Philadelphia that ' "We don't exist in a vacuum .... We're a very major corporation. We're not that insensitive to public opinion. That is a factor in our decision-making.... We have never been opposed to wider access. We have discounted our drugs. We've done everything we could (20/04/01)." ' As we have seen, when the case was withdrawn, activists had cheered and celebrated. But ominous signs were on the horizon, Achmat told *The Guardian* of London that ' "The difficult job starts now, to ensure our government mobilizes the resources it has to implement an appropriate treatment plan for Aids. We will use the law to protect people's lives. Within months to years we will have antiretrovirals in our public health service" ' (20 April 2001). Sadly, it would be over two years rather than a few months before the South African government would roll out combination ARV therapy in the public sector of the country's health system.

Conclusion

Activist opposition to the PMA's court case reveals key patterns in the development of the international HIV treatment access movement. The TAC's transnational nature – as manifest in the international activist alliances that the South African movement forged – proved vital in forcing the 40 major multinational pharmaceutical corporations to drop their case. This was also a critical moment in the founding and consolidation of the international HIV treatment access movement. As this chapter shows, the TAC contributed to a specifically South African form of moral capital to the international movement. When the international and domestic movements were first formed, the overwhelming 'development consensus' among donor governments, UNAIDS and the World Bank was that widespread provision of HIV treatment in resource-constrained settings failed the utilitarian test of 'cost-effectiveness' and that it was anyway unfeasible due to health systems-related issues and Africans' 'cultural differences'.

It was easy for South African and American activists to equate the industry's actions with those of the apartheid regime: the case was brought only a few years into South Africa's post-apartheid period; the country had one of the highest numbers of people living with HIV globally; the case was brought against the Mandela administration, and it was aimed at advancing the interests of a small, but powerful, constituency at the expense of the well-being of millions of poor patients. But the fact that South Africa also had the TAC – a new social movement of affected and aggrieved people led by an openly HIV-positive former anti-apartheid activist – lent additional credibility to international solidarity actions, including those of American activists. American activists effectively used the political opportunities presented by Gore's presidential bid to advocate for a change in US trade policy. This was an important early victory in the campaign against the pharmaceutical industry association's case, as it robbed them of critical political and diplomatic support from the US government.

Within South Africa itself, the movement was heavily shaped by its origins in anti-apartheid activism in ways which were also beneficial to the international movement. The TAC's growing credibility as a movement, which was evident in its expanding membership, depended heavily on the anti-apartheid backgrounds of key leaders such as Achmat. The movement's growth can also be attributed to organizers' treatment literacy activities, which popularized the science around the epidemic and their work to sew the TAC's advocacy onto the social and political quilt of township life which was tailored around the country's (apartheid and anti-apartheid) history.

In addition, the TAC had a deft legal strategy which involved invoking the socio-economic right to access to health care to be admitted as an *amicus*. This strategy was enabled by the new Constitution and it provided the TAC with an additional political forum to present its arguments against the PMA's case. International allies played a critical role in the case in that they provided vital expertise on drug pricing and innovation in America and the generic drug industries in India and Brazil.

The TAC's use of socio-economic rights-based legal arguments in this manner marked a critical shift in the history of South African AIDS activism. Whereas earlier activism in the country had prized the principle of the people living with HIV having a right to privacy (a concept grounded in negative freedom), the new AIDS activism encouraged voluntary openness about living with the disease. It did so to underline its campaigns which used the right to health, a concept grounded in a substantive understanding of freedom, to demand more state services and regulation of the pharmaceutical industry via health-advancing trade and patent policies.

The global HIV treatment access movement and the TAC had won its first important victory. But this would be far from the last time that the South African movement would take to the streets and appear in court making arguments based upon the socio-economic right to access to health care. Indeed, owing to the President's continued AIDS dissidence, in August 2001 another court case began to force the government to expand access to Nevirapine for PMTCT, as Chapter 6 discusses.

6
Radical Legitimacy: Rights and 'Reasonableness' in the TAC, 2001–2003

Busiswe Maqungo presented the Pretoria High Court with the portion she had been dealt of the collective human misery of AIDS in August 2001. Maqungo was a TAC activist who shared her story in court papers submitted by the South African AIDS movement in *TAC v. Minister of Health and others*.[1] She told the court that she was a 29-year-old woman who lived in Mfuleni township in the Western Cape. The young mother discovered that she was living with the virus which caused AIDS after taking an HIV test at Conradie Hospital in Pinelands in May 1999, where she had taken her one-month-old daughter Nomazizi after she became 'very sick' – indeed, her baby suffered from pneumonia, diarrhoea and dehydration.[2] The TAC activist said that she felt 'hurt for my child' when she found out that her baby girl was HIV-positive because she had unknowingly passed the virus on to her; prior to her own diagnosis she had never suspected that she could be living with the disease.[3] While pregnant, she knew that AZT could be used for PMTCT of the virus and recalled that 'I gave birth to a[n] HIV positive child and wondered why, if she could be treated with AZT'.[4] The grieving mother was plagued by thoughts of how easily things could have turned out differently. What if all South African hospitals, including the one she attended, had asked pregnant women if they would like to be tested for HIV? Then she would have taken the test and wanted adequate counselling on her results. And what if her doctors had then told her that she could use Nevirapine for PMTCT of HIV? Then she would have tried to have obtained it 'for the sake of my baby'.[5] Her baby daughter who was 'always sick' died at nine months of age.[6] She pleaded with the South African government to 'implement MTCTP [PMTCT] nationally so that women can be given a chance and children can be saved'.[7]

Maqungo's affidavit was part of the TAC's groundbreaking litigation based upon the socio-economic right to health. In the early 2000s, when it launched this litigation the South African movement used the law in a flexible and strategic manner to highlight the unreasonable nature of the government's position on ARVs. While it collaborated with 'cause lawyers' to force the Mbeki administration to provide Nevirapine for PMTCT of HIV on a universal basis, it later engaged in a peaceful civil disobedience campaign for a roll-out of ARVs for chronic use in combination drug therapy. The Mbeki administration's reluctance to comprehensively provide ARV drugs, including Nevirapine, in the public sector of the health system stemmed from its adherence to irrational AIDS denialism. The TAC argued its case for the universal provision of Nevirapine for PMTCT on the basis of the socio-economic right to access to health care, which was enshrined in the South African Constitution's Bill of Rights. The success of this case rested on proving that the government's policy had failed the Constitutional test of 'reasonableness'.[8] The use of expert scientific testimony was critical to this. Moreover, the movement also expanded its treatment literacy programme in this period. The choice of state provision of Nevirapine for PMTCT as a test case made sense given that it was a relatively cheap intervention. This chapter's main argument is that the TAC gained 'radical legitimacy' and, hence, popular support, through the following: its use of 'struggle symbolism'; marshalling of expert testimony to bolster its socio-economic rights-based legal arguments; and, via its successful efforts, to popularize the scientific knowledge of how the drugs worked.

But, as this chapter describes, some feminists such as Catherine Albertyn, Shamim Meer and Sisonke Msimang argued that in its Nevirapine case, the TAC did not comprehensively assert women's reproductive rights. Feminists within the movement were also critical of what they perceived as its failure to adequately confront its own internal sexism. Such gender issues would only be systematically and politically addressed after the period centrally examined in this book (as discussed in the Postscript). But because these issues were programmatically addressed by the TAC after the main period under discussion in the book, recounting them does not imply that the movement's female members were either passive victims or that it remained impervious to feminist entreaties for gender-related organizational change.

Despite these internal tensions, the movement's political legitimacy continued to grow. It drew on the very public support of anti-apartheid icon Nelson Mandela, who visited Achmat while he was ill at his home in Cape Town because of his drug fast in July 2002. In December 2002, the former president donned one of the movement's HIV POSITIVE t-shirts during a visit to an HIV clinic it jointly ran with MSF to provide combination ARV treatment to low-income township residents.

Once the Constitutional Court had ruled in the TAC's favour, sparing many mothers Maqungo's unbearable loss, the movement focused on the more ambitious goal of a state roll-out of ARVs for chronic use. As it launched its second civil disobedience campaign against the Mbeki administration, the TAC drew on the support of its international allies. Simultaneously, the domestic and international public profile of Zackie Achmat, its chairperson, continued to grow. Both Achmat's elevated global media profile and international solidarity actions in support of the movement increased diplomatic and foreign-investor pressure on the government to change its stance. Mandela's support for combination ARV drug therapy provision within the country proved invaluable in generating domestic legitimacy for the movement, because it lent the former president's powerful struggle symbolism to the TAC's cause and assisted the movement in combating claims that it was inherently 'anti-government'. This campaign reached its apex in March 2003, when the transnationally connected TAC launched its second civil disobedience campaign, where its international allies aided the South Africans in pressing for the Mbeki administration to adopt a National Treatment Plan. In August 2003, the government met this core TAC demand. By the end of 2003, the TAC had become a multiracial, multiclass movement with significant moral and political authority both within the country and internationally.

TAC v. Minister of Health

In 2001, Maqungo's story was being repeated many times across South Africa: the previous year's antenatal clinic prevalence survey found that 24.5% of pregnant women in the country were living with HIV (Department of Health 2000). With the Medicines Act case settled, in April 2001, the TAC returned to the issue of government provision of Nevirapine for PMTCT, resorting to legal action once more in July. This strategy's success depended on the TAC's lawyers' use of expert scientific testimony. At the same time, the movement achieved the desired reform via effective social mobilization around the case.

A great deal of legal literature has been produced on the topic of the TAC's Nevirapine cases. In this literature, legal scholars have argued that the TAC's effectiveness in pressing the government to roll out Nevirapine for PMTCT beyond the pilot sites depended upon *both* its clear demonstration that the government's policy on this issue failed the legal test of reasonableness *and* its effective social mobilization (Heywood 2003; Davis 2006; Kapczynski and Berger 2009). This chapter does not aim to add to this literature concerning the legal aspects of the cases: it rather focuses on the roles of doctors and scientists in providing expert testimony for the TAC's case and the ways in which its treatment literacy programme and use of struggle symbolism helped marshal public support for its demands within South Africa.

But, in order to understand the importance of such expert testimony and social mobilization to the TAC's success in accomplishing its goals through the case, it is worth briefly describing this legal literature. In the post-apartheid era, as cases involving socio-economic rights began to be brought to the high courts and the Constitutional Court, legal scholars began to debate the merits of the judgements offered in these matters.

Legal academics were generally in agreement that after the *Grootboom* judgement, the Constitutional Court had adopted the criteria of *reasonableness* to assess whether people's socio-economic rights had been violated by the government (Pieterse 2004; Wesson 2004; Bromley Chan 2006; Davis 2006; Steinberg 2006). There is general agreement among legal scholars that reasonableness is a concept which was taken from administrative law and applied to the socio-economic rights cases post-*Grootboom* (Bilchitz 2002; Wesson 2004; Kapczynski and Berger 2009). In relation to the evolving jurisprudence (legal theory) around socio-economic rights, Marius Pieterse has argued that the Constitutional Court's reasonableness approach can be defined as being an administrative law-like 'inquiry into the rationality, coherence, flexibility, evenhandedness and inclusiveness of state policy aimed at the progressive realization of socio-economic rights' (2004, p. 473).

It is important to note, in relation to the TAC's Nevirapine case that the court came to define it as the requirement for a socio-economic policy to be rational, flexible and to not exclude a significant, relevant sector of society (Bilchitz 2002; Pieterse 2004). What South African legal scholars who wrote on this issue in the period diverged on was whether this approach was sufficient to protect the rights of poor and socially marginalized people.

Some scholars argued that the Constitutional Court had failed to define a bare minimum, or *minimum core*, of goods and services that the state had to provide to realize socio-economic rights (Bilchitz 2002). Dennis Davis held that socio-economic rights were, thereby, reduced to 'paper' rights with little meaning for poor people (2006, p. 314). Conversely, other scholars contended that the Constitutional Court's reasonableness approach to adjudicating on such rights was sensible, because such judicial deference to the executive branch of government respected the separation of powers (Wesson 2004; Steinberg 2006). For our purposes, we simply have to note that in order to be successful in litigation against the state, the TAC's case had to demonstrate the government's failure to pass the legal test of reasonableness and that the movement also had to conduct political advocacy in addition to its legal action because of the court's refusal to outline a minimum core approach (Heywood 2003; Davis 2006).

It is also worth briefly outlining a few events which led up to the case. On 12–13 August 2000 the Department of Health met with scientists to assess the state of knowledge around PMTCT, including the new findings on Nevirapine from the HIVNET 012 trial (Heywood 2003, p. 286). After this meeting, the Health MINMEC council, which was composed of the national Minister of Health and nine Provincial Health MECs, met and decided that once Nevirapine was registered, it would launch two 'pilot' sites for research and training per province (Heywood 2003, p. 286).

The TAC remained dissatisfied with the restriction of national provision of Nevirapine to two pilot sites per province, with the notable exception of the Western Cape, which had engaged in a full-scale roll-out of the drug for PMTCT. Meanwhile, paediatricians who wanted the government to roll out Nevirapine for PMTCT had formed a new, emotively named 'Save Our Babies' coalition. According to Heywood, relations between activists and the government had reached their 'nadir' by July 2001 (2003).

On 17 July 2001, the TAC and its allies Save Our Babies and the Durban Children's Rights Centre (hereafter collectively referred to as the TAC in this section of the chapter) set the wheels of legal action in motion when they sent their first letter of demand to the National Minister of Health and the nine provincial MECs. The letter asked the government to make Nevirapine available at health facilities which were not pilot sites and that it allow doctors to prescribe the drug to their patients, where it was medically indicated (Heywood 2003). The Minister's response cited barriers such as the viral resistance which could arise from taking a single dose of Nevirapine, that a single dose of drug did not address risk of transmission through breastfeeding and that the roll-out would be unsustainable (Heywood 2003).

On 21 August 2001, the TAC launched a constitutional challenge to the government's PMTCT policy in the Pretoria High Court, asking for the policy of limiting provision of the drugs to pilot sites to be declared unconstitutional. They also requested that the government be ordered to make the drug available to all HIV-positive pregnant women who went into labour at public health facilities, where it was deemed to be medically indicated by the health professional in attendance (Heywood 2003).

The movement argued that the policy was unconstitutional because it violated two sections of the 1996 Constitution's Bill of Rights: the right to access to health care (contained in s27) and every child's right to basic nutrition, shelter, basic healthcare services and social services (contained in s28) (Heywood 2003).

But to garner wider popular support for its litigation the TAC needed to convey correct scientific information about HIV and Nevirapine to its supporters and members of the public in communities where the movement was active. In an interview with me, Mandla Majola, who was then the TAC's Western Cape provincial coordinator, recalled that treatment literacy efforts were scaled up around the movement's court cases to enable it to mobilize support for its litigation (3 April 2008). This was because many of the TAC's target audience were not aware of the benefits of Nevirapine prior to participating in its treatment literacy workshops and meetings. Having educated participants about scientific aspects of PMTCT, Majola found that it was possible to talk about the political reasons for bringing the case. He told me that 'once that education was there and we [the TAC] said to people this can happen, but government doesn't want to do this, and we don't know why, we had discussions with them [about the case]'.

In mobilizing support for the court action, TAC activists had to overcome perceptions that it was a white-dominated movement that was 'anti-government'. Thabo Cele was a Durban-based NAPWA member who had joined the TAC. Cele told me that he had encountered perceptions among many ANC supporters in Durban's townships that the TAC was formally aligned to the white-led opposition party, the Democratic Alliance (DA), and that it was therefore part of a 'white force to undermine the government' (Interview 25 April 2007). These allegations were apparently levelled with particular frequency in relation to prominent white movement leaders such as Heywood. Cele said that '[c]ouncillors and the ANC would say that people were not supporting TAC. Then when we were fighting for PMTCT people would say that Manto [Tshabalala-Msimang] was their "comrade" and that we were fighting against "our government" ' (Interview 25 April 2007). In response, the activists like Cele who were based in the city held treatment literacy meetings to 'educate' movement members and residents of communities where the TAC was active about how Nevirapine could be safely and effectively used for PMTCT and to correct political misconceptions about the movement. For instance, at meetings and workshops, TAC activists would set the record straight that Heywood had no links with the DA and was, in fact, an SACP member. Also, Cele and his 'comrades' would correct the inaccurate view that the TAC was white-dominated by pointing out that several of its key office bearers were black: its Chairperson, Zackie Achmat, was a coloured man and its National Deputy Chairperson, Sipho Mthathi, was an African woman. The TAC was, in fact, a black-led, multiracial movement.

There were similar obstacles in organizing support in Cape Town's townships. In an interview, Majola recounted how the president's questioning of HIV as the cause of AIDS also operated as a barrier to garnering greater support for the TAC's Nevirapine court case (3 April 2008). Some people at its workshops on PMTCT in these Cape communities would question the merit of the scientific information being shared by reiterating the president's dissident views: they would apparently say things like ' "[t]he president is saying this about HIV: the president is saying there's no HIV. How come you are saying there's HIV? Because the president is disputing that there's HIV." So you need to explain the science of HIV.' As in other regions, in Cape Town's African townships the people taking dissident positions were often 'close to the ANC leadership' or ward councillors (Interview 3 April 2008). But, Majola added, there were others who adopted these positions for more personal reasons, because they did not want to 'know the truth' or 'face reality' and use condoms.

The large turnout at the TAC's mass demonstrations indicated that in areas where its activists organized, thousands of ordinary members of the public were won over by their painstaking explanations of the workings of the virus and ARVs. One of the most important barriers to treatment literacy work was the need to explain a lot of the relevant scientific terms such as Nevirapine, viral load and CD4 cells. Key activists such as Majola were taught the meaning of these terms by doctor-activists like Hermann Reuter and would then go on to explain them in African languages using phrases and concepts which were comprehensible to community members. Majola described that 'people were educated and people went out to different communities to educate others in our own language. And simplifying it, because we are coming across people who are not educated at all' (Interview 3 April 2008).

Whereas previously people living with HIV had often felt robbed of hope, powerless and ill-informed, after they joined the TAC they often felt more empowered as citizens. In Majola's view, this was because people became 'more informed', less scared and 'a step ahead of the virus, of the illness' after attending treatment literacy workshops. In terms of movement building, it also meant that the TAC could get supporters to turn out in numbers at protests and rallies which were held in the major urban centres around the country in support of its case.

Scientific and expert submissions were also pivotal to the TAC's win in the Nevirapine case because the government defended its existing policy by contending that the medicine could lead to the development of drug-resistant strains of the virus. Several scientists submitted expert affidavits in support of the TAC's case: Robin Wood discussed the safety and efficacy of Nevirapine for PMTCT; Quarraisha Abdool Karim offered an affidavit on the epidemiology of HIV and mother-to-child-transmission.[9] A virologist stated in his affidavit that the government's submissions had misquoted him on the issue of Nevirapine and drug resistance. The TAC also obtained an affidavit by the principal investigator in the HIVNET012 trial. By contrast, as Heywood points out, the allegations of possible drug resistance to Nevirapine were made by Department of Health officials who were neither virologists nor pharmacologists (2003).

On 14 December 2001, High Court Judge Chris Botha found in favour of the TAC on all the key issues in the case and ordered the government to develop a nationwide PMTCT programme.[10] The judge also ruled that the government had to return to court by 31 March 2002 so that its plan could be subjected to further scrutiny.[11] Four days later, the government sought leave to appeal on the grounds that the judgement interfered with the separation of powers, which, it held, gave the executive branch control over policy making. In January 2002, the TAC launched a legal counter-offensive and obtained an execution order in the Pretoria High Court forcing the government implement the judgement. In March, the government was denied leave to appeal this execution order by the Constitutional Court.

In February 2002, former President Nelson Mandela joined the chorus of voices condemning the government's policy. By virtue of his long incarceration and role in the country's transition to democracy his political and moral stature as a South African was unparalleled both domestically and abroad. He told the *Sunday Times* that AIDS was a 'war' and that ' "We must not continue debating, to be arguing, when people are dying" ' (17 February 2002). Mandela also said that he planned to use an upcoming meeting with the ANC's leadership to discuss his support for state provision of ARVs for PMTCT. A few days later Mandela reportedly back-tracked from this statement and said that he supported the government's handling of AIDS but felt that it had communicated its approach poorly (*Pretoria News* 20 February 2002). However, the damage was done – South Africa's elder statesman had already pronounced a few days earlier that the government's PMTCT policy was morally and politically bankrupt.

Media coverage of the TAC's case was overwhelmingly positive. For instance, an article in *The Star* headed 'Do it now, Mbeki!' called for the president to 'Give ALL [article's emphasis] pregnant HIV mothers Nevirapine' and billed itself as 'a plea to the president to change the national Aids policy that is condemning about 100 babies a day' (*The Star* 20 February 2002). Meanwhile, the scandal over the president's dissident views did not abate. Indeed, a bizarre anonymously authored document came to light called 'Castro Hlongwane, Caravans, Cats, Geese, Foot & Mouth and Statistics: HIV/Aids and the Struggle for the Humanisation of the African' (Anonymous 2002). The March 2002 document bore all the hallmarks of AIDS dissidence and, at times, descended into outright fulmination against those who adhered to mainstream AIDS-related science, accusing them of holding racist views of African sexuality. Shortly thereafter, in mid-April, the *Mail & Guardian* claimed that this document had been authored by Mbeki since it bore his 'electronic signature' (19 April 2002).

The Cabinet began to distance itself from Mbeki's position on AIDS. On 17 April 2002 it released a statement through the Government Communication and Information Service (GCIS) which clearly stated that ARVs could 'help improve the condition of people living with AIDS if administered at certain stages in the progression of the condition, and in accordance with international standards'.[12] But despite this positive development, the National Minister of Health and the provincial Health MECs pressed ahead with their appeal at the Constitutional Court.

Moreover, the fight within the ANC for Mbeki to cease making public statements informed by AIDS dissidence also claimed political victims: feminist MP Pregs Govender left parliament in May 2002 after having resigned. Govender has written that she left because she was placed under intolerable pressure by male colleagues in the ANC, including Chief Whip Matthew Goniwe to cease pursuing her calls for the government to provide ARVs during her time as chair of the National Assembly's Joint Monitoring Committee on the Improvement of the Quality of Life and Status of Women (Govender 2009, p. 51).

William Mervyn Gumede, an Mbeki biographer, has attributed the cabinet's statement to 'economics rather than compassion' (2007). The president's public pronouncements on AIDS were threatening one of his most cherished projects: his diplomatic role pleading for African renewal and foreign investment on the continent on the international stage. The global business leaders who sat on Mbeki's International Investment Council apparently found the confusion over the government's approach 'unsettling and downright frightening' and argued that it was fuelling 'negative perceptions about South Africa as a potential investment opportunity' (Gumede 2007). Finance Minister Trevor Manuel and Reserve (Central) Bank governor Tito Mboweni were also reportedly starting to receive questions from foreign investors about the government's AIDS policy and started warning the president that his public pronouncements on the issue could have negative economic consequences.

On the first day of the Constitutional Court hearings, the TAC held 'Stand Up for Your Rights' marches across the country: a photograph from one of these marches is depicted in Figure 6.1. The posters for the demonstration showed a pregnant woman reading the Constitution with her one hand and cradling her abdomen with her other.

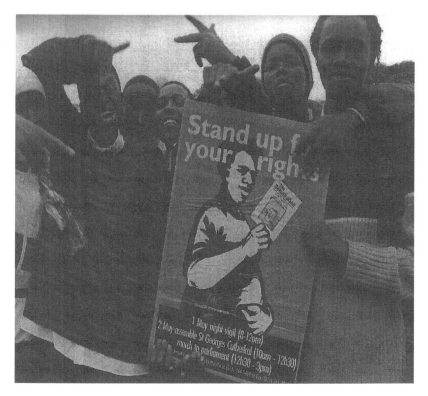

Figure 6.1   TAC supporters holding a 'Stand up for your rights' poster
Source: TAC (2008, p. 61).

In Johannesburg, 5000 people marched to the country's highest court to affirm their belief in the right to access to health care services, as enshrined in its Constitution. On 5 July 2002, judgement was handed down in the case. The judges had reached a unanimous decision that the government had not met its constitutional obligations to provide access to health services in a reasonable way, taking account of social needs.[13] It ordered the national and provincial governments to remove restrictions on the provision of Nevirapine outside pilot sites and to permit and facilitate its use where it was medically indicated, through a comprehensive and coordinated plan.[14] The court also found that there was no evidence to support the government's claims that Nevirapine was unsafe.

Jonathan Berger and Amy Kapczynski have cast the litigation as 'one of the most celebrated human rights cases in the world' (2009, p. 3). But the movement's approach in the case has subsequently been criticized by some feminists. For example, Sisonke Msimang published an article in the journal *Gender and Development* in 2003, which lauded the TAC as a movement 'begun by and for people living with HIV/AIDS' and one which had 'managed to mobilize national and international support for the idea of universal access to drugs for people living with HIV' (2003, p. 112). At the core of her article lay a critique of the failure of feminists in the global North to engage with AIDS as 'a critical issue' for women (Msimang 2003, p. 109). However, she also stated that the TAC's strategy needed to be 'vigorously debated and analyzed by feminists', because their case 'did not use arguments about reproductive and sexual rights' (2003, p. 112). Instead, she argued that the movement used a 'classic "woman as vessel" ' argument that the health of pregnant women mattered chiefly in as much as they were carrying foetuses (2003, p. 112).

Msimang went on to characterize the TAC as having subsequently 'been pushed by gender activists within the movement to ensure that the drugs do not stop when the baby is born' (2003, p. 112). This statement can be challenged with reference to the fact that from its earliest days the TAC always had the broader goal of access to combination ARV treatment in its sights (as discussed in Chapter 4). Indeed, most members – male and female – joined the movement with this bigger, ultimate goal in mind. As Kapczynski and Berger have pointed out, 'the TAC always conceived of the case as a stepping stone towards the provision – at state expense – of comprehensive HIV treatment services' (2009, p. 26). This interpretation is also reinforced by reading Maqungo's affidavit, where she described to the court her pain, as a mother, in disclosing that she was living with HIV to her other, older child who 'kept on crying and was afraid that I would die and leave him alone'.[15] Maqungo knew that HIV was a 'controllable' disease and, therefore that she 'would want to have access to treatment when I need it at a later stage'.[16] She also added that 'The government should give people with HIV anti-retroviral drugs because they need it.'[17] In this part of her affidavit, the

TAC activist was clearly referring to combination ARV therapy for chronic use, as she did not urge the government to simply give them to pregnant women or children, but *people* living with the disease, in general.

Similar feminist assessments of the case have been presented in the work of Cathi Albertyn, a legal scholar, and Shamim Meer, a researcher. Albertyn and Meer have claimed that although the TAC's Nevirapine court case may have advanced 'redistributive' gains for poor women, it did little to promote their 'recognition' (2008, p. 27).[18] Moreover, Albertyn and Meer have stated that 'women's agency was compromised' (2008, p. 28). What they are contending here is that the case undermined women's power to act and that women were primarily 'constructed' as 'bearers of children and as patients' instead of as equal citizens possessing an array of reproductive choices, including abortion (Albertyn and Meer 2008, p. 28).

Their critique is driven by the fate of another *amicus* brief which was submitted to the court by the RRA. As we have seen, the Reproductive Rights Alliance was formed by feminists who advocated for the legalization of abortion (as discussed in Chapter 3). It was also part of the women's movement, which barely addressed AIDS in the early 2000s and where feminists working on different issues operated in separate silos. When the government acceded to the RRA's main demand by liberalizing the country's abortion laws in 1996, the alliance mostly shifted to assisting in implementing the new law (Albertyn and Meer 2008, p. 37). As Albertyn and Meer report, the RRA did not initially take a public stance on the issue of PMTCT, partly because it was fearful of alienating the 'pro-choice state' (2008, p. 38). They hold that the ALP's earlier reproductive choice arguments were discarded following a conversation between Mark Heywood, the legal NGO's head and a TAC leader, and Geoff Budlender, the advocate who represented the AIDS movement. Budlender was, in their account, concerned to offer the court human rights-based legal arguments that he thought would 'work'. Furthermore, he allegedly believed that presenting the state's policy of limiting the number of clinics providing ARVs for PMTCT in the state sector as irrational would prove more convincing than those that it constituted unfair gender-based discrimination against the HIV-positive pregnant women. The TAC's advocate apparently admitted that 'he did not understand the [reproductive] choice arguments that were put to him at the time, and felt that if he did not understand them, he would be unable to persuade a judge about them' (Albertyn and Meer 2008, p. 39).

'Feminist lawyers' in the RRA then decided to file a preliminary *amicus* brief casting the government's failure to provide Nevirapine was a 'violation of women's reproductive rights' (Albertyn and Meer 2008, p. 40). These feminist lawyers were worried about the implications of the right to treatment being located in children's rights: that policies could be created to force women to take Nevirapine, could thereby create a 'slippery slope' to a reversal of the liberalization of abortion. The TAC had mentioned reproductive

choice in its papers but 'not argued it extensively and the RRA's preliminary *amicus* application was, therefore, opposed by the state and rejected by
the High Court' (Albertyn and Meer 2008, p. 41). At this stage, the TAC's
lawyers asked the RRA's lawyers not to proceed to making oral arguments
for fear of causing a postponement. The TAC's lawyers promised to make
reproductive choice arguments, but, apparently, 'No further collaboration
took place [with the feminist lawyers] on the legal arguments' (Albertyn and
Meer, p. 41).

But the legal arguments the TAC used in its Nevirapine case also need
to be viewed against the bigger sweep of the history of South African AIDS
activism. TAC activists had obtained their first favourable judgement finding
that the socio-economic right to access to health care was indeed justiciable
(something upon which courts could rule). The ruling also forced the state
to develop a programme sparing many poor women the agony of having to
bury children born with AIDS. It is also important to recognize that while
poor women were represented in court by more powerful male lawyers, such
as Budlender, who may not have fully articulated the importance of their
rights to make every conceivable reproductive health choice, it did offer
them one more option, in addition to abortion, which was already legal.

Furthermore, it is unclear whether the more extensive inclusion of reproductive rights-based *legal* arguments would have altered the underlying
political gender-power dynamics within the movement itself. As Albertyn
and Meer recognize, there were many problems afflicting the wider women's
movement in the period and, like many women's organisations, the RRA did
not develop a public voice on AIDS in the late 1990s (Klugman 2011).

Ultimately, the TAC and its lawyers certainly could have focused more on
women's reproductive rights, and the movement did not have a comprehensive gender policy in place during this period. But in the TAC, poor and
marginalized women like Maqungo found an accessible advocacy vehicle
which they could use to speak out on an issue they viewed as being among
their greatest concerns. Therefore, Albertyn and Meer's critique that such
TAC women's agency (capacity to act) was compromised in this period needs
to be softened: women activists such as Maqungo spoke out and marched
alongside men, but they did so in a way which did not necessarily entrench
their power, as a caucus, within the movement – something I elaborate on
later in this chapter.

In the final analysis, these published feminist critiques of the TAC's
Nevirapine litigation, while flawed, do point to wider gender-power disparities within the movement. But, they do not substantially detract from the
profound influence of the Nevirapine judgement on domestic and international legal thinking and the case's role in strengthening the movement's
overall political power. Indeed as Heywood argued an interview with me, the
constitutional case 'consolidated TAC into a movement' because it 'brought
a whole new layer of people into TAC. It created a visibility around people

with AIDS that hadn't existed before...I think it was really successful as a mobilisation' (Interview 15 April 2008).

The TAC's attempts to negotiate with the government for a national treatment plan in 2002

In late June 2002, shortly before the Constitutional Court would announce its judgement (in early July), the TAC already had its eyes on a bigger prize: along with its allies, including COSATU, it publicly stated that it wished the government to include combination ARV therapy in its 2000–2005 Strategic Plan (*The Sowetan* 26 June 2002). Both the TAC and COSATU demanded that 250,000 people in South Africa be placed on combination ARV therapy in the upcoming year at a projected cost of R500 million. The AIDS movement and trade union confederation also argued that the government would spend more money – R4 billion per year – on treating opportunistic infections in people living with HIV than if such combination ARV therapy were provided.

The South African media's attention on Achmat's persona escalated, partly because he was an outspoken AIDS activist, but also because of his extraordinary personal drug-fast pledge. In July 2002, his health was deteriorating, and it was reported that his doctor had recommended that he commence combination ARV drug therapy (*The Star* 4 July 2002). Discussing the portrayal of Achmat in the film *It's My Life*, a *City Press* reporter described him as the 'hero' of the HIV/AIDS war (7 July 2002).

Achmat's health became front-page news in South Africa when he was visited in his Muizenburg home by Mandela on 27 July 2002. Mandela hugged Achmat and promised to 'acquaint' the President with 'his [Achmat's] position' (*Sunday Times* 28 July 2002). The former president was publicly promising to conduct advocacy on Achmat's behalf with Mbeki – his successor. The internationally fêted leader told Achmat that he was a ' "loyal and disciplined member of the ANC" ' and that his actions were ' "not against the ANC, nor against the government" ', something that Mandela would explain to Mbeki. The support of a powerful struggle icon gave the TAC enormous legitimacy and an air of moral authority both in South Africa and abroad: *The Guardian* of London reported that Mandela described Achmat as 'a role model' whose drug fast was 'based on a fundamental principle we all admire' (29 July 2002). Mandela's visit enervated the ANC's leadership who personally attacked Achmat and accused him of benefitting from the suffering of black people (*The Guardian* 26 August 2002).

Kgosi Letlape of the South African Medical Association (SAMA) also visited Achmat and urged him to begin treatment (*Cape Times* 1 August 2002). The TAC's ties with the country's medical profession were reinforced when Achmat was granted life membership of SAMA 'for pricking the medical profession's conscience about the AIDS pandemic'. But Achmat remained defiant and tried to use his own deteriorating health to shame the government into rolling out the drugs. ' "It's very simple" ', he said, ' "If the government announced an intention to treat people with antiretrovirals tomorrow, I would reconsider my position [drug fast] immediately." '

A few weeks later Mandela again expressed his disagreement with the South African government's AIDS policies when he revealed to the Johannesburg-based *Sunday Times* that one of his nieces and two sons of a nephew had died of AIDS (*The Guardian* 26 August 2002). The former president's growing international stature on the issue was demonstrated by the fact that his revelation was also picked up by *The Guardian* of London (26 August 2002). Mandela said that he had visited his niece in hospital during a trip to the Eastern Cape province, and a few days after his return to Johannesburg he had learnt of her death. He added that he had only become aware that his nephews' sons were living with HIV after their deaths. In Mandela's eyes, the disease was 'devastating' South Africa. The elder statesman called upon South Africans to 'stand up and make sure this matter is widely publicized'. 'We must be supportive of our relatives and encourage them by all means not to lose hope', he added. Because the 'determination to live', said Mandela (alluding to ARV drugs), was 'as important as the medicines prescribed by the doctors'. Mandela added that there was 'no shame' in disclosing that one was suffering from a terminal illness, sharing that while in prison he had suffered from tuberculosis and after his release he had battled prostate cancer and had disclosed that he had suffered from both illnesses without being 'shunned'. Instead, he said, people living with HIV deserved to be embraced and loved.

While the South African government remained the main target for the TAC's advocacy, it continued to pursue domestic remedies for the high prices charged by multinational pharmaceutical companies for ARVs which it also viewed as a barrier to wider HIV treatment access. In September 2002, the TAC launched a complaint against multinational pharmaceutical companies Boehringer Ingelheim (BI) and GlaxoSmithKline (GSK) with the Competition Commission – a South African antitrust, or antimonopoly, body. It took this action because Indian drug manufacturer CIPLA and MSF (one of the TAC's critical allies) had requested voluntary licences to produce generic drugs, a request which the multinational pharmaceutical companies had declined. The TAC argued that GSK and BI had used their patents to command prices that only a small minority of patients could afford and that they were, thereby, 'directly responsible for premature, predictable and avoidable deaths of people living with HIV/AIDS, including both children and adults'.[19] Their actions in this regard were deemed by the TAC to be in violation of the Competition Act which prohibited dominant firms from charging 'excessive' prices, defined as those which were elevated beyond the commodity's 'reasonable economic value' in a way which harmed consumers.[20] Hazel Tau, a TAC activist living openly with HIV, was also a complainant in the case because she could not afford ARVs, and the government had yet to provide them.[21]

Meanwhile, the TAC's government-focused advocacy continued in earnest. From October to November 2002, in concert with COSATU, the TAC experimented with yet another strategy (TAC 2003b). It tried to negotiate a treatment plan with the government and private sector at the National Economic Development and Labour Council (NEDLAC). The Council was a government-run forum for corporations, government and unions to discuss social and economic policy in South Africa. At NEDLAC the various sectors managed to develop 'A framework agreement for a national HIV/AIDS prevention and treatment plan'. Originally, it had been hoped that the agreement could be finalized in time for World AIDS Day (1 December 2002), but, the government and corporate sector requested more time to work on the agreement.

In December 2002, Mandela paid a visit to the Khayalitsha clinic run by MSF and the TAC, a clinic which was providing combination ARV treatment. As we have seen, the clinic was crucial in demonstrating that such treatment could be successfully provided in resource-poor settings within South Africa (Nattrass 2007; Orbinski 2008). Clutching the former President's hand, Achmat welcomed ' "the greatest African leader to Khayalitsha" ' (*Cape Times* 13 December 2002). Then 'Matthew Damane, the first HIV/Aids patient to be treated at the clinic, stepped forward to present Mandela with a white t-shirt with the words "HIV-positive" emblazoned in purple across the chest. To loud cheers Mandela removed his trademark Madiba shirt and donned the t-shirt' (*Cape Times* 13 December 2002).

In this period, there were also new studies on the spread and demographic impact of South Africa's epidemic that added an extra sense of urgency to advocacy on the issue – including one which was co-sponsored by the Mandela foundation. As discussed, the annual antenatal clinic surveys had shown a dramatic escalation in HIV infection in the 1990s, a trend which continued into the early 2000s (Department of Health 2002). For instance, by 2002, the Department of Health's annual survey found that 26.5% of pregnant women were HIV-positive (2002, p. 6). AIDS had also been identified as South Africa's leading cause of death by a Medical Research Council (MRC) study in 2001 (Dorrington et al. 2001).

In December 2002, the first major systematically sampled, nationwide household survey of HIV prevalence in South Africa was conducted by the Human Sciences Research Council (HSRC) in collaboration with the Nelson Mandela Foundation (Bezuidenhout et al. 2002). While antenatal surveys were an internationally recognized method for measuring HIV prevalence among the sexually active and for enumerating cases in a stable and identifiable segment of the population, they had their flaws: only women were tested, and they may have over-estimated the rate of infection in younger women because participants were by definition engaging in unprotected sex

(AVERT 2012). Lastly, because the antenatal clinic surveys only included pregnant women using public health facilities, HIV prevalence of wealthier women using private health facilities may have been underestimated by these studies.

Unlike the antenatal clinic surveys, the Mandela/HSRC household survey involved the testing of blood samples for HIV taken from people of both sexes and with a wider spectrum of ages (Bezuidenhout et al. 2002). However, it is also important to note the limitations of the Mandela/HSRC household survey. One was that only 73.7% of those approached to participate in the study agreed to do so, and of those who agreed to be interviewed for the survey only 88.7% also agreed to give a blood specimen to be tested for HIV (Bezuidenhout et al. 2002, p. 11). It is unclear whether the non-responders were more or less likely to be living with HIV (AVERT 2011). Another limitation was that the study did not include participants under two years of age or who were in hospitals, military barracks, old age homes, schools or university hostels (AVERT 2012). Nevertheless, this new study was significant because it was the first national, household survey of HIV prevalence which it pegged at 11.4% (Bezuidenhout et al. 2002, p. 45).

Despite their various limitations the three sets of studies, taken together, pointed to the high rate of South Africa's HIV prevalence and its devastating demographic impact. They, therefore, only added to the TAC's case for a roll-out of combination ARV drug therapy.

'Dying for Treatment': The second civil disobedience campaign

By mid-January 2003, the TAC was threatening to start a second civil disobedience campaign to press the government to roll out ARV drugs for use in chronic therapy (*The Citizen* 14 January 2003). This threat was repeated two weeks later in a media article drawing attention to the reasons for the delay: the Minister's AIDS denialism, which was indicated by her decision to invite AIDS dissident Roberto Giraldo to address a meeting of health ministers from neighbouring Southern African Development Community (SADC) countries (*Leader* 31 January 2003). The stakes were high: the TAC estimated that 200,000 people would die of AIDS-related illnesses if they did not access ARV treatment that year (*Pretoria News* 11 February 2003).

The TAC organized a massive demonstration on Parliament on 14 February 2003. Mandela's image began to be used more prominently in the TAC's organizing materials. This was in line with its strategy of deploying 'struggle symbolism' to bolster its domestic and international legitimacy. A poster advertising the march, depicted in Figure 6.2, urged the public to 'Stand Up For Our Lives' and the South African government to 'Treat the People!' (TAC 2003c). To the right of the poster was a large image of Mandela smiling and waving while donning his HIV POSITIVE t-shirt during his 2002 visit

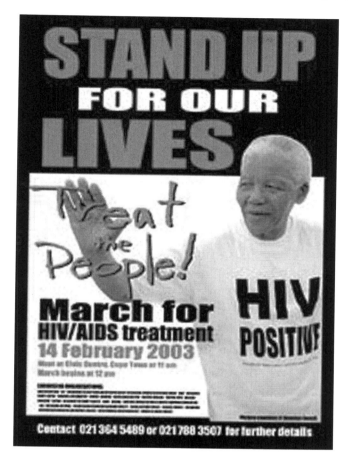

Figure 6.2 A TAC poster advertising its 14 February 2003 march to parliament

to Khayalitsha. This image was placed on the back of an 'edition' of the HIV POSITIVE t-shirts activists wore during the civil disobedience actions. It was also used on ACT UP New York's website to organize its solidarity actions in this period (ACT UP 2003). The TAC activists wore the Mandela t-shirt with pride and were ready to get arrested, if need be, to make their point. Cape-based township activist Majola remembered that 'with Mandela coming out [in support of the TAC], you know with Tutu coming out it was exciting and we felt strongly that we are getting support from the elders and legends. At least something could be done, we could push for this policy to be put into place' (Interview 3 April 2008).

Mandela's support for the TAC was studded with historical symbolism. In 1952, he had led the Defiance Campaign Against Unjust Laws, the country's first major anti-apartheid civil disobedience campaign. His image had been banned from publication within South Africa throughout the apartheid years, so before he was released from prison most South Africans (and people around the world) had no idea what he even looked like. The television image of him being released from prison was a defining, global news event of the 1990s and, arguably, of the late twentieth-century. Even as a retired, greying president, wearing his trademark batik shirts, he was usually reverently referred to using his isiXhosa clan name Madiba or *tata* (father). He was in every sense viewed by many as 'the father of the [new] nation' who embodied the newly liberated country's constitutionally enshrined values, such as dignity and equality.

On 14 February 2003, 10,000 TAC supporters marched on parliament in Cape Town. By early 2003, the TAC's mobilization efforts were paying off, as their marches grew in both size and radicalism. An article in the Cape-based *Saturday Weekend Argus* conveyed the movement's growing support:

> Health professionals, church leaders, community organizations and trade unionists voted with their feet, the majority wearing t-shirts bearing the HIV-positive slogan.

> But there were also the little Aids orphans marching quietly at the rear .... Tiny white 'coffins' were a shocking reminder of children dying of Aids .... A sea of hands was raised when Achmat asked who was prepared to go to jail, if necessary, to secure an HIV/Aids treatment programme for the country (15 February 2003).

But Mbeki and Tshabalala-Msimang remained defiant in the face of such demonstrations of popular support for the movement. This was despite growing foreign-donor assistance for African ARV drug roll-outs and international reductions in the prices of the drugs (as discussed in Chapter 7). They told the press that there was ' "no agreement" ' to supply the drugs, despite the TAC and COSATU's insistence that senior officials in the department such as Nono Simelela (head of the Department of Health's HIV/AIDS/STI and TB directorate) and Ayanda Ntsaluba (the Director-General of Health) had participated in negotiating the framework agreement (*Cape Argus* 18 February 2003). At the end of February, and in an unexpected move right before the campaign's launch, COSATU withdrew its support for the TAC's use of civil disobedience tactics. The trade union confederation declared that it concurred with the government that no national AIDS treatment plan had been agreed to at NEDLAC, and 'apologized to President Thabo Mbeki for having drawn him into the controversy over whether or not there was agreement on the treatment plan' (*The Sowetan* 28 February 2003). This contradicted earlier media statements where the union confederation had expressed its dismay about government's claims there was no such agreement.

As the TAC's threat of a second civil disobedience campaign loomed, the government embarked upon a public relations exercise. In an article in the *Mail & Guardian*, Tshabalala-Msimang argued that the government did have an AIDS plan: the 2000–2005 Strategic Plan (6 March 2003). A joint task team from the Treasury and Health Department were looking at the cost implications of rolling out combination ARV therapy. The Health Minister said that the government placed 'poverty squarely on the Aids agenda' which was not an 'indication that they were reluctant to tackle the issues of treatment'.

The TAC, however, continued to stand its ground on the need for a national treatment plan and, as it did so, its domestic and international legitimacy grew. Achmat started to receive a stream of high-profile awards and accolades. In March 2003, the University of Natal awarded him an honorary degree in recognition of his legal struggles for the rights of lesbians and gay men and people living with HIV (*Natal Witness* 7 March 2003). Significant outpourings of international solidarity for the movement continued: protests were planned in support of the TAC's civil disobedience campaign in the United Kingdom, Latin America, Jamaica, the Philippines and several African countries, mostly outside South African embassies (*Cape Times* 17 March 2003).

The rhetorical flavour of some of the international solidarity is evident in a picture of an AIDS vigil which was held by ACT UP, Health GAP, Gay Men's Health Crisis and African Services Committee outside the South African consulate in New York City on 13 February 2003 (ACT UP 2003).[22] The picture shows that one of their placards depicted a bloody hand (an old ACT UP symbol from the 1980s and early 1990s) and asked the South African government to 'Treat the People!' and provide 'HIV/AIDS Treatment for South Africans'. Another stated that HIV prevention was 'not enough' and called on the public to 'Demand AIDS Treatment Now' in South Africa. A large black banner urged the South African government to 'Stop AIDS Apartheid!'. These American AIDS activists were, thereby, accusing the post-apartheid ANC-led government of treating people living with HIV in South Africa as second-class citizens in the manner of the segregationist system. This was withering normative and political criticism of a democratic government which was led by African nationalists. The American activists could credibly level such a charge because of the anti-apartheid background of the some of the TAC's key leaders and Mandela's expression of support for its goals.

Such expressions of international support for the TAC were also covered by the South African media. The South African Press Agency (SAPA) reported that the American activists attending the solidarity demonstration outside the country's consulate in New York City had 'played drums, sang TAC protest songs and presented a memorandum to consulate officials' (14 February 2003). Similarly, a Cape Times article on the first International Treatment Preparedness Summit in Cape Town (discussed in Chapter 7) quoted Filipino activist Gina Davis as having stated that activists in the Asia-Pacific region supported the TAC's demands (17 March 2003). The article added that Marie Mendene of Camaroon said that African activists also endorsed 'all the actions implemented by the TAC'.

As international relations scholars Margaret Keck and Kathryn Sikkink have pointed out, such expressions of international solidarity by activists based abroad can prove especially important when channels of influence have broken down between a state and activists based within the same country (1998). This is because the solidarity actions by activists overseas can create a 'boomerang pattern of influence' which enables the internally based activists to circumvent their own state and bring external pressure to bear upon it (Keck and Sikkink 1998, p. 12). Differently put, international allies can add their voices to those of the internally based activists in ways which influence a state's actions in its domestic arena. As we have noted, Mbeki was enthusiastic about his diplomatic work and one of his administration's signature projects was the promotion of an African Renaissance. His administration's awareness of – and sensitivity to – the views of foreign diplomats meant that it could not remain utterly impervious to domestic and foreign media coverage of such international solidarity actions.

The TAC officially launched its second 'Dying for Treatment' Civil Disobedience campaign on 20 March 2003, the eve of Human Rights Day: a South African public holiday commemorating the infamous Sharpeville massacre of anti-apartheid protestors in the 1960s (*Mail & Guardian* 27 March 2003). In an interview, Heywood described the movement's decision to start the second civil disobedience campaign as having been 'politically tough because it was really confronting the ANC and confronting the policies squarely . . . even though TAC has mobilized people, it has mobilized people that are still thankful to the ANC and see the ANC as the party of liberation . . . so to go into an out-and-out campaign in opposition. . . . Looking back it was defiant to do that' (15 April 2008).

In a last-minute bid to avert the protests, the government placed advertisements in South Africa's major Sunday newspapers which government spokesperson Joel Netshitenzhe said were aimed at 'putting the facts about the government's AIDS programme before the public'; he 'accused TAC of deliberately distorting the facts' (*Cape Argus* 24 March 2003). Achmat dismissed the adverts as ' "a wish list, not a plan" '.

On the first day of the protests, the TAC went to police stations around the country and attempted to lay culpable homicide charges against the Ministers of Health and Trade and Industry for 'failing to prevent 600 deaths every day' (*Mail & Guardian* 27 March 2003). The Minister of Trade and Industry was also a target because the TAC had unsuccessfully negotiated with his ministry for months for local, state-manufacturing of generic ARVs in the manner of other middle-income countries such as Brazil, India and Thailand who had already been producing such affordable HIV medicines for many years. One hundred and sixty TAC activists were arrested in the civil dis-obedience protest actions attempting to lay the charges at police stations in Gauteng and Cape Town (*Sunday Times* 30 March 2003).

In Durban, TAC activists who participated in the non-violent campaign were met with police brutality. Many of these activists who had participated in the Durban action had only joined the TAC weeks or months before. One of these new TAC activists was Lihle Dlamini who had been diagnosed with HIV and joined a support group in Durban's Lamontville township which had shortly thereafter become a TAC branch (Interview 8 April 2008). She told me that her branch had participated in the civil disobedience campaign at the urging of TAC activist Thabo Cele.

Sindi Blose was another TAC activist who joined the civil disobedience demonstration in Durban. Blose was an Umlazi-born, working-class town-ship resident. Her decision to become an AIDS activist emerged from her direct personal confrontations with the disease. By the early 2000s, her fam-ily members had begun dying of AIDS-related illnesses and 'even though it was not said [that this was the case] those assumptions were made' (Inter-view 11 July 2011). But for her it grew even more direct when she 'became sexually active and apparently my first partner had cheated on me with another woman who had a history of dating men who used to steal cars'. In Blose's experience, car thieves were 'very popular because they had money and they would flash it and they were known for having multiple partners' and 'if a woman dated such a guy, automatically she was diagnosed as HIV-positive'. It was under these circumstances that Blose had her first HIV test in the year 2000, and when 'it became more real for me'.

In 2001, having left school, Blose was unemployed and spent most of her days at home 'looking for something meaningful' to do with her life. While braiding a friend's hair, Blose learnt about an HIV treatment counselling course which was offered by an NGO called Netcomsa, which immediately piqued her interest because of her own fear of the very real possibility that she could become HIV-positive in future. While attending the course she learned about ARVs and was 'amazed' to find out that effective HIV treatment existed at a time when a member of her family was extremely AIDS-ill. Her faith in the safety and efficacy of combination ARV therapy was anchored in the people she met on the course who were living with HIV and taking treatment for the disease at the AIDS Healthcare Foundation's Ithemba Labantu clinic in Umlazi township. Some of these HIV-positive patients had experienced the 'Lazarus effect', and all continued to enjoy relatively good health. These real people who had survived AIDS with com-bination ARV therapy showed her that effective HIV treatment was 'not a fairytale': it was 'real', and the drugs truly did work. Her elation at learn-ing about effective HIV treatment was rapidly deflated by the reality that it was unaffordable and unavailable to people in her family and community. When she queried why this was the case, her instructors told her, ' "Well, government says they don't have money".' But Blose said that this response failed to satisfy her and that she was then referred by the NGO to the TAC, where she met Thabo Cele, among other activists.

Blose joined the TAC at the age of 18 in November 2002 – a mere four months before the civil disobedience action. She told me that she had worked as a volunteer with TAC organizers in Durban helping to establish new branches of the movement by outlining their take on 'the political environment in South Africa and the provision of health care'. The activists would inform new branch members on how ARVs and treatments for opportunistic infections worked and also 'raise political issues' linked to those drugs. According to Blose, their main critique of the 2000–5 Strategic Plan was that it did not incorporate treatment, that 'it didn't save anyone's lives'. The eve of the civil disobedience campaign was 'a very emotional time' for Blose, as she had tried and failed to get a relative onto ARV drugs through a free programme at Helen Joseph Hospital in Johannesburg. This member of her family had, consequently, died a preventable death from AIDS-related illnesses.

The night before the action, TAC activists in Durban who wanted to join the protest received civil disobedience training, including what to do if they were arrested. The example of Mahatma Gandhi was discussed at the training to illustrate the concept of non-violent, symbolic violation of laws to highlight unjust policies. The activists knew that the action could have dire consequences, not least being arrested, or beaten, or prosecuted and given criminal records. However, Blose remembered that they 'were angry and tired of waiting and wanted change. It was change or nothing.'

On the day, as per the plan, the Durban TAC activists marched inside C. R. Swart Police Station, demanding that the police arrest Manto Tshabalala-Msimang (the Minister of Health) and Alec Erwin (the Minister of Trade and Industry) for culpable homicide for failing to prevent 600 AIDS deaths per day by not developing a plan to roll out combination ARV therapy. The police responded brutally, using teargas, batons, horses and water cannon against the demonstrators. Blose was outside in the parking lot preparing to deliver food to the activists staging the sit-in inside the police station and remembers that 'the comrades came out soaked. There were old women like Mam'Zodwa who they hit on the feet with sjamboks [a South African type of whip]. They also hit me on the feet. I spun around on the floor and had a blue eye.'

*   *   *

I remember what happened next very well. During the period of the civil disobedience campaign, I was working as a Research Assistant at the Centre for Civil Society at the University of KwaZulu-Natal (UKZN) in Durban. I was also the Secretary of the TAC's UKZN branch which I had co-founded with a group of concerned faculty and students at the Howard College and Westville campuses. I chose not to participate in the action as I could not risk arrest because I needed to be able to get a visa to give lectures on my research on Mbeki's AIDS denialism at the University of Minnesota in Minneapolis in the United States. I was sitting in my office in the Memorial Tower Building of the University's Howard College campus which I shared with Andy Gibbs – a visiting British academic – when I received a cell phone call which filled me with dread. Mandla Majola, who was then a key organizer in Durban, was on the other line telling me that the police had beaten up activists at CR Swart police station. 'Could you come down and help us get people to the doctor?', he asked me.

Andy Gibbs and Mark Hunter (another British academic) and I immediately set to work: we telephoned Nathan Geffen at the TAC's national office in Cape Town about the grim turn of events and fired off a short press release about what had happened. We then piled into Hunter's rusty, second-hand car and he drove us as fast as he could to C. R. Swart. He parked, and we were horrified by what confronted us in the parking lot outside the police station. The activists were all wet. Thabo Cele's arm had been broken by baton-wielding police. Another activist had difficulty seeing because tear-gas had been sprayed in his eyes. A visibly pregnant activist was extremely worried because she had been beaten with a baton in the stomach. Activists had black eyes, cuts and bruises, and some were crying and wincing in pain. We tried to ascertain who needed medical attention most urgently and those activists were given lifts to the TAC's offices in Smith Street, where they were seen by a doctor who had volunteered his services in the event of the police responding violently to the protest. On the doctor's advice, certain activists were admitted to McCord's Hospital and we waited for them to receive further medical attention. By the time we were finished dealing with the immediate fall-out from the police violence against our fellow activists, it was nine o'clock at night. Hours had passed helping friends and colleagues in crisis. I suddenly realized I was extremely thirsty and I had not yet had lunch. A few of us ate dinner together at a restaurant, too tired to talk much – one of the worst days of my young life had come to an end. In the following days and weeks we learned that none of the demonstrators had suffered any serious, long-term adverse health effects as a consequence of police action.

About a week later, the TAC returned again to show the police that they opposed police brutality and also highlight their demand for the government to adopt a national treatment plan. The second time around, I was there among the activists wearing the 'Nelson Mandela' edition of the HIV-POSITIVE t-shirts (an activist in the far left of the photograph in Figure 6.3 with her back turned to the camera is wearing the t-shirt). As the picture also shows demonstrators carried red posters featuring Ministers of Health and Trade and Industry, who were 'Wanted' by the TAC for failing to prevent 600 preventable AIDS deaths every day. One marcher had modified one of these

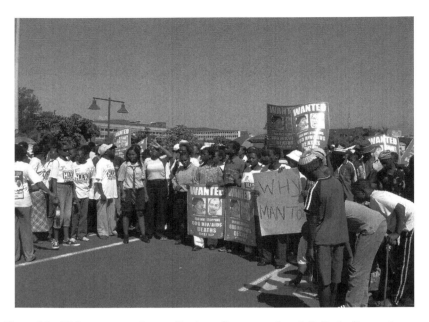

Figure 6.3   TAC protest against police brutality at a prior civil disobedience demonstration, Durban 2003
Source: © Mark Hunter.

by turning it around, having written on the back 'WHY MANTO?' Achmat, who had flown up from Cape Town, addressed the marchers and asked for a police representative to come out of the building to shake the hand of Thabo Cele's unbroken arm to show that the police did not discriminate against people living with HIV: eventually a senior officer emerged and this happened. The long wait for this to happen suggested that HIV-related prejudice may have been behind at least some of the violence the police unleashed at the first demonstration. But this time around, the demonstration was peaceful, doubtless, in part, because of the statements by Human Rights Watch and the TAC's international ally Health GAP which had condemned the violence at the earlier demonstration (Health GAP 2003).[23]

*   *   *

Meanwhile, the TAC remained focused on obtaining its main goal of forcing the government to adopt a national treatment plan. Heywood told me in an interview that the TAC saw the importance of 'retaining the moral high ground' over the course of the campaign (15 April 2008). The first day of the civil disobedience campaign coincided with the US invasion of Iraq, which muted the media coverage it received both within South Africa and globally. To maximize the domestic and global impact of its campaign, the TAC sought solidarity from its international allies and continued to robustly defend it in the media. Achmat wrote in the *Mail & Guardian* that the use of the tactic was a 'last resort' because 'exhaustive efforts at engagement' had 'not worked' (10 April 2003). International approval was also growing for the movement. In late April, TIME magazine voted Achmat one of thirty six heroes who reminded people of what it meant 'to make a difference' (28 April 2003). The outpourings of international solidarity for the movement continued.

The TAC e-mailed its allies abroad calling an 'International Day of Action' on 24 April 2003 (Health GAP 2003). Activists on five continents responded. ACT UP Paris held a die-in 'zap' outside the South African embassy in the French capital (ACT UP Paris 2003). Activists in Los Angeles, Washington DC, London and Milan placed 600 pairs of shoes on the pavements outside South African embassies and consulates: each pair of shoes symbolized a person who had died a preventable death from AIDS in South Africa that day (Health GAP 2003; ACT UP Paris 2003). In Japan, activists released 600 paper cranes representing the number of estimated daily AIDS deaths in the country at the South African embassy. Dutch activists distributed 600 red tulips. Kenyan doctors held a press conference on the issue in Nairobi, and Latin American AIDS activists published a joint statement of support for the TAC.

But it is important to also be mindful of the tensions and inequalities within the movement at that time, not least, those related to gender. Speaking of this period, Blose told me that women TAC activists in Durban were not only beaten by the police just like male activists at CR Swart but also faced sexism at home and, at times, in their activist work in the movement (Interview 11 July 2011). During an interview with me she recounted a time when she moved between her home and the TAC's Durban office every day, with an eye which had been blackened by police brutality. This was also a period when she had to face other struggles, which related to being woman in a patriarchal society. She found that

> Being a young woman and part of any struggle has more layers too. You are dealing with organizational problems while fighting for common things. You are dealing with sexual harassment. At home another struggle, you are a young girl, dishes need washing and cleaning and you are not being paid. There's this idea among family members that you are running from housework.

She tried escape from her domestic drudgery through her work with the TAC, but found that some male 'comrades' at the Durban office expected women to adhere to traditional gender roles. In particular, she told me about two particular workplace incidents in this period that she found troublesome as a woman. One day she was in a meeting which was running into lunch time, and participants were getting hungry, so a male activist suggested that women in the meeting should have left to prepare food for the group. Blose refused to do so and remembers the male colleague as having replied, 'Then what are women for?' She replied, 'I did not come here to make tea and wash dishes. I came here for the political agenda and to advance our issues around HIV and AIDS. My interest is in the meeting and so I'm staying in the meeting.'

Sexual harassment could also, at times, prove challenging for women activists at the Durban office. If a male proposed love to a woman she was expected to take it as a compliment: 'You are supposed to feel flattered because they are craving you, but that's not how some of us felt.' Another common scenario was that a woman activist would hug a male colleague 'as a comrade', and then they would 'start rubbing their hand around your back', and the woman would ask him to stop, which would not be taken seriously. Some men would ask women if they wanted to date them 'and if you [the woman] refused somebody who's in a position of power, you would in some way be marginalized'. Matters reached a head when a group of women in the Durban office reported a male activist to the national office for sexual harassment, and they felt their complaints 'were not taken seriously' by some members of management 'because they thought it was a personal thing'. Blose supported the complaint because 'I thought if it was supported by me it would have more voice and more power and yet it was seen that I was creating conflict and I was told not to waste managers' time', which made her feel 'deeply, deeply hurt and just powerless in that situation'.

These intra-movement gender conflicts need to be viewed against the backdrop of the sexism which South African women faced both in the 'AIDS world' and wider society (discussed in Chapter 3). In this regard, Ida Susser has noted that there has been a paradoxical 'repeated disappearance of women's experience from research and public discussion' around the AIDS despite the fact that they have been continually 'counted, monitored and tested' to generate better scientific understanding of the epidemic and disease, not least to prevent and reduce its incidence in infants (2009, p. 217).

Within the civil society sector in the country, this problem was far from unique to the TAC. In 2005, Cha-Cha Connor, and I studied 50 South African women AIDS activists from a variety of advocacy-orientated NGOs. All of our informants asked to remain anonymous, because they feared that negative professional repercussions might stem from their interactions with us. Several of the women shared experiences very similar to those mentioned by Blose. One woman told us that in her organization 'To get a hired position, you must sleep with the male supervisor.... If you break the relationship you will be harassed. Until the woman has to resign, leave the job, and go back home to die' (Interview 18 April 2005).

As we have seen in Chapter 3, in the early 1990s, AIDS organizations were frequently led by gay men and these NGOs did not always provide safe spaces for women to discuss their experiences of living with and being affected by HIV, *as women*. Blose's account of her experiences of sexism in this later period points to the persistence of such gender-disparities in AIDS activism. The fact that the TAC was largely led by men in its early years meant that its male leaders had more policy-advocacy experience on the issue, more media visibility and more international links than their female counterparts. But the fact that male activists such as Achmat, Geffen and Heywood were more frequently quoted in the media can be attributed to more than mere internal organizational sexism: newspapers, the television and the radio were also reflecting the dominant gender norms within South African society, that women should not exercise political leadership. In this regard, one woman AIDS activist informant in mine and Connor's study told us in 2005 that

> Women have been participating in AIDS organizing since the beginning of the epidemic. But ... a woman who does home-based care and a woman who's caring for orphans gets credited and thanked. And then a man ... who speaks on behalf of everybody, gets prestigious recognitions ... I think that needs to change, because women are doing similar kinds of work. It's like we are good if we are doing domestic and caring types of HIV/AIDS work ... but then if you do political stuff, you get marginalised. No recognition whatsoever.
>
> (Interview 27 April 2005)

Blose's testimony further demonstrates that they were also not immune to sexual harassment within their organizations or having to face the 'double shift' of paid work preceded and followed by their disproportionate share of unpaid housework in the home. Denise Walsh has written about these issues in relation to women in the TAC and COSATU, and has pointed out that civil society has often been conceptualized in the theoretical literature as separate from the 'private sphere' of the family (2009). She also argues that South African women trade unionists' and activists' domestic obligations, such as the greater demands on them *as women* to perform housework and engage in child rearing, have acted as a barrier to their public political participation (Walsh 2009).

This combined with internal organizational sexism meant that women in civil society often had more limited experience and skills to be eligible for promotion and that there was frequently a lack of institutional support for them in the rare instances where they ascended to leadership positions (Walsh 2009). But it is also important to recognize that by successfully pushing for a state-sector ARV roll-out, the TAC also struck a blow against societal sexism by fighting for an end to the externalization of the social cost of caring for people living with HIV on to women through 'home-based care'. In this regard, Connor and I interviewed a female home-based care worker who told us that she would visit the sick and wash them, all the while being hungry herself because she was not being paid (Interview, 26 April 26 2005; Mbali and Connor 2007). Olagoke Akintola has argued that women disproportionately bore the burden of domestic care for the AIDS ill because social norms dictated that they should perform this job in the home (2004). While gender tensions remained unresolved within the movement, it made further progress in its advocacy for a public sector roll-out of ARVs.

The TAC suspends its civil disobedience campaign

On 30 April 2003, the TAC's National Executive Committee (NEC) decided to temporarily suspend the civil disobedience campaign, following a meeting with Deputy President Jacob Zuma who had agreed to take up the need for a South African treatment plan with the National AIDS Council (TAC 2003d; Heywood 2004). Heywood told me that this decision was far from unanimously well received within the movement, with some supporters feeling 'let down' by it (Interview 15 April 2008).

While the TAC suspended civil disobedience as a tactic, it continued to engage in lawful protest actions. On 5 May 2003 the TAC-aligned SAMA urged doctors who wanted a roll-out of combination ARV drug therapy to wear 'HIV POSITIVE' t-shirts to work for a day (*Cape Times* 6 May 2003). But no sooner had the TAC suspended its civil disobedience campaign than signs began to emerge that the government was less than serious about developing a treatment plan. Tshabalala-Msimang failed to release the findings of the Joint Treasury and Health Task Team on a roll-out of ARVs at her Ministry's budget vote in parliament, as expected (*Cape Times* 14 May 2003).

The TAC held its second national congress in early August 2003, immediately before the first South African National AIDS Conference in Durban. At its Durban Congress, the movement vowed to 'intensify its struggle to force the government to roll-out ARV drugs to people living with HIV/AIDS' (*City Press* 3 August 2003). Achmat also finally agreed to start combination ARV therapy because he vowed that he would not allow Tshabalala-Msimang and Mbeki to kill him (*The Star* 5 August 2003). Peter Dwyer, a visiting British academic, wrote that

> Over the three days of the congress, 'positive Muslims', 'health care workers united against AIDS', trade unionists and the unemployed, socialists and priests who make up TAC's united front campaign, hugged, danced, sang, cried and laughed (in frustration with the ANC government). The

congress unanimously vowed to continue their struggle for treatment and embark, once again, on civil disobedience.

(*Green Left Weekly*, 24 July 2011)

Stephen Lewis, the UN Special Envoy for HIV/AIDS in Africa, addressed the Congress and compared it with some of the most important and influential social movements of the twentieth century and the global justice movement in the twenty-first century.

Lewis's public expression of direct support for the TAC was hardly the norm in the diplomatic community. He shared with me in an interview that diplomats of Western countries regularly shared their befuddlement and exasperation at Mbeki's position on AIDS with him behind closed doors. According to Lewis, Kofi Annan, Jimmy Carter and Bill Clinton all privately tried to persuade South Africa's President to repudiate his AIDS dissidence, but there was relatively little direct, public diplomatic condemnation of the government's flawed AIDS policy in these years. The Canadian former diplomat added that in his view such private approaches were often defended in accordance with the rationale that 'we don't have the right to criticize a country publicly' (Interview 26 August 2011). But, he added, this did not apply in the cases of countries such as Iran, North Korea or Myanmar which were overwhelmingly, in Western diplomats' eyes, at least, 'bad countries'. In an interview with me, Peter Piot, the then Executive Director of UNAIDS, also pointed to Western governments' realist calculations that South Africa's status as a regional power meant that it was of strategic importance to them in terms of its African continental peacemaking and peacekeeping (Interview 7 October 2011). Piot and Lewis presented me with a coherent picture of Western governments continuing to advance their interests through their diplomatic relations with the country, irrespective of the moral nature of the health policies adopted by the country's government.

When Tashabalala-Msimang gave an address at the opening of the South African National AIDS Conference the next day, TAC activists protested silently and other delegates booed her. She was followed by Jacob Zuma, who struck a conciliatory note and said that the government was finalizing international agreements to ensure access to medicine for people living with HIV and said that the government did not question the existence of HIV and AIDS (BBC 3 August 2003; IRIN 2003). The Deputy President also praised advances in scientific research in South Africa and a 'very strong and vocal civil society response to HIV and AIDS' which he saw as complementing the work of the government (BBC 3 August 2003).

The South African government sent another signal at the Durban conference that it was beginning to relent on the treatment activists' demands – Ayanda Ntsaluba, the Director-General of the Department of Health, announced at a press conference that the government would conclude an agreement with the Global Fund to release the KZN monies the next day:

a denialism-fuelled controversy which is described in Chapter 7 (*BuaNews* 6 August 2003). Ntsaluba blamed the delay on legal paperwork and glitches but read alongside Zuma's conciliatory speech it was clear that this about-turn was influenced by a policy rethink which was finally underway in the government. On 7 August, South African national government signed an agreement with the Global Fund for monies to be released – a clear signal that the government would no longer block international assistance for the provision of ARVs for use in chronic care (IRIN 7 August 2003). Richard Feachem – the Global Fund's Executive Director – hailed the agreement as 'a turning point' and a 'signal of hope for those living with HIV and for all Africans working to turn the tide against HIV and AIDS'. But the government continued to send mixed messages on ARVs. Just a week before the conference, the country's drug regulatory agency – the MCC – had controversially announced that it was examining the clinical trials of Nevirapine for PMTCT in Uganda because the drug company that had manufactured it was withdrawing an application for its approval for its use for this purpose, a controversy which dominated the meeting's proceedings.

The South African government relents and develops the operational plan

On 8 August 2003, shortly after Jacob Zuma's conciliatory speech at the National AIDS Conference, the South African cabinet made a dramatic announcement. It had met to discuss the findings of the Joint Treasury and Health task team on ARVs and 'decided that the Department of Health should, as matter of urgency, develop a detailed operational plan for an antiretroviral treatment programme' (GCIS 2003a). The Cabinet would be assisted in this task by 'experts' from the CHAI. It was 'expected that this detailed work would be completed by the end of September 2003' (GCIS 2003b). This news was reported in the media on 10 August 2003 and was well received. In South Africa, the *Sunday Times* reported that Mandela was 'overjoyed' at the announcement (10 August 2003). The announcement won the government international praise and foreign leaders congratulated the government (*Globe and Mail* 13 September 2003).

But this was not the first time that international expertise had been offered to assist South Africa's government in providing free drugs to the country's poor people living with HIV. As discussed in Chapter 7, the Global Fund and other middle-income countries in the global South had offered such assistance for many years. Clinton, like Mandela, had already tried to convince Mbeki to alter his views on AIDS.[24] What had changed by the time the Clinton Foundation finally stepped in to assist was that the Mbeki administration had been forced to accede to the TAC's demands for a roll-out of ARV drugs. As a government task team hammered out the national ARV roll-out strategy, the TAC and Achmat received more awards, including the Nelson Mandela Award for Health and Human Rights (*This Day* 7 October 2003). On 19 November 2003, the cabinet announced that Tshabalala-Msimang had, as instructed, presented it with the main features of the new 'Operational Plan for Comprehensive Treatment and Care for HIV and AIDS' (GCIS 2003b). According to media reports, the government planned to spend R12 billion on combination ARV therapy over the following five years (*The Star* 20 November 2003). Within a year there would be at least one ARV service point in every health district across the country and within five years one in every local municipality. The TAC was elated and its spokespersons Rukia Cornelius and Nathan Geffen were quoted as saying that 'This is brilliant, we're very happy. It has been a long five years that we've been fighting with the government for the rollout. We could not have done this without the help of all the NGOs, unions, churches, volunteers and health-care workers who helped us in this struggle' (*The Star* 20 January 2003).

The government's planning to roll out HIV treatment was also aided by developments at the Competition Commission. In October 2003, the Competition Commission found that Boehringer-Ingelheim and GlaxoSmithKline had abused their market dominance in terms of South African anti-trust/competition law. It asked the Competition Tribunal to allow any entity to manufacture generic versions provided they offered the patent holders fair royalties. This pushed the drug companies into negotiations with the TAC, MSF and CIPLA for a settlement.

As Sean Flynn has noted, the TAC had, thereby, successfully and innovatively used competition law to circumvent the 20-year patent period prescribed under the WTO's TRIPS Agreement. While the TRIPS Agreement harmonized intellectual property, there was no equivalent international treaty dealing with competition law and South Africa's Competition Act incorporated developmental objectives (Flynn 2010, p. 467). Following the TAC's example, AIDS activists in Thailand and the United States also used competition-based legal strategies to press for wider access to medicines. The strategy proved especially deft because it allowed access-to-medicines advocates to re-frame the debate from one centred around the pharmaceutical corporate 'persons' intellectual property 'rights' to one of monopoly regulation. An intellectual property rights-based framing was weighted in favour of the corporations who claimed them. By contrast, a corporate monopoly framing presented consumers such as Hazel Tau as the wronged party. The strategy can also be viewed as an example of 'regime shifting', that is, moving law making and regulatory activities from one venue into another (Flynn 2010, p. 466). In shifting their claims to the regime of the Competition Commission, the TAC found a forum sympathetic to its cause.

Flynn has referred to Competition Law as existing on the 'flip side' of the economic liberalization (neoliberalism), which, paradoxically, also enforced global harmonization (uniform tightening) of intellectual property restrictions (2010, p. 467). This dominant Western model of liberalized 'free markets' was undergirded by contract and property rights. In this model, the efficiency of deregulated industries was ensured by competition law which prevented price-fixing and other abuses of monopoly power (2010, p. 467). In a deeper sense, it can, therefore, be said that its Competition Commission complaint, the TAC successfully exploited the inherent contradictions within neoliberalism in South Africa and globally.

The Clinton Foundation also announced that it had concluded deals with CIPLA, Ranbaxy and Matrix (Indian generic pharmaceutical companies) and South African generic drug producer Aspen Pharmacare to provide substantially discounted ARV drugs to countries with high HIV prevalence (Clinton Presidential Centre 2003). These Clinton foundation brokered generic drug deals subsequently played a significant role in reducing the prices of ARV drugs in developing countries, including South Africa (Waning et al. 2009).

The American Quaker Society of Friends nominated Achmat and the TAC for a Nobel Prize (*Cape Times* 3 December 2003). They did not, in the end, win the prize but it was an important international moral endorsement of the TAC's work, including its second civil disobedience campaign. As 2003 drew to a close, the TAC's push for the implementation of the Operational Plan also received a boost from the competition-related settlement it obtained in December 2003 with GlaxoSmithKline and Boehringer Ingelheim – the multinational pharmaceutical companies would allow South African and Indian generic producers to make cheaper versions of first-line ARV drugs (Creamer 2003; Flynn 2010).

At the close of 2003, daunting challenges lay ahead for the government in commencing a national roll-out of ARV drugs: only 20,000 South Africans were privately purchasing ARVs yet, according to a government study, half a million needed them immediately (*The Observer* 23 November 2003). The government did not match this need initially: it only planned on placing 100,000 people living with HIV on treatment in the roll-out's first year. The TAC would go on to fight many other battles over the tardy and half-hearted implementation of this plan, but it was now a fully fledged social movement with a significant measure of international influence and domestic political clout.

Conclusion

In August 2001, the TAC provided Busiswe Maqungo with a platform to speak out about how the government had failed to prevent her daughter's death through its irrational limitation of Nevirapine-provision to a few state health facilities. The grieving mother's testimony formed a part of the movement's innovative socio-economic rights-based litigation, a strategy it deployed alongside its treatment literacy programme and street protests using struggle symbolism.

This type of litigation was only an option for AIDS activists in the *post-apartheid era* as South Africa's new Constitution was novel in the country's legal history in its inclusion of socio-economic rights. The country's Constitutional Court adopted an administrative law-like 'reasonableness' approach to assessing whether government policies were progressively realizing these rights, which meant that scientists played an especially important role in the case. Indeed, their expert testimony to the Court that the government's reservations about widening access to Nevirapine for PMTCT were not based on the best available research were vital to the success of the TAC's suit.

But, while the TAC's litigation received international praise, it was not without its feminist critics who argued that it made inadequate reference to women's reproductive rights. There are valid gender critiques of the TAC's work in this period; however, the most salient ones relate to other aspects of the movement and come from a different source. The TAC did not simply view pregnant women as valuable in as much as they were mothers: its longer-term goal was to press for a roll-out of combination ARV therapy for all people living with HIV. This, in turn, was vital to challenging the patriarchy embedded in 'alternatives' such as 'home-based care,' which was unpaid work, largely performed by women. TAC women told me that, for them, the most pressing gender issue in the movement in the period was that it had too few women leaders. Moreover, those who were starting the 'break through the glass ceiling' were struggling with issues such as sexual harassment and for the creation of programs to develop their skills and experience *as women leaders*. In these respects the TAC was not unique: like other AIDS civil society groups, its internal sexism reflected the patriarchy in wider South African society.

In its first five years, the TAC's stature grew immensely both internationally and in South Africa. Mandela's support for the movement was critical in shaping domestic public opinion in the TAC's favour because he lent his humanitarian credentials to the issue and showed that the TAC did not have party-political motives in making its demands. The anti-apartheid background of some of the movement's most visible leaders also conferred legitimacy upon it. Its international support expanded in this period: the TAC's civil disobedience campaign for a National Treatment Plan led to solidarity protests outside South African embassies in several countries abroad. Many campaigns lay ahead but the TAC was now entrenched as an internationally recognized mass-movement for local and global health justice and a 'household name' in South Africa.

7
'The Durban Effect': The TAC's Impact on Global Health Diplomacy and Governance, 2001–2003

In late June 2002, the TAC's openly HIV-positive chairperson – Zackie Achmat – fell ill with a lung infection, and he still declined ARV drugs, despite the fact that his doctor had recommended that he take them. The TAC's Nathan Geffen told the press that ' "Zackie doesn't want to make too much of his illness because there are thousands of people in South Africa in a much worse position than him" ' (*The Star* 4 July 2002). ' "He is not at death's door" ', he added, ' "He has a lung infection, but there are no signs of pneumonia at the moment" '. It was in this dramatic context that Achmat – who remained too ill to travel – delivered a taped address which was shown to delegates at the Barcelona International AIDS Conference on 11 July 2002. Achmat's drug fast was garnering international media attention, and his bedside lecture added a sense of moral urgency to the cause of universal HIV treatment access.

The ill activist said that 'The global community decided to campaign for affordable medicines and ARV access for poor countries and communities in the wake of the Durban 2000 conference', a phenomenon he referred to as 'The Durban Effect' (Achmat 2002). He framed his appeal for universal access to HIV treatment in moral terms, by railing against the dominant dichotomy between prevention and treatment, and by emphasizing that the development of programmes with both aims in mind was a moral imperative. Rolling out treatment was 'not only a matter of cost to the state', at stake were 'the lives of women, the lives of children, [and] the lives of men'. He went on, 'Just because we are poor, just because we are black, just because we live in environments and continents that are far from you, does not mean our lives should be valued any less.' The TAC leader ended his speech by thanking his international allies such as Health GAP, MSF, Gay Men's Health Crisis, Pela Vidda in Brazil and 'people across Asia and Europe' who had made the South African movement's work 'much easier'.

Achmat's address sheds light on what the TAC offered the international HIV treatment access movement – a uniquely South African form of moral capital which was scientifically informed, emphasized the numbers of poor people living with the disease who lacked access to treatment and which significantly deployed anti-apartheid symbolism. Differently put, the TAC contributed a unique dimension to the international movement's ethical 'meaning work' – that is, to its reframing of HIV-related global health inequalities in moral terms (Tarrow 2005, p. 75). The TAC activists wearing HIV POSITIVE t-shirts, including Achmat – its articulate spokesperson – put numerous 'human faces' to the cause of universal HIV treatment access in developing countries.

Achmat came to be characterized by the TAC's international activist allies and the media as what Raymond Smith and Patricia Siplon have termed the 'Gandhi of the AIDS movement' (2006, p. 87). In more affluent countries, the international HIV treatment access movement's campaigns began to generate historic levels of political will and foreign development aid to widen access to ARV medicines in developing countries. Smith and Siplon have usefully characterized the period discussed in this chapter as one in which activists won 'major victories' in terms of reductions in the prices of HIV medicines and increased foreign aid for global AIDS (2006, p. 82). But they have not elaborated in detail upon the exact role of the South African activists in the events leading up to these developments.

In a deeper sense, with the TAC as a vital participant, the international movement changed the politics of global health, which can be measured in their influence over the creation of new models of global health governance and diplomacy. In this chapter, I use the term 'global health governance' in the manner of international relations specialists to describe the broadening webs of institutions and social sectors which have been making and implementing international health policies since the 1990s (Hein et al. 2007; Rushton and Williams 2011). By contrast, I use the term 'global health diplomacy' to describe state–state interactions around international health policy. Whereas there had previously been a singular emphasis in global health on low-cost infectious disease prevention, transnational activist pressure drove a new additional push in international policy-making arenas for both donor and developing countries' governments to act to expand access to chronic HIV care. Transnational AIDS activists, including those in the TAC, 'externalized' their claims onto foreign governments and the institutions governing global health in the sense suggested by sociologist Sidney Tarrow and also continued to press for vastly expanded foreign aid to combat the pandemic, which came to be chiefly provided to developing country governments in the form of grants, as opposed to loans (2005, p. 32).

In 2001, the UN held its first general assembly special session on the issue of AIDS (UNGASS). The declaration that emerged from UNGASS echoed the

TAC's framing of access to HIV medicines as a critical element of realizing the human right to health.

While it was American academics who proposed the creation of a new Global Fund to Fight AIDS TB and Malaria, the international HIV treatment access movement's advocacy added political ballast to the idea. The new Global Fund to Fight AIDS, TB and Malaria offered a novel approach to global health funding. The Global Fund started offering very large grants in April 2002, monies which – while still inadequate – played a critical role in the dramatically expanded access to treatment, internationally. But, the first major country-level crisis in the life of the new Global Fund occurred over the disbursement of a grant to the KwaZulu-Natal province of South Africa, which was substantially stalled by the Mbeki administration from 2002–3, an issue upon which the TAC campaigned. This crisis can be viewed as one which can be traced back to the multisectoral governance structure of the Global Fund and its use of technical criteria to assess proposals – both of which meant that it was able to take a position on the KZN proposal which was independent of that taken by Mbeki and his Health Minister Tshabalala-Msimang.

There was also progress on drug pricing, partially as a result of transnational activist pressure, developments which the South African government failed to immediately capitalize upon. In response to such activist pressure and deft diplomatic negotiations by the Brazilian government, the WTO produced the Doha Declaration, which was aimed at clarifying the wording in the TRIPS Agreement. The Doha Declaration did not facilitate trade in generic drugs between developing countries. It was nevertheless, important in terms of the politics of global health because, in it, most of the world's governments had collectively recognized the impacts that patent-strengthening trade agreements could have upon human health. On a practical level, it also gave generic-ARV-producing, middle-income developing countries a rhetorical tool when negotiating drug prices with pharmaceutical companies. Even more significant in reducing HIV drug prices, internationally, was the Clinton Foundation's decision to start negotiating cheaper fixed-dose combinations of ARV drugs.

But, it is also important not to overstate the influence of the TAC and its international activist allies' influence over bilateral global health diplomacy in the period. In his 2003 State of the Union address US President George W. Bush announced the formation of a new Emergency Fund for AIDS Relief (PEPFAR) which would spend US$15 billion in 15 heavily affected African and Caribbean nations over five years. The creation of PEPFAR was a result of pressure from other more conservative and elite advocacy groups, such as evangelical Christian organizations and a world-renowned rock musician (Bono). However, it is doubtful these events would have occurred in the absence of the consistent visibility of activists in the international HIV treatment access movement, which contributed to shifts in public opinion in both the United States and European countries in favour of increased foreign aid to combat global AIDS. The international movement shaped public opinion through street protests, a savvy global media strategy and its increasingly deft uses of the Internet.

Similarly, the TAC's efforts to contribute to the consolidation of the international HIV treatment access movement enjoyed mixed success. The South African activists benefited from their alliances in the global North and worked hard on strengthening their ties with their colleagues in the global South, including with AIDS activists in other African countries. The TAC certainly exercised a strategic influence over AIDS activism in other countries in the global South: there was Tarrowian 'diffusion' of its tactic of making and wearing HIV POSITIVE t-shirts (2005, p. 32). By contrast, its efforts to cultivate African advocacy networks were hindered by the continent's underdeveloped infrastructure and South Africa's wider diplomatic role in the region.

The creation of the global fund and the HIV drug price war

Achmat's bedside appeal to the delegates who had gathered in Barcelona included a call for rich countries to support the new Global Fund. He pointed out that the fund had not received the necessary US$7–11 billion which had been requested by UN Secretary-General Kofi Annan and urged countries such as the United States, Europe, Japan, South Africa and Brazil to donate more money to the Fund. The TAC leader then called for delegates to 'step up the activism in your countries to ensure that the global fund has the money that it needs' (2002). But what sort of entity was this new Global Fund and how did it come about? And, how did it come to play such a critical role in massively expanding access to combination ARV therapy? While it was chiefly the brainchild of prominent academics, the sense of political urgency behind its creation and consolidation was certainly facilitated by the international HIV treatment access movement's advocacy.

As we have seen, from the Durban AIDS Conference onwards, activists in the international HIV treatment access movement had called for radical increases in foreign aid to provide the new ARV drug regimens. Simultaneously, Jeffrey Sachs, a Harvard economist, started making vocal appeals for a new international aid effort to combat the global AIDS pandemic. In the 1980s, and early 1990s, Sachs had been better known for his anti-inflationary and pro-privatization policies in Latin America and the post-communist countries of Eastern Europe (*TIME* 6 November 1989; Sachs 2005). Sachs's reputation as an economist working on international health issues became cemented in early 2000, when the WHO Secretary-General Gro Harlem Brudtland appointed him to chair the international medical body's Commission on Macroeconomics and Health.

At the Durban Conference in 2000, Sachs urged UNAIDS to 'manage a *global fund* [his emphasis] of some $4 Billion per year, with project funding based on independent scientific review, monitoring and evaluation' (Sachs

2000, p. 10). In his Durban speech, Sachs added that HIV interventions should 'combine prevention, MTCT and patient care including combination therapies' (2000, p. 11). This was significant because, as we have seen, the prevailing orthodoxy of the day among governments and development foundations in the global North was that in developing countries HIV prevention programmes deserved prioritization over those aimed at widening access to treatment.

Just over a week after the Durban AIDS conference, the leaders of the Group of Eight industrialized countries (the G8) met in Okinawa, Japan. The G8's final Okinawa communiqué picked up on many of the themes of Sachs's Durban address: the leaders of the affluent countries 'welcomed' the success of the Durban AIDS conference (G8 2000). They also committed themselves to work towards reducing the number of HIV-infected young people by 25% by 2010. Furthermore, the assembled leaders agreed to mobilize 'additional resources', 'support innovative partnerships' with NGOs, the private sector and multilateral organizations and work to make 'existing cost-effective interventions, including key drugs ... more universally available and affordable in developing countries'.

Meanwhile, Sachs's vision of a dramatically scaled-up global response to AIDS continued to evolve, partly in dialogue with some of his colleagues at Harvard. Paul Farmer, a Harvard anthropologist and professor of medicine, had run a clinic providing combination ARV therapy in Haiti – one of the poorest nations on earth – since 1998. Farmer had obtained marvellous clinical results in his Haitian patients. These thriving HIV-positive patients in rural Haiti were able to take their drugs every day, as specified. Farmer's patients maintained high levels of ARV drug adherence because they were encouraged by *accompagnateurs* – people living with HIV who were trained to offer psychosocial support to others who were also on the drugs (Behforouz et al. 2004). This *accompagnateur* model built upon an existing Directly Observed Treatment (DOT) programme for Farmer's patients with tuberculosis.

Sachs found that a trip to visit Farmer's clinic in Haiti allayed any further doubts he had previously about the feasibility of providing ARV drugs to patients in resource-poor settings. He then collaborated with his Harvard colleagues Bruce Walker, a professor of medicine; Max Essex, a public health specialist and Farmer on producing a document which aimed to show 'that treatment of dying AIDS patients was possible and could be scaled up to millions of people within a few years' (Sachs 2005, p. 206).

In February 2001, CIPLA – an Indian generic pharmaceutical company – announced that it would make a triple cocktail of ARV drugs available to MSF for US$350 (CIPLA and MSF 2001). By contrast, up to that point, patent-holding pharmaceutical companies had charged US$10,000 for a year's course of such therapy (Kapczynski 2009, p. 1585). This development sparked what *The Wall Street Journal* dubbed as an AIDS drug 'price war', involving CIPLA and its Indian competitors Ranbaxy and Hetero Drugs Limited (*Wall Street Journal* 7 March 2001). According to the same report, patent-holding pharmaceutical company Merck also announced that it would reduce the prices of its AIDS drugs by 40–55% in African countries.

Such radically expanded global HIV funding could, theoretically, now benefit an ever larger number of poor patients in developing countries. James Orbinski, the then president of the International Council of MSF, delineated the humanitarian dividends the international NGO obtained by capitalizing upon such drug price reductions in its programmes in 2001–2002 in his memoirs which stated that '[a] year after starting treatment the majority of the 150 AIDS patients in Khayalitsha had gained at least 10 kilograms of weight and 84% of patients were alive and well. We expanded the Khayalitsha program and started similar programs all over the world' (2008, p. 362).

HIV treatment activists' calls for cheaper ARV medicines were also partially, but in the long term, significantly, met by the work of a foundation formed by one of the most successful politicians of the late twentieth-century – a newly retired former US president, Bill Clinton. Shortly after leaving office, he established the William J. Clinton Foundation, and one of its core elements was the CHAI. As we have seen, AIDS activists had criticized his administration's policy responses to the global pandemic. After his departure from the Oval Office, his foundation began to design an AIDS initiative in mid-2001. His foundation's staff began to work closely with Dr. Jim Yong Kim, a public health specialist who had collaborated with Paul Farmer in founding Partners in Health (Takiff 2010). Kim was part of a group of public health experts who met with Ira Magaziner of the Clinton Foundation. Magaziner was an old friend of the former president's from his time at Oxford and a former student activist and business consultant who had run Hillary Rodham Clinton's health care task force in the mid-1990s.

In this period, Kim shared his view with Magaziner that under WTO agreements it was legal for developing countries to purchase generic HIV medicines from their middle-income counterparts such as India. He also briefed Magaziner on MSF's progress in obtaining single pills (referred to as fixed-dose combinations) which combined three ARVs for the mere cost of US$350 per patient per annum. Kim told Clinton biographer Michael Takiff that Magaziner then resolved to reduce this price by just over a half (Takiff 2010, p. 406). Magaziner apparently had a sense that the generic companies would accept these further price reductions because the trend of increasing levels of foreign aid to fight AIDS meant they had guaranteed new markets and so could profitably sell more drugs at lower prices.

The AIDS drug price war suddenly made the unthinkable possible: a sustained and far-reaching global effort to scale up the provision of HIV treatment. Meanwhile, the Harvard academics' document was finalized and came to be called the 'Harvard Consensus Statement'; a document which was signed by 133 academics based at the prestigious university. The statement outlined: the medical evidence of the efficacy of the new treatment regimens; the public health rationale for scaling up access to them (their benefits for prevention programmes) in developing countries; and, most importantly, their affordability in the event of significant reductions in the prices of HIV drugs. As the statement pointed out, such advocacy for widened access to HIV treatment was necessary because 'the very mention of AIDS treatment has often been avoided by donor agencies in wealthy countries, for fear that raised expectations would increase the financial and operational demands upon them, and detract from prevention efforts' (Harvard Faculty 2001, p. 4).

The Harvard academics went on to state that the 'disparity in access to effective treatment between wealthy countries and developing countries' was 'neither scientifically nor *ethically* [my emphasis] justified' (2001, p. 4). HIV treatment and prevention programmes were not necessarily mutually exclusive: instead, the academics said, they had to 'go hand in hand' (2001, p. 4). They argued that in the absence of access to effective treatment, individuals who suspected they were living with HIV had limited incentives to be tested to see if they were infected because it was a lethal and heavily stigmatized disease. They also contended that combination ARV therapy could reduce the viral loads of people living with HIV which limited the probability of the transmission of the virus.

Their assertion of the economic feasibility of widening access to combination ARV treatment depended on three developments which were conceivable with the exercise of adequate political will, namely: a 90% reduction in the prices of AIDS drugs; an increase in foreign aid to finance their provision; and, the ongoing need for scaled up prevention programmes to limit the numbers of patients requiring treatment. Given the reductions in drug prices which had recently occurred, the Harvard academics conservatively estimated that the pills in a 'typical' combination ARV drug regimen would cost US$500 per patient per year (2001, p. 14). But, as they pointed out, such drug price reductions were necessary, but hardly sufficient, to widen access to the medicines. Increases in foreign aid would also be required by African countries such as Ghana, Tanzania and Nigeria, if they were to provide ARVs as they had per capita gross national products of under US$400 and spent US$8, or less, annually, per person on health (2001, p. 15).

Given the scale of HIV prevalence and the poverty of heavily affected countries, foreign aid would have to be given as *grants*, not loans: which was a then common approach to development and global health financing, as evident in the operations of the World Bank. The scholars estimated that scaling up HIV treatment would cost US$1,123 per patient, per year in Sub-Saharan Africa (2001, p. 15). This estimate included the cost of the drugs, operational expenses, monitoring and evaluation and the fees for clinical supplies such as diagnostic tests. The Harvard academics projected the total cost of placing three million patients onto ARV therapy at about US$4.2 billion by year five: it was hoped that US$3.3 billion of this figure would be generated by donor assistance (2001, p. 15). Their proposals had radical implications: raising and spending such vast sums of money to treat a single infectious disease on a chronic basis in developing countries in such a short space of time was unprecedented in the history of global health. In this context, the academics argued that it required a new kind of global financing institution. The Harvard Consensus statement incorporated Sachs's proposal for the creation of an 'HIV/AIDS Prevention and Treatment Trust Fund' and called upon 'wealthy countries to provide financial and scientific leadership and poor countries to provide necessary political and institutional support at both the national and community levels' (2001, p. 18).

Back in South Africa, shortly after its release, the TAC hailed the Harvard document as being 'the first major authoritative statement and practical vision from academics and scientists' in the United States 'on the necessity and possibility of HIV treatment' provision in resource-poor settings (2001b, p. 1). The South African activists characterized the signatories of the statement as having offered an 'ambitious' plan to treat a million people in three years, and outlined the 'minimum set of demands' which had to be put to the international community (2001b, p. 1). The TAC statement added that both middle-income countries and those with major epidemics (such as South Africa) had to interrogate the plan in terms of its 'sustainability' and the 'economic dangers of dependency on development assistance to keep a substantial proportion of its population alive' (2001b, p. 4). Such caution was warranted by 'the ephemeral nature of compassion from governments in developed countries' (2001b, p. 4).

The TAC called for more detailed costing analyses to be done on country-by-country bases. It also argued that the drugs' high prices remained the most significant barrier to their wider availability. They agreed with the Harvard academics' assertion of the need for wealthy countries to provide financial and scientific leadership and poor countries to provide political and institutional support. But the TAC said that there was also a need to recognize that 'political leadership' had many forms 'including mass mobilization by civil society organizations such as religious bodies and trade unions' and also business (2001b, p. 5). There was also still 'much work to be done' in rich and poor countries alike to ensure wider access to HIV treatment (2001b, p. 5). Yet again, the movement criticized the South African government as having 'displayed a remarkable unwillingness' to face up to the 'realities' of the pandemic (2001b, p. 5). It urged the group of Harvard academics to pressure the US government to implement the plan or something akin to it immediately.

The global fund idea gained further traction at an Organization of African Unity (OAU) conference on HIV/AIDS, TB and Other Infectious Diseases, which was held in Abuja, Nigeria, from 26 to 27 April 2001. UN

Secretary-General Kofi Annan gave a keynote address on the first day of the meeting where he joined the African leaders in calling for the creation of the fund. The African leaders produced the 'Abuja Declaration on HIV/AIDS, Tuberculosis and Other Related Infectious Diseases'. In this declaration, Africa's presidents, prime ministers and monarchs pronounced that AIDS was causing a 'State of Emergency' on the continent (OAU 200). They committed themselves to taking 'personal responsibility' and providing 'leadership' for the activities of their National AIDS Councils. In future, they pledged that 15% of their annual budgets would be allocated for 'the improvement of the health sector'. The African leaders urged donor nations to give 0.7% of their Gross Domestic Product (GDP) as Official Development Assistance (ODA). Finally, they expressed their support for the creation of a new global fund, which would, among other things, assist their governments in widening access to ARV drugs.

Sachs and Amir Attaran published a paper in *The Lancet* which further fleshed out the Global Fund proposal. Drawing on data submitted by wealthy countries' governments to the Organization for Economic Cooperation and Development (OECD), the academics estimated that from 1996 to 1998 the financing from all rich countries to sub-Saharan Africa for AIDS control projects averaged at US$69 million annually and that total donor spending on AIDS was twice that at most over the whole period (Attaran and Sachs 2001). By 1998, foreign aid to combat AIDS in sub-Saharan African was equal to US$3 per person living with HIV in the region (Attaran and Sachs 2001, p. 57). They proposed that unlike much previous foreign aid for health, the proposed Global Fund would give grants, not loans. Such funding would have to rise to US$10 billion per annum which would be administered by the new global fund (Attaran and Sachs 2001, p. 60). The putative global fund would accept proposals drawn up by affected countries themselves, including civil society and be judged by scientific experts. The monies would also 'fund concurrent needs' including HIV prevention and the provision of ARVs for chronic use and for PMTCT (Attaran and Sachs 2001, p. 57).

The international community's growing focus on AIDS was also evident at the July 2001 G8 summit in Genoa, Italy, where leaders of wealthy nations joined UN Secretary-General Kofi Annan in launching the Global Fund and made pledges amounting to US$1.2 billion (*Toronto Star* 21 July 2001). A few days later, the UN General Assembly held its first Special Session on AIDS (UNGASS) from 25 to 27 June 2001. This meeting produced a Declaration of Commitment on AIDS, which framed the AIDS pandemic as 'a global emergency' (UNGA 2001, p. 6). It also endorsed the idea of forming a Global AIDS and Health Fund, which had already by that stage received US$1 billion in pledges.

As we have seen, the long, inflexible product patents enabled under the WTO's TRIPS Agreement had been a notable barrier to developing countries producing, exporting and importing generic medicines. From April 2001, governments began preparing their positions for the WTO's fourth ministerial meeting in Doha, Qatar, which was scheduled to be held in November 2001. At this meeting, there was a special session on the TRIPS Agreement's stance in relation to affordable access to essential medicines in developing countries. In the deliberations leading up to the November meeting, the United States took a position which was firmly in line with that of the patent-holding multinational pharmaceutical companies, which called for compulsory licensing to only be permissible under extremely limited circumstances and for parallel importation to be forbidden (Nunn 2009, p. 37).

But its negotiating position on this issue changed following a menacing and unexpected turn of events in the United States: anthrax was found in letters to senators and news media offices in that country one week after the atrocities of 11 September 2001. The US and Canadian governments took swift action to contain the public health threat posed by the biological attacks: in order to guarantee an affordable stockpile of Ciprofloxacin, an anti-anthrax drug, they threatened its manufacturer Bayer that they would issue compulsory licences to produce generic copies of the medicine. For many supporters of access to essential medicines in developing countries, such as TAC-ally MSF, the American response to the anthrax scare highlighted the 'hypocrisy' of Western governments 'invoking the threat of compulsory licensing in the face of anthrax while denying the same right to the developing world in the face of HIV and AIDS' (Orbinski 2008, p. 372). Bayer responded to the US government's compulsory licence threat by lowering the price of Ciprofloxacin. In the end, the anthrax attacks caused five deaths whereas AIDS took the lives of millions every year.

Given this turn of events, the US Trade Representative entered the negotiations at the WTO's fourth ministerial conference in Doha, Qatar, politically weakened in defending its former hard-line stance on compulsory licensing. Legal and trade policy scholar Amy Kapczynski has usefully characterized the Doha meeting as having represented 'the high point in health activists' engagement with the WTO' (2009, p. 1585).

It is also important to note that health NGOs worked in tandem with some developing countries' governments to obtain this breakthrough. In her book on Brazilian HIV treatment policies, Amy Nunn recounts that she was told by 'several diplomats and experts present in Doha that the final text of the Doha Declaration was negotiated behind closed doors between the US and Brazilian delegation', and the Americans finally accepted a text which had been proposed by a coalition of developing countries (2009).[1] The WTO published its 'Doha Declaration on the TRIPS agreement and public health' on 14 November 2001. The Doha Declaration clarified 'flexibilities' under the TRIPS Agreement: member states now had the right to obtain compulsory licences in the event of a self-defined national health emergency, including those related to HIV/AIDS, tuberculosis and malaria (WTO 2001). In this Declaration the WTO gave least-developed countries the deadline of 2016 as the year by which they had to grant or enforce pharmaceutical product patents (t'Hoen 2009, p. xvi).

For Brazil, a middle-income country, whose leaders had adequate political will and which had the industrial capacity to manufacture generic HIV medicines, this represented substantial progress because it clarified TRIPS flexibilities in a way which strengthened its hand in negotiations with pharmaceutical companies (Nunn 2009). But the governments of developing countries with generic pharmaceutical manufacturing capabilities had to make use of the agreement in order for it to generate the desired reductions in preventable AIDS deaths – unlike its middle-income counterpart Brazil, South Africa tragically failed to take advantage of these even-clearer TRIPS flexibilities to produce ARVs because of its government's AIDS denialist policies.

While activists in the international HIV treatment access movement were, in general, ebullient about the Doha Declaration's clarification of the legality of using compulsory licences in health emergencies, they were also critical of its failure to enable developing countries without pharmaceutical manufacturing capabilities to import generic drugs manufactured in other countries. For example, ACT UP Paris noted that 'the majority of people with AIDS ... live in countries where there is no sufficient drug-production capacity', which meant countries like Brazil and India should have been free to export generics to countries such as Zambia and Malawi (ACT UP Paris 2001). Nevertheless, trade policy and legal scholar Ellen 't Hoen has characterized the declaration as having 'signalled a sea change in thinking about patents and medicines' and having been at 'the root of a cascade of activities aimed at reformulating intellectual property protection as a social policy tool for the benefit of society as a whole' (2009, p. xvi). In particular, in the post-Doha period, between 2001 and 2007, 52 developing countries and least developed countries issued compulsory licences to make generics, took advantage of government-use provisions or did not enforce pharmaceutical patents ('t Hoen 2009, p. xvi). Another tactic was added to these Doha-enabled measures when the TAC used South African anti-trust law to force patent-holding pharmaceutical companies to negotiate voluntary licences in return for reasonable royalties (discussed in Chapter 6).

Another, generally positive development in the period was that the new Global Fund to Fight AIDS, Tuberculosis and Malaria came into existence in January 2002. The Global Fund was independent of the United Nations, but worked in close collaboration with some of its agencies, including the World Bank. It financed evidence-based AIDS, tuberculosis and malaria programmes. All proposals which were sent to the Global Fund were assessed in terms of public health and medical criteria by experts who belonged to an independent Technical Review Panel (TRP).

The Global Fund was governed by a Board which was notably multisectoral – it included representatives from donor and recipient governments, NGOs (including organizations representing people living with the three diseases), corporations and foundations. While UN agencies were represented on the Global Fund's Board, they did not have any voting rights. All lower-income and lower-middle-income countries, as defined by the World Bank, were eligible to apply for Global Fund monies – this meant that South Africa was eligible to apply for its grants. Each country was asked to designate a Country Coordinating Mechanism (CCM), which included all key stakeholders in programmes around the three diseases. These CCMs decided upon who the 'Principal Recipients' would be for proposals they submitted to the Global Fund – that is, who in their country could apply for its money. The Global Fund's secretariat managed its grants and implemented policies as set by its board. Accounting firms, or 'Local Funding Agents' (LFAs), conducted annual audits to ensure that Global Fund monies were being correctly spent and that selected programmes were delivering on their targets. The World Bank managed the Global Fund's money according to the secretariat's specifications. The Global Fund's board approved its first round of grants in April 2002. In July 2002, it appointed Richard Feachem, a seasoned British scholar of global health, as its founding Executive Director.

Political scientists Amy Barnes and Garrett Wallace Brown have usefully characterized the Global Fund as fashioned to avoid 'politicization', that is, to prevent the development of situations where decisions were purely determined by powerful and wealthy actors (2011, pp. 53–4). They quote a 2005 PBS Frontline (American TV current affairs show) interview with Feachem where he argued that in contrast to the UN it was 'a very apolitical organization' by design (2011, p. 53). Wealthy countries such as Japan, those in the European Union and the United States had pushed hard at UNGASS for the Global Fund to be independent of the UN and managed by multiple sectors. In this context, the Global Fund's designers in its Transitional Working Group hoped that the financing mechanism would avoid perceptions of a lack of representativeness, efficiency and effectiveness, and corresponding deficits in its legitimacy. The Global Fund's designers envisaged that it would avoid these pitfalls by being independent of the UN, multisectoral and through assessing proposals using solely technical criteria.

It is, however, important to avoid overstating the extent to which the Global Fund was actually financed in this period. At the time of its founding, it had only obtained US$2 billion in pledges, half of which would be available in its first year (*The New York Times*, 13 February 2002). The United States had only pledged US$500 million to the Global Fund, a fifth of which would be available in the financing mechanism's first year (2001). Donor pledges received for the Global Fund by mid-February 2002 had fallen far short of the US$7 billion a year which UN Secretary-General Kofi Annan had requested. By contrast, Paul Zeitz of the Global AIDS Alliance reiterated

Sachs and Attaran's call for US$10 billion a year to be donated to the Fund because the virus which caused AIDS was 'outpacing the response' to it (*The New York Times* 13 February 2002).

The global fund's first dispute about a South African proposal

While Achmat's Barcelona address mentioned the need for the Global Fund to be given 'all the money' it needed, one thing it did not mention was its first major controversy – over a South African grant. A mere six months into the fund's existence, the South African government refused to allow the KwaZulu-Natal (KZN) provincial administration to accept a US$72 million five-year grant which had been allocated to it by the Global Fund, which was supplemental to the US$93 million which had been awarded to the country as a whole (*Business Day* 11 April 2003). As we have seen, KZN was a region which had been consistently found to have an exceptionally high rate of HIV infections since 1990. In the early 2000s, KZN was governed by the opposition Inkatha Freedom Party (IFP), which had already broken with the national government over the issue of Nevirapine for PMTCT.[2]

This was not the first time that foreign assistance for a roll-out of ARVs had been refused: a few months earlier in January 2002, the Thai government had offered to share free technology with their South African counterparts to enable them to manufacture 300 different generic drugs. This was an offer that the Thais claimed the South African government had declined because of 'a lack of political will' (*Mail & Guardian* 18 January 2002).

The Global Fund monies had been awarded to the Enhancing Care Initiative in KZN (ECI KZN). This consortium's formation was spearheaded by a group of medical academics based at the Nelson R. Mandela Medical School at the University of Natal. The partnership also included the provincial department of health, the Durban Chamber of Commerce and Industry and various NGOs in the province. The KZN Global Fund consortium's establishment had been supported by the Enhancing Care Initiative (ECI) led by Richard Marlink and Sophia Gruskin, two Harvard public health researchers. ECI was funded by Merck Company Foundation, a charitable arm of the multinational pharmaceutical firm (ECI 1998). As we have seen, civil society, medical academics and the corporate sector were represented on the Global Fund's board. It was, therefore, unsurprising that they chose to fund a similarly diverse public–private entity to provide combination ARV therapy to patients in the most heavily affected province of South Africa – especially in a context where the national government refused to provide ARVs for such therapy. Also, while the Global Fund preferred to allocate grants through CCMs, under certain circumstances, such as those which prevailed in South Africa, it would consider direct applications by civil society entities or provincial governments.

South Africa's Minister of Health, Manto Tshabalala-Msimang, soon expressed her fury that the KZN consortium had approached the new Global Fund for monies directly (*Financial Mail* 14 June 2002). Most controversially, for the Mbeki administration, KZN's Global Fund proposal included the provision of ARVs for use in combination drug therapy, in contrast to the other successful proposals by loveLife and Soul City, two NGOs whose work focused heavily on prevention (*The Daily News* 11 April 2003).

Umesh Lalloo – the professor of medicine who had led the province's bid – was summoned by Tshabalala-Msimang and Essop Pahad to a meeting along with the Ben Ngubane, the premier of KZN and Zweli Mkhize, the Member of the Executive Council (MEC) for Health (*Financial Mail* 14 June 2002). Tshabalala-Msimang then asked the province to retract the bid which was impossible, given that the funds had already been allocated. Thereafter, the national government consistently tried to position the South African National AIDS Council (SANAC) – chaired by Deputy President Jacob Zuma – as meeting the requirements of a CCM, worthy of managing South African Global Fund proposals. But since its formation in 2000, this body had enjoyed extremely limited credibility in the eyes of many AIDS activists and researchers in the country. Indeed, that year, Mark Heywood of the TAC had attacked SANAC in the *Sowetan* because it had excluded some of the country's top medical and public health researchers and activists campaigning for state provision of ARVs. Like many other AIDS activists, Heywood feared that the council was 'not angry enough, not informed enough, not determined enough and not representative enough' (*The Sowetan* 25 January 2000).

The TAC soon began to criticize the government for its role in delaying the disbursement of the Global Fund monies to KZN. In mid-July, in an interview from the Barcelona International AIDS Conference with the Johannesburg-based *Mail & Guardian*, the TAC's Heywood characterized the KZN Global Fund project as 'a well-thought-out proposal for prevention, care and treatment' (12 July 2002). He went on to accuse the health minister of ' "trying to block the grant" ', stated that the matter was ' "urgent" ' and demanded that the situation ' "be resolved quickly" '. The TAC also threatened legal action if the government failed to release the funds within two weeks.

The same report mentioned that Tshabalala-Msimang had engaged in 'a tense stand-off with UNAIDS director Peter Piot' the previous Sunday, where the South African health minister reportedly said that the country could control and finance its own AIDS programmes ' "without outside interference" '. The report added that she had told a journalist the day before that Nevirapine was poisoning ' "her people" '. The South African government was allegedly being criticized by senior UN representatives for its obstructionist stance in relation to HIV treatment. Perhaps most damningly, the report quoted Piot as having made comments which were obviously directed at the South African government. He apparently said that it was possible donors would be obliged to fund civil society initiatives over those which were state-led in countries where governments impeded the funding of treatment and care projects, ' "as happened under apartheid" ': withering criticism of the ruling party, an entity that had historically fought against the former, racist regime.

Later that month, Mbeki told the media that Tshabalala-Msimang had won her 'battle' for the KZN monies to be merged with those awarded to other, national proposals (*The Star* 26 July 2002). But the conflict simmered on: both activists and the Global Fund found it to be unacceptable for the province not to receive the monies which it had been duly granted to provide humanitarian assistance to people living with HIV.

AIDS activists and academics continued to address the media in this regard. Religious and academic leaders and civil society organizations issued a joint statement on the issue on 1 August 2002: in addition to the TAC and their NGO allies, this group included Njongonkulu Ndungane, the Anglican Archbishop of Cape Town; Professor Jerry Coovadia, a prominent paediatrician and AIDS specialist; and epidemiologist Quarraisha Abdool Karim. The academics and civil society leaders said that the KZN consortium's proposal was evidence-based. Moreover, the projects that the group wanted to implement could become 'a necessary part of the implementation of a treatment plan for HIV/AIDS and ... the comprehensive provision of antiretrovirals in the province and countrywide' (TAC 2002). They added that the dispute over the disbursement of the funds was 'unnecessary' and it was 'damaging South Africa's reputation with the Global Fund and the international community'. Most importantly, the delay in implementing the projects could have caused 'further unnecessary AIDS deaths and new HIV infections'. The statement ended by calling on the government to enable Global Fund monies to be released to KZN and to reconstitute the National AIDS Council as a 'legal, functioning, independent entity that truly represents the interests of people living with HIV and ... all sectors of South African society with a real interest in alleviating the HIV/AIDS epidemic'.

In a similar vein, the next day, Nathan Geffen of the TAC told the *Cape Times* that the movement objected to KZN not receiving the funds it had been awarded because it was at 'the epicentre of the epidemic' (2 August 2002). Geffen also characterized the decision not to allow the monies' release as having been 'basically an action by Aids denialists to block the funds'. When Tshabalala-Msimang met with Feachem, the Global Fund's Executive Director, in Geneva in early September, they failed to reach an agreement on the disbursement of the funds to implement the KZN proposal (*The Star* 9 September 2002).

The controversy dragged on later that month and activists perceived the government as attempting to exclude representatives of civil society, scientists and health care workers from a workshop scheduled for early October to 'restructure' the National AIDS Council (*Mail & Guardian*

27 September 2002). Both the TAC and COSATU – the main national trade union confederation – called upon the government to restructure SANAC to make it more representative. Polokgolo Ramathwala, a TAC spokesperson in Gauteng, lamented civil society's lack of knowledge about SANAC's operations. He also told the *Mail & Guardian* that ' "If we, the people who represent those living with HIV are excluded [from the workshop] then this means Sanac will be reviewing itself".' The confusion which reigned at SANAC even extended to the academics who had applied for the KZN grant. The University of Natal's Deputy Vice-Chancellor David Maughan Brown said that the higher education institution had been unsuccessful in trying to develop a 'dialogue' with SANAC as it was ' "unclear" ' who in the Council was ' "dealing with Global Fund applications" ' (*Mail & Guardian* 27 September 2002).

On Friday 1 November 2002, Dr. Robert Pawinski a co-leader of the provincial consortium which wrote the Global Fund proposal addressed a meeting of health workers and AIDS activists in KwaDabeka township in Durban (*Sunday Times* 3 November 2002). He told them that he expected the Global Fund monies to be released by December and that the ARV roll-out would begin in two months. He also pointed out that two-thirds of the money would go to PMTCT, home-based care and voluntary counselling and testing programmes. The Global Fund had rejected the health minister's demand that the KZN money be distributed equitably across all provinces. The consortium's plan was that KZN's roll-out of ARVs would start with infected health care workers and their families and then extended to patients with tuberculosis and other opportunistic infections.

This controversy has some interesting implications in terms of the small, but growing, literature on public–private financing mechanisms and global health governance. Simon Rushton and Owain Williams have usefully characterized the Global Fund as being a new kind of institution in global health governance, which they refer to as a 'global health partnership' (2011). They argue that because global health partnerships such as the Global Fund are run by both public and private actors, they represent a 'private turn' in the institutions managing international health, with critical implications in terms of their guiding norms and rules (2011, p. 2). They critique such institutions as having, on occasion, been guided by neoliberal economics and the interests of the wealthy and rich countries. I am not disputing their overall critique of global health partnerships, it is certainly true that private foundations and the corporations have, at times, wielded disproportionate influence over their disbursement of foreign aid, the initial exclusive funding of patent-holders' drugs by PEPFAR being a prime example (2011, p. 11).

But the KZN Global Fund debacle shows that the business and civil society sectors have at times offered important critiques and counter-models to state-led health policy-making and implementation, especially in an instance where a national government fails to develop policies based upon scientific consensuses. The debacle over the KZN proposal also demonstrates that the Global Fund could not be insulated from politics in recipient countries merely by virtue of its multisectoral management and use of technical criteria.

In making this argument, I am building upon Barnes and Brown's observation that the idea that the Global Fund can or should be 'apolitical' is fiction: health policies, whether global or national, are made in political environments. Moreover, as they have argued 'it can only be through some form of political discourse, and public-reason formation that a system of global health governance can claim to determine legitimately "who gets what, when and how?" These concerns are inherently normative political questions, as much as they are questions of technology and science' (Barnes and Brown 2011, pp. 73–4).

In an ideal world, developing countries like South Africa would not have had to choose between preventable mass death and foreign aid provided by public–private partnerships. But the South African activists resided in the real world where such neoliberal thinking dominated global health governance and so to save lives in the short term they capitalized on the resources and political opportunities which were provided by the Global Fund. Even though it was a public–private partnership, the Fund enabled counter models to irrational state-led health policies in a high HIV-prevalence setting.

Moreover, the independence of the Global Fund from the UN was not purely rhetorical, as the KZN proposal issue showed. Its board included civil society and business representatives and while individuals from UN agencies were also present at its meetings, they did not have voting rights, which meant that it did not have to be bound by the same diplomatic protocols governing the operations of bodies such as the WHO, which, as we have seen in Chapter 6, have often been circumspect about directly, publicly challenging a sovereign state's national health policies. In a sense, the Minister's complaints at the Barcelona conference that South Africa's sovereignty was being undermined were hardly surprising or disingenuous. States' power over the multisectoral institution was limited by its design, but this was deemed by the Global Fund's creators to have been necessary to encourage the private sector and rich countries to donate unprecedented sums of money to it.

The controversy over the Global Fund's KZN proposal dragged on into 2003, despite the TAC's best efforts to press for the government to release the monies to the provincial consortium. Moreover, the crisis would only be resolved when its underlying cause was eliminated – the national government's refusal to develop a plan to provide ARVs for use in chronic care (discussed in Chapter 6).

Advocacy by the TAC and its allies for increased US foreign aid

International solidarity actions in support of the TAC's demands in relation to affluent countries' governments also grew in radicalism in this period. American allies 'drowned out' US Health and Human Services Secretary Tommy Thompson's speech at the 2002 Barcelona AIDS Conference with cries of 'Shame! Shame!' and carried placards saying 'Wanted: Bush and Thompson for murder and neglect of people with AIDS' (Kaiser Network 2002). At this conference, the US government offered a US$500 million mother-to-child-transmission programme and promised to increase its contribution to the Global Fund by US$2.5 billion by 2005 if it saw 'results'. At that time, Sachs, who had by then moved to Columbia University, commented that the protests merely reflected the Bush administration's 'utter confusion' on global AIDS spending (Kaiser Network 2002).

On 9 October, the TAC also held protests at US consulates in Johannesburg and Durban demanding substantial increases in foreign aid for the Global Fund. The US was targeted because of its ability to act as a global leader on the issue – without a significant American donation to the Global Fund the South African activists feared that the future of the fund was in jeopardy and with it 'the lives of millions of poor people' (Xinhua 9 October 2002).

Influential, conservative US legislators' attitudes were, however, changing – developments which can be substantially attributed to advocacy of an entirely different political stripe. Moreover, the US$500 million the United States had allocated for PMTCT can be attributed to this shift. In this period, one of the PMTCT programme's greatest champions was Jesse Helms, a conservative Republican who chaired the US Senate's Foreign Relations Committee. As discussed in Chapter 2, Helms had previously been unsympathetic to people living with HIV (a disease he associated with homosexuals) and foreign aid, which he viewed as being ineffective. But Franklin Graham, evangelist Billy Graham's son and the president of Samaritan's Purse – a Christian charity – had convinced Helms that morally 'innocent' children were also being affected by HIV in developing countries, a framing which led him to change his position on the issue (Messac 2011, p. 18).

In the same period, Health GAP – one of the TAC's American allies – began to call for the creation of a 'Presidential AIDS Initiative', which they envisaged would provide dramatically elevated levels of foreign aid – US$2.5 billion for the 2004 financial year – to combat global AIDS, half of which would be allocated to the Global Fund and the other half to debt cancellation (Smith and Siplon 2006, p. 130). To underscore their demands, in late November 2002, the American activists demonstrated in front of the White House and delivered mock body bags representing poor people in developing countries who had died from AIDS-related illnesses, due to being unable to afford HIV treatment. Thirty-one of the protestors, including the heads of two NGOs (Africa Action and Housing Works), chained themselves together for a die-in, and they were subsequently arrested (Smith and Siplon 2006, p. 130).

Inside the White House, out of sight from the media and AIDS activists, important conversations on these issues were also taking place. African and American HIV specialist clinicians were meeting with representatives of the Bush administration to hash out a detailed plan for steep increases in US foreign aid for global AIDS. The plan would dramatically scale up the number of people living with the disease who were taking combination ARV therapy in Africa and Caribbean countries. In Bush's words, he had decided to 'make confronting the scourge of AIDS in Africa a key element of my foreign policy' (Bush 2010, p. 335). His administration was exploring setting up a new US AIDS initiative because by early 2002, he had grown resistant to financing the Global Fund because he thought that it had inadequate monies and took a long time to act (Bush 2010, p. 337).

Peter Mugyenyi, an Ugandan paediatrician and HIV clinician, was invited to one of the planning meetings at the White House by Anthony Fauci whom he had already met in Kampala. Fauci was the Director of the National Institute of Allergies and Infectious Diseases (NIAID) at the NIH and played a significant role in presenting the Bush administration with the medical and public health case for providing ARVs in high-prevalence, resource-poor settings. Mugyenyi recalled in an interview with me that he, Paul Farmer, Eric Goosby and Bill Pape were brought into the West Wing to address 'a think-tank' made up of members of the Bush administration and the visiting doctors did 'a presentation to explain why it was imperative that AIDS to be treated in Africa' (28 March 2011). Each of the visiting medical specialists demonstrated that it was feasible to provide HIV treatment in resource-poor settings: Paul Farmer and Bill Pape had done it in Haiti; Eric Goosby in Rwanda and Mugyenyi in Uganda. They set out to counter the 'prevalent view at that the time, that AIDS treatment in Africa was impossible'. In Mugyenyi's view, this was not an easy task in those days because there were sceptical 'experts' and those who took a 'hard line' on the issue and who thought that 'all that could be done was prevention and not treatment'.

On 28 January 2003, President Bush gave his annual State of the Union address on Capitol Hill. With Mugyenyi seated next to the First Lady, Laura Bush, and with both looking proudly on, half way through his speech, Bush unveiled his AIDS plan. The US president spent seven paragraphs expounding upon the devastating humanitarian impact of the global AIDS pandemic and his thoughts on America's response to it.

To illustrate the human impact of the pandemic, he raised the plight of a rural doctor in South Africa without access to HIV medicines; of hospitals where doctors and nurses routinely told patients: ' "You've got AIDS. We can't help you. Go home and die" '; words, he said, no patient should have had to have heard in 'an age of miraculous medicines' (Bush 2003). Bush then announced an important new diplomatic initiative: to meet a 'severe and urgent crisis abroad', he proposed the creation of an Emergency Plan for AIDS Relief. The US President conceived of his plan as being 'a work of mercy beyond all current international efforts to help the people of Africa'. He asked the US Congress to vote for the budgetary allocation of US$15 billion over five years for prevention and treatment programmes in 15 heavily affected African and Caribbean nations – he proposed that two-thirds of this would be 'new money'. The rest of his speech largely focused on the reasons why the United States and its allies planned to invade Iraq if its president, Saddam Hussein, failed to 'disarm'. Goals of Bush's Emergency AIDS Plan, which were later published in the media, included placing two million patients on ARV drugs, preventing seven million new HIV infections and providing 'medical and other care' to AIDS orphans and people living with the disease (*USA TODAY* 30 January 2003).

American AIDS activists and researchers were generous in their praise of Bush's announcement: even some of his greatest activist critics expressed their enthusiasm for his administration's radical increase in foreign aid to fight AIDS. Paul Davis of Health GAP who had been arrested demonstrating outside the White House two months before told the *Washington Post* that while he was disappointed that Bush had not announced further financing for the Global Fund, 'we [the activists] applaud the president for acting to address the plague of AIDS in Africa, and we are particularly encouraged by his focus on getting treatment for 2 million people' (*Washington Post* 29 January 2003). Bush's initiative was 'a significant step', and 'a credit to the president', echoed Jamie Drummond of NGO Debt AIDS Trade Africa (DATA), a group led by Bono of rock band U2 (*Washington Post* 29 January 2003). Bush's initiative later became the PEPFAR which he signed into law on 27 May as the US Leadership Against HIV/AIDS, Tuberculosis and Malaria Act of 2003.

The TAC's American allies – Health GAP and GMHC activists – had been caught totally off guard by Bush's announcement. Gregg Gonsalves, who was closely involved in collaborating with the TAC's treatment literacy ini-tiatives in South Africa and who was then working with Gay Men's Health Crisis in New York City, told me in an interview that for him PEPFAR 'just sort of came out of left-field' (19 May 2011). Gonsalves said that many of the American AIDS activists with whom he worked most closely did not play a significant role in hatching the plan because it was 'a Republican initiative, happening in the White House' and in those days the TAC-allied American activists' relationship with the Bush administra-tion was 'incredibly hostile, mutually'. This can be significantly attributed to the fact that many American AIDS activists – including Gonsalves – had backgrounds in gay rights activism, which meant that they were dia-metrically opposed to the 'abstinence-only' approach to HIV prevention, which was then favoured by the Bush administration. Instead, it came through 'another channel', which Gonsalves characterized as 'right-wing civil society'.

In neither Bush's campaign nor his first year in office did he demonstrate that he had any substantial belief in the importance of foreign aid for AIDS in Africa. Indeed, as historian of medicine Luke Messac has argued, 'For Bush, the personally resonant frame relevant to his shift on AIDS spending was his belief in God's power to forgive, and the consequent Christian duty to help heal the hurt inflicted by sinful habits', a theme which chimed with the President's own life experiences as a recovering alcoholic (2011, p. 20).

Gonsalves and Messac's interpretations also mesh well with Bush's assertion in his autobiography that he had been influenced by Bono's religious appeals to act on the issue (2010, p. 348). Messac has convincingly demonstrated that 'security' and 'economic' arguments were far less effective in influencing the former president and powerful, conservative US legislators' shift on the issue than religious assertions that global AIDS constituted a moral crisis (2011, p. 8).

But Bush's announcement of the creation of PEPFAR had not totally assuaged South African activists' criticism of US foreign policy. Marchers in the TAC's February 2003 demonstration on South Africa's parliament also passed the US consulate in Cape Town to protest against that state's 'militarism', its high defence spending and to urge it to redirect such funds to address 'real threats to global human security: poverty, environmental degradation and ill health' and provide further monies to the Global Fund (TAC 2003a).

The TAC and the consolidation of the international HIV treatment access movement

The TAC was very aware of the important role its international allies had played in helping it to accomplish its goals, as Achmat's Barcelona speech showed. The South African movement's international allies had provided valuable expressions of solidarity for its domestic campaigns (as discussed in Chapter 6). Its international allies also grew in strength and number in this period, particularly those from the global South and on the continent of Africa. South Africa's TAC was especially influential in exporting its model of encouraging openness about living with HIV to combat the stigma and discrimination related to the disease. But the TAC's leaders also perceived that it also had something to gain from strengthening these alliances, especially in terms of gaining bargaining power at African intergovernmental forums.

In an interview with the Pretoria-headquartered Medical Research Council's *AIDS Bulletin* in September 2002, South African judge Edwin Cameron, a vocal advocate for universal HIV treatment access, described the international movement as having issued 'both a simple moral statement and a call to action'.[3] He believed that such action would be 'infectious throughout Africa' and that it would have 'an international impact' and 'the sort of treatment breakthroughs on a mass scale' that people were then 'talking about'.[4] Cameron went on to equate injustices around AIDS with those of apartheid, a familiar trope in South African and global HIV treatment access advocacy. For Cameron, such AIDS activism was 'comparable to the activism that surrounded the race issue before and after the Second World War'.[5] Moreover, Cameron averred that the 'same' thing was 'happening in the AIDS debate' where the 'big shift' had been to Africa.[6]

Efforts to consolidate the international movement were ongoing in this period. For instance, the TAC played a critical role in co-founding the International Treatment Preparedness Coalition (ITPC). According to Gonsalves, the transnational Treatment Coalition's origins can be traced back to a few months before the Barcelona Conference, when Deborah Zwedie of the World Bank's AIDS Program and Piot of UNAIDS approached GMHC – a TAC ally – in New York and asked how the American NGO could assist in getting communities ready for treatment (Interview 19 May 2011). The treatment activists' thinking on how to proceed in this regard only truly developed at their further meetings at the Barcelona Conference, where they decided to convene again in the coming months to discuss how to scale up HIV treatment literacy and advocacy in affected communities in the global South.[7]

As a result of these deliberations, the TAC co-hosted the first International HIV Treatment Preparedness Summit of 125 AIDS activists from 67 countries which was held in Cape Town in March 2003 and was arranged by the South Africans, GMHC and TAG. At the conference, AIDS activists from other developing countries got to meet their South African counterparts in the TAC, which certainly consolidated its South–South international alliances. While this summit represented an important milestone in terms of the consolidation of the international HIV treatment access movement, there were also, at times, tensions between organizers from different countries. For instance, Gonsalves recalled a moment at the summit where Achmat accused two American activists of failing to 'manage' their own 'imperialism' (Interview 19 May 2011).

As we have seen, the TAC's earliest international allies were American, European, Thai and Brazilian. In late August 2003, the movement developed its international footprint further by strengthening its ties with African HIV treatment activists. This was a period in which HIV treatment activism was emerging in new countries and where activists who were still relatively new to the issues learnt about, and emulated, the TAC's model.

The TAC also hosted the founding meeting of the Pan-African HIV Treatment Access Movement (PATAM) in Cape Town from 22 to 24 August. Seventy activists from 21 African countries were in attendance. 'We are angry. Our people are dying', began the strongly worded declaration of action that the African activists produced at the meeting (PATAM 2002). They were concerned that 28 million people were living with HIV/AIDS on the continent who would 'die predictable and avoidable deaths' over the following decade, which constituted 'a crime against humanity'. The activists called on their governments, multilateral institutions, the private sector and civil society to 'intervene without delay to prevent a holocaust against the poor' on the continent and urged them to implement the WHO's goal to place 3 million on HIV treatment by 2005 (the 3 × 5 initiative). ARV therapy was 'not only an ethical imperative' but would also among other things, 'strengthen prevention efforts'. In this vein, the African activists argued that a 'successful response' to HIV had to be based upon a 'recognition' of the human rights to life, dignity, equality, freedom and access to public goods, including health care. PATAM called upon African governments to radically scale up access to ARVs.

They also urged donor countries to provide the Global Fund with their fair share (measured as a proportion of GDP) of US$10 billion and implement the Doha Declaration to enable access to generics. The donor countries were called upon to 'Immediately stop pressuring developing countries to focus primarily on prevention', use patent-holding pharmaceutical companies' drugs and 'scale-back proposals to the GFATM'. PATAM pressed multilateral institutions including relevant UN agencies and the Global Fund 'develop a strategic plan including specific targets and time-lines' to achieve the 3 × 5 goal. Africa's emerging HIV treatment movement added that the pharmaceutical industry needed to reduce the prices of drugs and cease blocking generics.

According to Friedman and Mottiar, the TAC decided to focus on developing its African ties in this period because it was especially keen to share the lessons it had learnt on civil society coalition building with activists in other African countries. The South Africans thought this to be necessary because they saw AIDS organizing in other countries on the continent as often having been limited to people living with HIV, which had rendered it politically and socially isolated. They cast the TAC as perceiving this regional network as beneficial because it enabled collective advocacy at meetings of the Southern African Development Community (SADC) and African Union (AU), a successor organization to the OAU. Indeed, such work had the potential to boost the TAC's bargaining power, by 'creating new momentum toward treatment in South Africa as well as other countries' (2005, p. 548). Moreover, such a regional focus assisted in advocacy on trade negotiations, as the Southern African Customs Union (SACU) – a regional body to which South Africa belonged – sometimes negotiated trade agreements with the EU and United States as a block (Friedman and Mottiar 2005).

HIV treatment activists in several other Southern African countries were struggling with apathy and, at times, outright suspicion among their governments in relation to rolling out ARVs. There was a strong perception among international civil servants that the South African government's problematic stance on AIDS was adversely influencing the policies of its neighbours, which also had entrenched and serious epidemics and desperately needed to roll out ARV drugs. Piot, the then Executive Director of UNAIDS, told me that in those days he was deeply concerned about South Africa's efforts to influence the SADC health ministers to be hostile towards ARVs (Interview 7 October 2011). As discussed in Chapter 6, AIDS dissident Dr. Roberto Giraldo was invited by Tshabalala-Msimang to address SADC Health Ministers in January 2003. In Piot's recollection, Tshabalala-Msimang was trying to 'undermine' any discussion of treatment access at a regional level. He attributed the relative inaction of the governments of Swaziland, Zimbabwe, Mozambique and Namibia to the negative influence of the South Africans as they followed their more powerful Southern neighbour's lead in failing to provide their people with ARVs, even as they were becoming cheaper.

Stephen Lewis, the then UN Special Envoy on AIDS in Africa, recalled that many African government officials with whom he interacted in his travels were 'resistant' to Achmat and the TAC because they were 'stirring rebellion and opposition to government policy in other countries' (Interview 26 August 2011). But, for him, that also 'showed the power of Zackie [Achmat] and the TAC: that governments were uncomfortable when, suddenly, within their environments, people who associated and indentified with the TAC, and who were HIV-positive, started demanding their rights'.

Eric Goemaere who was then the head of MSF's programme in South Africa recounted in an interview with me that when he had recently travelled within the continent and found that 'everybody knows about TAC, TAC is a model. Activists in Congo, in Lesotho, in Kenya, in Zimbabwe... everybody has met some TAC activists and everybody is proud to wear a similar t-shirt' (Interview 20 December 2010). This was doubtless critical in terms of stigma-reduction, which was, in turn, necessary to widen demand for HIV treatment. But, as Friedman and Mottiar have pointed out, while African AIDS activists in some other countries started to engage their parliamentarians on health policy in this period, the odds of them enjoying 'a productive relationship' – one which could be influence policy – depended upon 'the degree of democratisation in particular countries' (2005, p. 548). While more African countries held multiparty elections than ever before in the early 2000s, they frequently lacked press freedom, judicial independence, legal trade unions and strong traditions of civil society activism (Mbembe 1992; Mamdani 1996; Iliffe 2007; Reid 2008; Adebayo 2010). The TAC's domestic policy victories depended on democracy and rule of law, political attributes which were not in evidence in many states in the region.

It is also important to further qualify some of Friedman and Mottiar's optimism about the TAC's pan-African work by noting that it also faced many challenges. Mugyenyi observed that there was a tendency for the TAC 'and other organizations in Southern Africa to work alone' when the pandemic really needed to be tackled 'on a continental basis' (Interview 28 March 2011). Mugyenyi asserted that South African groups such as the TAC 'seemed to be more pan-African than they really were' because South Africa remained 'Africa's richest country' where many people flocked from the rest of the continent as either economic migrants or refugees or people in need of medical treatment. This meant that for him, in Africa-wide terms, 'South Africa was more than South Africa' in the post-apartheid period.

This paradox has also been succinctly described by Adekeye Adebayo – a scholar of African diplomacy – who has stated that: 'South Africa is the most pan-African and least pan-African country in Africa' (2010, p. 119). Adebayo goes on to explain that this is because it has been ruled by self-defined *African* Nationalists since 1994, many of whom spent long periods of exile in neighbouring states. However, a tragic legacy of the apartheid era has been many South Africans' ongoing characterization of their country as an extension of Europe. In the post-apartheid period, many South Africans' lack of identification with the continent as a whole has been an underlying factor behind the widespread xenophobic prejudice and discrimination against African migrants in the country. South Africa was without doubt a regional power and aspired to 'global middle power status', but the unfair labour practices of some of its corporations and its less-successful diplomatic efforts in its own backyard did not always generate goodwill among its neighbours (Adebayo 2010, p. 118). In this context, South African AIDS activists' relationships with their regional counterparts cannot be said to have been unaffected by the prevailing perceptions of the country's wider, comparatively powerful, role on the continent. In addition, all such pan-African civil society contact was impeded by the continent's sheer geographical vastness and the relative expense involved in travelling between different African countries, language barriers and poor infrastructure (especially the poor roads and Internet bandwidth in many countries).

But, the TAC doubtless made a significant and measurable contribution to the consolidation of the international HIV treatment access movement in this period. Gregg Gonsalves described it to me in the following terms: 'Do you know that you'll find HIV POSITIVE t-shirts all over the world? But more importantly, you see that it's been transformative for people' (Interview 19 May 2011). Gonsalves also said that TAC became 'the grandmothers or grandfathers, they became a catalytic force for AIDS activism in many, many, many places' partly through their role in co-founding the ITPC and PATAM.

Conclusion

South African AIDS activists were critical in catalysing what Achmat termed the 'Durban Effect' – a powerful network of scientific, civil society, diplomatic and global health financing initiatives, all aimed at providing medicines to prevent AIDS deaths among the world's poor. A mere two years after the Durban conference, a global roll-out of HIV treatment was already underway. By the Barcelona conference cheaper generic ARVs were available and the WTO's Doha Declaration further enabled their production. The new Global Fund was also offering unprecedented financial assistance to roll out HIV drugs for chronic care. The international HIV treatment access movement effectively framed a global ARV roll-out as a moral imperative. This helped to generate adequate political will in donor countries to bring initiatives to accomplish this goal to life. The visibility of South African activists like Achmat in the international movement gave credibility to the idea that there was a global medical apartheid, where poor people were being denied access to medicines. The TAC gave the international movement legitimacy in asserting this both because it represented large numbers of people living with HIV in one of the world's most affected countries, and because many of its leaders had anti-apartheid backgrounds.

But it is also important not to overstate the global political influence of the TAC and its allies in this period. The transnational activists successfully threw their weight behind the creation and financing of the Global Fund. However, the debacle of the distribution of Global Fund monies to the KZN province of South Africa showed that neither its use of technical criteria to assess proposals nor its independence and multisectoral governance structure could insulate it from the 'politicisation' of its activities. Similarly, the movement had little sway over the generation of Bush's PEPFAR initiative. Instead, Bush's initiative was shaped by elite, faith-based advocates who framed the issue in ways which chimed with the US president and many Republican legislators' conservative Christian beliefs. This demonstrates that, in certain contexts, moral frames other than human rights or those equating HIV-related discrimination with racism could prove influential in advancing social justice in relation to the global AIDS pandemic.

In the post-Durban period, the TAC also strengthened its South–South international alliances. The South African activists' model of encouraging openness about living with HIV's spread was exemplified in the transnational diffusion of its HIV-positive t-shirt. Similarly, TAC activists – who co-founded the ITPC and PATAM – networked and exchanged their experiences of domestic coalition building with allies in the global South. It is also critical to avoid over-stating the extent of such networking. Indeed, by the end of the period, African coalition building remained very much a work-in-progress owing to varying levels of democratization across the continent and negative perceptions in neighbouring countries about South Africa's role as a regional power.

Transnational HIV treatment activists faced many other challenges, but they had permanently altered the politics of global health. Achmat's speech at the Barcelona conference symbolized the global voice and reach of the South African movement. HIV treatment activists, including those in the

TAC, had consistently amplified the idea that the global AIDS pandemic was a moral crisis – one which world leaders eventually felt obliged to tackle. The provision of token sums of AIDS-related foreign aid, solely for HIV prevention, would no longer suffice. Governments in the global North were now committing unprecedented sums of foreign aid to combat global AIDS, and they were also funding HIV treatment in developing countries. New global institutions had been created to distribute this money. A multilateral trade agreement had been clarified in a way which aided generic ARV production. Seven years after scientists announced that combination ARV therapy was effective in medically managing HIV, global efforts were finally well underway to roll the drugs out to poor patients in developing countries.

Postscript: Recession and Reinventions

On World AIDS Day (1 December) 2011, Nonkosi Khumalo, the chairperson of the TAC, issued a statement on the 'crisis in global health'. Khumalo's World AIDS Day statement went out into cyberspace from London, where she was conducting a speaking tour which included an address to the All Party Parliamentary Group on HIV/AIDS at Westminster. Khumalo delivered a straightforward message to the world that day: global health needed a 'bail out' (2011). The Global Fund had just announced that it would not consider any fresh grant proposals until 2014. Spain, Italy and Ireland had all failed to give monies they had pledged to the Global Fund, forcing it to cancel its 11th round of funding. This meant that the fund could only provide money to existing programmes. Yet, Khumalo wrote, millions were still waiting for life-saving treatment in Southern Africa. For the TAC chairperson, the crisis in global health financing was a clear example of how the world's most marginalized were being 'made to pay' for the financial crisis started by the banks and hedge funds. If Germany could bail out corrupt banks, Khumalo reasoned, surely it would 'be morally and ethically right for them [the German government] to bail out the Global Fund too'. The provision of adequate financing for the Global Fund was all-the-more urgent given the findings of a new NIH-funded study, which showed that combination ARV therapy could reduce HIV transmission by 96%. in sexual relationships where only one person was living with the virus. Given this new finding, she said, universal access to ARV therapy, combined with other proven interventions, could help end AIDS 'within a generation' (2011).

Khumalo's statement can be used to highlight both the continuities and changes in the TAC's history since its first five years (post-2003). Her invitation to London was a product of the South African movement's moral authority within the international HIV treatment access movement and in wider networks of global health policy makers. As we have seen, the movement developed this moral legitimacy in its early years, and it had three main components – the TAC's success in popularizing and defending the science behind HIV treatment; its effective socio-economic rights litigation and its use of 'struggle symbolism'. Moreover, the vastly increased foreign aid for global health which Khumalo was defending could be partly, but significantly, attributed to the advocacy of the international HIV treatment access movement, which included the TAC. By the time Khumalo gave her speech in London, there had also been changes in both South Africa's political leadership and that of the TAC itself – changes that had occurred since the movement's 2003 achievement of its main initial domestic goal to force the government develop an ARV treatment roll-out plan. The TAC had only been led by women since 2008. Mbeki's time at the helm of the South African state was long gone and his successor, Jacob Zuma, had the political capital to press ahead with dramatic reforms to promote equity in the country's health system.

This postscript, written in March 2012, analyses the TAC's history since its first five years in terms of two major themes – the transnationally connected movement's ongoing articulations of the need for global health justice in an era of recession and the ways in which it can be said to have reinvented itself within South Africa, partly in response to major changes in the country's politics. Firstly, it discusses how the entire international HIV treatment access movement – including the TAC – has conducted vigorous advocacy opposing recession-era reductions in AIDS-related foreign aid and against renewed pharmaceutical industry attacks on the production of affordable generic medicines, especially in India. In the contemporary economic context, the TAC's moral capital has been as important as ever in the international HIV treatment access movement's ongoing campaigns for the maximal global extension of ARV provision. Secondly, this postscript explores the TAC's domestic political 'reinventions', in terms of its greater engagement in struggles for gender and sexual orientation equality and its more cooperative relationship with the two post-Mbeki administrations. It also discusses the implications of these developments for the movement's domestic moral and political standing.

The TAC and global health politics

The recession and global health financing

Since 2008, many countries in the global North have experienced recessions sparked by the 'credit crunch' and, more recently, the sovereign debt crises in many Eurozone countries. In November 2011, the Global Fund cancelled Round 11 of grant proposals in which it would have started releasing monies for new projects in 2012. Behind this cancellation lay the fact that, as discussed, several of the 2010 donor pledges remained unfulfilled. It also related to Italy and Spain having made no pledges for 2011–2013 and Denmark's reduction of its pledge for 2011–2013 (Global Fund Observer 2011). US President Barack Obama and his Secretary of State Hillary Clinton recently announced that the main aim of their government's AIDS policy is the end of the global pandemic. But the Obama administration's budget request for Fiscal Year (FY) 2013 was critiqued by many American AIDS activists in MSF and Health GAP for having 'raided' PEPFAR, which he proposed to reduce by US$542.9 million to fund a 26.9% increase in monies for the Global Fund which also funds AIDS, TB and malaria programmes (to a proposed total of US$1.65 billion) (Lubinski 2012; *TB Online* 2012). Moreover, this may not necessarily be the last reduction in US foreign aid for global AIDS in 2012. Since November 2010, fiscally conservative Republicans have controlled the US House of Representatives. In 2011, House Speaker John Boehner (R-OH), Senate Majority Leader Harry Reid (D-NV) and President Obama agreed to a 0.2% cut to global AIDS programmes in their budget deal (Lubinski 2011). If 2011 is anything to go by, the best probable outcome is for a bipartisan agreement to be reached in terms of the FY2013 US budget which will not make any further cuts to global health programmes, in addition to those already made.

Furthermore, emerging powers have not yet made up for many large donor countries' cuts to foreign aid for global health. At the time of writing, China is the world's second-largest economy, but it has yet to contribute substantial foreign assistance for global health. The Asian economic power-house pledged US$5 million to the Global Fund in 2012, compared to the American pledge of US$1.05 billion, Germany's US$263.6 million and the United Kingdom's US$237.7 million (Global Fund 2012).

South Africa remains a middle-income country better able to weather the downturn in global health financing than many of its poorer neighbours; however, it will still require foreign aid to combat AIDS for some time to come. Many African countries are still not spending the 15% on health that they pledged at the Abuja summit in 2001 (mentioned in Chapter 7). South Africa, for instance, only allocated 11.5% for health in its 'first R1 trillion budget' for 2012/13 (*The Sowetan* 22 February 2012).[1] A recent economic study projecting the long-term costs of South Africa's public-sector ARV roll-out argued that 'external support from sources including PEPFAR, the Global Fund and others will [still] be needed to fill the gaps in domestic funding' (aids2031 2010, p. 9). In the past few years, the global health financing crisis has also adversely affected groups like the TAC, which has faced large budgetary deficits, and its further future negative impacts AIDS NGO-funding remain uncertain (SAPA 30 November 2008; *The Star* 11 March 2012).

As we have seen, when the international HIV treatment access movement – including the TAC – first called for universal access to combination ARV therapy, the dominant 'development consensus' among donors was that such demands were not 'cost-effective' and, therefore, not justifiable from a utilitarian standpoint. In recent years, and since the onset of the 'age of austerity', these ideas have experienced a revival in academia and among international health civil servants based in the global North. This is a development which is difficult to analyse in isolation from renewed calls from centre-right parties in Europe and in the United States for fiscal austerity measures. From 2008, health economist Mead Over of the Centre for Global Development (CGD), a think-tank which comprised many former World Bank economists, expressed his fears that a new global 'entitlement' had been created to US-funded HIV treatment, which, he held, could jeopardize the donor country's health-related foreign aid for other diseases (2008). Instead of universal access to HIV treatment, Over called for limited access to donor-funded ARVs and for a renewed focus on prevention.

Ezekiel Emanuel – the Chair of the NIH Clinical Centre's Department of Bioethics and a Special Advisor to the Director of the Office of Management and Budget in the White House – became the focus of intense criticism by American AIDS activists in 2010. Like Over, Emanuel suggested that funding HIV treatment in developing countries was not cost-effective and that too much money had gone to PEPFAR (Denny and Emanuel 2008; Gonsalves 2010). Instead, Emanuel called for the monies to be redirected to deal with respiratory and diarrhoeal diseases and maternal and child health (Denny and Emanuel 2008). Emanuel went back to his job at the NIH in January 2011.

The false dichotomy between HIV prevention and treatment was only definitively laid to rest in May 2011, when the dramatic results of the NIH-funded HPTN 052 study alluded to by Khumalo were released. This study found a substantial reduction in HIV transmission in sero-discordant couples where the partner living with the virus was taking combination ARV therapy. To date, many existing cost-effectiveness studies have only focused on the benefits of combination ARV therapy for patients themselves and have not taken into account this new finding that it also has a population-wide benefit in terms of preventing new cases of the disease (Nosyk and Montaner 2012). Science has determined that HIV treatment *is* prevention. While the economic implications of this finding have yet to be fully articulated – in addition to being socially unjust – it is now also scientifically illogical for economists to describe combination anti-retroviral therapy as less cost-effective than 'prevention'.

Despite a more compelling scientific rationale than ever before for universal access to ARVs, foreign aid for such programmes continued to decline in 2011 with dire humanitarian implications, especially in Southern Africa. Swaziland, a state neighbouring South Africa, is one of several African countries which have struggled to deal with the recession-era cuts to global health aid. The Kingdom of Swaziland has the highest HIV prevalence rate in the world (UNAIDS 2010, p. 28). Since 2008, the country's government has experienced a serious fiscal crisis, which is partly due to declining revenue from the Southern African Customs Union (SACU). The Southern African country's government chose not to apply for aid for ARV drugs in the Global Fund's Round 10 of grant disbursements and, as we have seen, the international aid body refused to accept new proposals in Round 11

(IRIN 15 November 2011). Swaziland's drug stocks grew perilously low in 2011 and MSF and the Swaziland Network of People Living with AIDS continued to fear that a similar crisis could develop in 2012 (IRIN 15 November 2011; *Mail & Guardian* 27 February 2012). Unfortunately, the inadequate financing of HIV treatment programmes in such heavily affected countries continues even in an era when their expansion could end the global AIDS pandemic within decades.

The new politics of patents

In recent years, multinational pharmaceutical companies have continued to launch litigation redolent of the Medicines Act case and to influence US and EU bilateral free trade negotiations in ways which have blocked generic competition. Since 2006, Swiss pharmaceutical firm Novartis has pursued various court cases against the Indian government aimed at forcing it to alter its Patents (Amendment) Act of 2005. Most controversially, for the Swiss corporation, the legislation contains provisions aimed at curtailing a practice industry critics refer to as 'evergreening' (t'Hoen 2009, p. 57). A pharmaceutical company is accused of evergreening when it tries to extend the life of a patent on a drug on a frivolous basis, that is, in cases where it has created a slightly different chemical form of a drug about to come off-patent, or where no new knowledge has been obtained in relation the drug's efficacy or fundamental properties.

The dispute can be traced back to 2005, when the Indian government passed a new Patent Act, in order to harmonize its intellectual property laws with the WTO's TRIPS agreement. Once this Patent Act had been passed, India's parliament quickly amended it to limit patentability criteria in order to prevent evergreening. According to Kapczynski this was following 'pressure from local industry [which mostly consisted of generic firms] and activists' and was aimed at leaving 'substantial scope for competition in the pharmaceutical sector' (2009, p. 1616).

Novartis first embarked upon litigation against the Indian government when it refused to grant a patent for cancer drug Glivec (marketed in the United States as Gleevec) on the grounds that it was salt form of a drug that already existed. The Swiss company's litigation has aimed to have the controversial anti-evergreening section (3d) of the amended Patent Act struck down. At the time of writing, this litigation was still ongoing as Novartis has launched numerous appeals all the way up to India's Supreme Court. The stakes are extremely high in the case as India is the 'pharmacy of the developing world': indeed, Indian generics constitute 80% of donor-funded ARVs which are provided in low- and middle-income countries (Waning et al. 2010). Groups such as the TAC, Oxfam, ACT UP Basel and Paris, Health GAP, ITPC and MSF have joined the Asia Pacific Network of People living with HIV (APN Plus) and Indian groups such as the Lawyers' Collective in calling upon Novartis to drop their case. The transnational activism around the case has included two Internet petitions. AIDS activists have also protested in New Delhi, Mumbai, outside company's shareholder meeting in Basel, Switzerland and at its corporate headquarters in New York and in Washington DC and Cambridge, MA.

This corporate litigation to prevent the production of generic cancer drugs has come at a time when the WHO and UN have been increasingly focused upon 'Non-Communicable Diseases' (NCDs). The term NCDs refers to non-infectious and chronic diseases such as cancer. In September 2011, the UN held its first High Level Meeting on NCDs in New York. The global history of AIDS suggests the generic medicines will prove crucial in widening access to treatment for NCDs. For the foreseeable future it is, however, probable that the patent-holding pharmaceutical companies will continue to litigate to delay the production of generic NCD medicines in middle-income countries.

Demand for affordable medicines for NCDs can only grow as the number of cases of these diseases continues to rise in the developing world.[2] Moreover, the Novartis case has indicated the willingness of AIDS activists to also challenge inflated drug prices for such non-infectious chronic diseases. It is still early days, but AIDS activists may be watering the green shoots of advocacy networks which could develop into a new global NCD treatment access movement.

In addition to litigation, patent-holding pharmaceutical companies have also used bilateral trade negotiations to advance their interests. At the time of writing, the EU was negotiating a Free Trade Agreement (FTA) with the Indian government. According to the MSF and its allies, leaked text from the FTA negotiations in 2009 indicated that the EU has pressed for the inclusion of clauses that would reduce access to generic medicines. One of the EU's proposed clauses would enable exports of generic medicines to be blocked at India's ports. Another would enforce data exclusivity, that is, the secrecy of clinic trials' data to delay registration of generic medicines (Donttradeourlivesaway 2011; MSF 2012).

In recent years, MSF has also critiqued the US Trade Representative's continued use of the Special 301 Trade Watch list (mentioned in Chapter 5) to block generic competition. MSF has been especially critical of the list's deployment to press developing countries to adopt data exclusivity and change their patentability criteria to in ways more favourable to patent holders (2011). In a wider sense, as Amy Kapczynski has observed, developing countries' abilities to capitalize on the Doha Declaration have been constrained 'by resource disparities, transnational legal culture, and the persistent threat of unilateral retaliation' (2009, p. 1631). This has meant that in the post-Doha period, access-to-medicines activists have still had to fight trade-related battles on a country-by-country basis: developments which suggest that the WTO may no longer be such an important theatre in their struggle for affordable drugs.

A different civil society approach emerged in a new non-profit entity called the Medicines Patent Pool (MPP) which was formed in December 2009 – this new initiative provides a one-stop shop which makes it easier for patent holders to issue voluntary licences for AIDS drugs to generic drug producers in developing countries. The NIH and Gilead (an American pharmaceutical firm) have already 'jumped in' to the pool (MPP 2011). Recently, activists with strong ties to MPP and MSF have called upon Johnson & Johnson (another American company) to license two of its AIDS drugs, darunavir and etravirine, into the pool. But at the time of writing, the MPP is still a new entity and its deal with Gilead has been criticized by the ITPC for having been reached with limited input from people living with HIV and affected 'communities', enabling the MPP to receive a proportion of Gilead's royalties, and, for excluding middle-income countries (2011). The history of South African AIDS activism recounted in this book points to the importance of amplifying the voices of affected patients from developing countries in civil society advocacy for cheaper medicines. Hopefully, groups representing people living with HIV in developing countries will be included more meaningfully in the MPP's operations in future. This will be especially necessary in order for it to accumulate and retain adequate moral capital to pressure pharmaceutical companies to facilitate access to generic HIV medicines in low- and middle-income countries.

AIDS activism and the South African state

Conflict over the HIV treatment roll-out in South Africa, 2004–2008

In the second five years of its history (2004–2008), the TAC faced ongoing struggles to force the South African government to roll out ARVs at a pace which matched the grave extent of AIDS-related sickness and deaths in the country. As the movement remained steadfast in demanding a speedy and effective public sector ARV roll-out, it retained the moral high ground in its ongoing disputes with the government. The TAC's continuing advocacy in relation to the ARV roll-out was necessitated by the government's suboptimal implementation of the Operational Plan in most provinces, with the exception of the Western Cape (Nattrass 2007). Manto Tshabalala-Msimang, the Minister of Health, continued to sow confusion about the efficacy and safety of combination ARV therapy and instead supported a highly selective set of vegetable-based nutritional interventions and unproven vitamin-based and traditional remedies as 'alternatives' (Geffen 2010). In August 2006, the sheer irrationality of the South African government's approach to AIDS was again put on display to foreign HIV researchers and activists at the Toronto International AIDS Conference. The South African government festooned its stall at the Toronto conference with lemons, beetroots, African potatoes and garlic cloves. Angry TAC supporters and their allies from the international HIV treatment access movement subsequently 'trashed' the stall (Thom 21 August 2006; *Economist* 24 August 2006).

While the Secretaries-General of the UN and WHO remained silent on the matter of South Africa's bizarre position on AIDS, they retained subordinates who spoke out on the issue, despite pressure from the country's Health Minister, for them to be dismissed. For instance, Stephen Lewis, the UN Special Envoy on AIDS in Africa, was forthright in his public statements on the need for greater political leadership to hasten South Africa's ARV drug roll-out (Interview 26 August 2011). Dr. Jim Yong Kim, who was then the Director of the WHO's HIV/AIDS department, also spoke his mind on the issue. He told me in an interview that he viewed Mbeki's position on AIDS as having been a 'major obstacle' to the accomplishment of the 3×5 goal (to have 3 million people on HIV treatment, globally, by 2005) (Interview 21 November 2011). At the Toronto conference, Kim had shared his fears with Canadian journalists that Mbeki appeared to understand neither the science of HIV medicine, nor 'the social justice implications of treating people living with HIV'. During his time at the WHO (2004–2006) the Harvard-trained infectious disease clinician also spoke to journalists at South African newspapers, informing them that beetroot and garlic were ineffective in treating HIV, even when eaten together: people living with HIV rather needed to take combination ARV therapy, as prescribed.

There were, however, also those within government who were critical of Tshabalala-Msimang and Mbeki's approaches to AIDS from 2003 to 2008. One of these dissenters was Nozizwe Madlala-Routledge who was appointed Deputy Minister of Health after the 2004 election. For a brief period from October 2006 to June 2007 when the Minister of Health was ill with liver and lung diseases, Madlala-Routledge played a more prominent role in the ministry which she used to publicly espouse scientifically mainstream views on AIDS. In this period, she also played a leadership role in negotiations for the 2007–2011 National Strategic Plan – which contained ambitious and clear targets for the widening of ARV treatment access. She was also pivotal in relaunching the South African National AIDS Council (SANAC), which became more representative of civil society. Perhaps most symbolic of this shift was the election of the TAC's Mark Heywood as Deputy Chairperson of SANAC in May 2007. Madlala-Routledge was, however, controversially fired by President Mbeki in August 2007. But tectonic plates were shifting within the ANC itself. As 2007 wore on, Mbeki grew increasingly politically weak because of his contest with Jacob Zuma for the leadership of the ANC – a contest which he dramatically lost at the party's Polokwane Conference. Following Judge Nicholson's ruling that there had been politically motivated, executive interference in the corruption investigations conducted by the National Prosecuting Authority (NPA) against the former Deputy President (Zuma), a broad coalition of Zuma's allies in the party conspired to force Mbeki to resign as South Africa's head of state in September 2008.

Kgalema Motlanthe, the country's 'caretaker' President, then appointed Barbara Hogan as his Health Minister in September 2008. Hogan clearly endorsed the mainstream science around AIDS and, thereby, signalled a departure from her predecessor's pseudo-scientific approach to AIDS policy (2008). When Jacob Zuma was elected as President of South Africa in 2009, he appointed Aaron Motsoaledi as his Minister of Health. The new Minister – a graduate of the Natal Medical School – also adhered to the scientific consensus when making AIDS policy.

The resurgent politics of gender and sexuality in AIDS activism

In recent years, as the TAC's initial demands have been met, feminists and gay rights activists have been more energetic in asserting their interests and needs within the movement. This trend has led to greater HIV services for men who have sex with men (MSM) in some areas of the country, and the TAC is now led by women. Gay rights and feminist AIDS activists' agendas have overlapped in relation to their demands for greater government action to end violence against women, including lesbians.

Until relatively recently, the epidemiological knowledge on same-sex HIV transmission in South Africa had remained virtually static following studies conducted in late 1980s (discussed in Chapter 2). This became an issue of growing concern to AIDS activists in the mid-2000s. To address this concern, researchers such as myself and representatives from OUT, the Equality Project (a successor organization to the NCGLE), the TAC, and the Triangle Project participated in a joint activist and scholarly conference on 'Gender, same-sex sexuality and HIV/AIDS'. This conference was held by the Human Sciences Research Council in Pretoria from 9 to 11 May 2007. At the conference, it emerged that in recent years only a few small, community-based prevalence studies had been conducted by South African organizations representing Lesbians, Gay Men, Bisexuals and Transgender and Intersex persons (hereafter, LGBTI people) (Reddy et al. 2009). Activists at the conference told the Department of Health representatives present that they wanted the South African government to fund larger epidemiological studies on same-sex HIV transmission and to assist LGBTI NGOs more in their provision of HIV prevention and health services tailored to the needs of same-sex practising people.

As a consequence of pressure from gay rights activists in the Joint Working Group, the government came to see the need to do more to address the HIV-related needs of MSM, which was reflected in the 2007–2011 and 2012–2016 National Strategic Plans (NSPs). Three new clinics specializing in providing HIV services for MSM have recently been established by the Anova Health Institute's Health4Men project in the Western Cape and Gauteng provinces with funding from USAID, PEPFAR and the South African Department of Health (Rebe et al. 2011). An area where gay rights activists have experienced more limited success is in their demands for firmer governmental action in relation to a spate of homophobic hate crimes against lesbian women, one of whom was an AIDS activist.

Tragically, Gugu Dlamini (mentioned in Chapter 3) was not the last woman AIDS activist to be murdered. In 2007, lesbian and AIDS activist Sizakele Sigasa was murdered in a homophobic hate crime. Sigasa had worked with Positive Women's Network – a group founded by Prudence Mabele, which is also discussed in Chapter 3 (IOL 13 July 2007). Sigasa was among a group of LGBTI activists who were instrumental in pressing for the inclusion of targets for the provision of services for gay men in the 2007–2011 National Strategic Plan. She was murdered with her friend Salome Masooa in Meadowlands, Soweto, in July 2007. The two women's killings were hardly unique: in April 2008, Eudy Simelane, a lesbian activist and former member of *Banyana Banyana*, the national women's soccer team, was murdered in KwaThema township in Gauteng. As scholars of the phenomenon have pointed out, it is critical to frame these murders as being hate crimes, that is, as unlawful acts motivated by prejudice, based upon the victim's identity or membership of a particular social group (Nel and Judge 2008). The widespread nature of such crimes has been suggested by a community-based survey of homophobic victimization in Gauteng which found that 15% of black lesbians interviewed said they had been physically assaulted or abused and that 10% claimed to have been sexually abused or raped because of their sexual orientation in the preceding 24 months (Joint Working Group 2007, p. 2). Many homophobic hate crime victims and their families have often also experienced 'secondary victimisation' when reporting incidents to police officers who have expressed antagonism or disinterest towards them – a problem which has also led to under-reporting of hate crimes (Reid and Dirsuweit 2002, p. 107; Nel and Judge 2008, p. 28)

Lesbian activists are, sadly, not the only group of women activists who have faced gender-based violence. Furthermore, a TAC activist has also featured among the ranks of women activists who have been murdered. On 13 December 2004, Lorna Mlofana, a TAC activist in Khayalitsha, was killed. Mlofana had been in a tavern with friends and a group of men proceeded to rape her. When she disclosed that she was living with HIV they also decided to take her life.[3] In response to Mlofana's murder, the TAC developed a comprehensive advocacy campaign against violence against women (Peacock et al. 2008). This campaign raised awareness about rape in the community and applied pressure for an effective investigation of Mlofana's murder and a thorough prosecution of the suspects, who were convicted in December 2005 and sentenced in February 2006.

In addition to calling for a specific hate crimes law, activists – including those in the TAC – have called for the criminal justice sector to work harder in investigating and prosecuting those suspected of homophobic hate crimes and to deal with their victims in a more respectful manner (Reid and Dirsuweit 2002; Joint Working Group 2007; Nel and Judge 2008; Mkhize et al. 2011). At the time of writing, activism for greater government action on homophobic hate crimes against lesbians is still ongoing and several demands – such as the development of specific hate crimes legislation – remain unmet.

As Chapter 3 showed, women activists' experiences of violent victimization shaped the political history of AIDS activism. Moreover, in addition to being morally repugnant and illegal, the murder of female activists can be said to further politically disempower women as a group, in general. This is because the murder of women activists deprives the movements to which they once belonged of their political skills and experience and, ultimately, of suitable female candidates who could be nominated for leadership positions.

There had been a steady growth in feminist epidemiological research on AIDS in the country since 1992. But sexism within mixed-gender organizations has persisted as a barrier to women's exercise of leadership in AIDS-related civil society entities, including the TAC, in the post-2003 period. As Chapter 6 described, in 2003, the TAC's initial failure to deal with its own internal, organizational sexism detracted from its moral authority in the eyes of some women members. Around the same time as the movement began conducting advocacy on violence against women, female TAC activists forced the movement to adopt sustained and far-reaching political remedies for its own organizational sexism.

In the post-2003 period, feminist allies of the TAC from South African and international NGOs also began to critique the absence of women from the movement's top leadership positions. Foreign feminists' mentoring of, and engagement with, women in the TAC is another, albeit later, example of the ways in which South African activists were influenced by their participation in the international HIV treatment access movement. Activists such as Blose played a key role in such women-empowerment-focused initiatives within the movement. They were encouraged in their efforts by feminist allies from outside the TAC. Such allies included Dawn Cavanagh and Vicci Tallis (of the Gender AIDS Forum in Durban), Everjoice Win (of ActionAid in Johannesburg) and Cindy Clark (of Just Associates in Washington, DC).

According to Blose, women's limited representation in the TAC's top positions was brought into sharp focus within the movement when its national organizer Linda Mafu conducted an audit of its members showing that over 70% were female (Interview 11 July 2011). Mafu also told Janine Stephen, a journalist, that criticism she had received from feminist groups at an international conference about women's underrepresentation in the TAC's leadership motivated her further to act on the issue (2009). By 2005, I observed that feminists in transnational networks such as the Association for Women's Rights in Development (AWID) were finally becoming more vocal in championing women's rights in relation to the global AIDS pandemic. Finally, Sisonke Msimang's 2003 call for more solidarity on the issue from colleagues in the global North – referred to in Chapter 6 – was being answered. At the TAC's 2005 Congress, its women members called for more females to be elected to the movement's leadership positions, and a woman activist, Sipho Mthathi, was elected as its General Secretary. Subsequently, feminist pressure within the movement led to a 50% quota system being implemented in relation to the movement's district and provincial-level leadership positions and the launch of its 'Women in Leadership' programme.

But even as TAC women started to ascend to the movement's leadership positions, they could still not count on the support of more powerful female politicians such as the Tshabalala-Msimang, or women civil servants in the Commission for Gender Equality or Human Rights Commission. Instead, as TAC and ALP activist Marlise Richter remarked, there was still no 'blazing feminist' response to AIDS by the country's women's movement (*Mail & Guardian* 9 December 2005). As Richter questioned, could this be explained by AIDS remaining 'too political' or 'too controversial' for the South African women's movement to deal with? Or was it, as Pregs Govender learned, still extremely difficult for many of South Africa's women politicians to take independent, feminist positions in a Proportional Representation (PR) system? Especially as such a PR system meant that if such women were at odds with male party grandees they could lose their position on a party's list, the main determinant of the odds of their election to office.

In the final analysis, getting women into leadership positions, either in government or civil society, was only part of the battle for gender equality in South Africa. As Stephen has crisply commented, women's ascendency to the HIV treatment movement's top leadership positions made it 'unfair to say that TAC wasn't trying to tackle gender divides' but 'false to pretend they didn't exist' (Stephen 2009, p. 167). One such area of disagreement within the TAC was over how to deal with former Deputy President Jacob Zuma's rape trial which went from March to May 2006 (Stephen 2009). Zuma was accused of raping a lesbian HIV-positive AIDS activist and the woman who made the allegation against him was intimidated by some of his supporters during the trial. A One-in-Nine NGO coalition was formed to support the right of both Zuma's accuser and others, in general, to seek prosecution in cases where they alleged sexual assault had taken place. Furthermore, for many feminist critics, the persistence of gender tensions within the organization was also suggested by the resignations of Mthathi, Mafu and three other women from the TAC in May 2007 (Stephen 2009).

The TAC's first female chairperson – Nonkosi Khumalo – was only elected in 2008. But even though women have broken through the 'glass-ceiling' to lead the TAC, not all those outside the movement have always recognized their political authority within it. Khumalo and the movement's new female General Secretary, Vuyiseka Dubula, have become its official spokespersons. Yet, according to Stephen, some journalists seeking comment on the TAC have still remained keen to speak to Achmat – who relinquished his position as Chair in March 2008 (2009). In a similar vein, Stephen has pointed to the reality that some ANC and COSATU representatives are still more comfortable negotiating with Heywood or Achmat because 'They don't want to speak to a woman' (2009, p. 169). Moreover, women's captaincy of the mixed-gender movement has not been universally welcomed by its male members. This is unsurprising, given the persistence and prevalence of sexist attitudes within wider South African society. In this regard, Peacock et al. usefully have pointed to the ongoing need for 'more structured opportunities for men and women in the organization to discuss gender equality' (2008, p. 98).

Social justice and the South African National Health Insurance (NHI) scheme

Political debates over the right to private property versus the right to access to health care have recently arisen again in South Africa in relation to the government's proposal to introduce a National Health Insurance (NHI) scheme. As discussed above, South Africa clearly needs to mobilize additional resources to fund the public sector roll-out of ARVs and improve its overall policy response to AIDS. But the country has to do so in an environment where international development aid for AIDS is shrinking, necessitating further domestic resource mobilization. In 2010, Costs and Financing Working group of aids2031 – a group of health economists – worked closely with the South Africa Department of Health and Treasury to project some of the future fiscal challenges which may be posed by the country's public sector ARV roll-out (aids2031 2010). The health economists forecast that between 2009 and 2015/16 there would be an up to two fold increase in the resources required for South Africa's AIDS response from R16 billion to R28–35 billion (aids2031 2010, p. 6). The group concluded that the South African government, therefore, needed to develop a 'strong and effective financial mobilization strategy' and to consider introducing an NHI scheme as 'a source of expanded public funding' (aids2031 2010, p. 9).

In 2011, the government proposed that such an NHI scheme be introduced, where everyone in South Africa would have state health insurance and would, therefore, be eligible for free health care services at the point-of-delivery. As discussed in Chapter 1, proposals for a health system providing services free at the point of delivery date back to the Gluckman Commission of the early 1940s. But these proposals never came to pass post-1948 because they did not fit with apartheid ideology. Instead, the country's segregated public health system provided unequal care. Moreover, from the late 1970s, the government also promoted private sector provision of health care funded by medical aids (private health insurance schemes), a privilege mostly enjoyed by whites.

These inequalities have persisted well into the post-apartheid era. According to the government, 8.3% of South Africa's GDP was spent on health in 2010 – 4.1% in the private sector and 4.2% in the public sector. Differently put, almost half of all health spending in South Africa was by the 16.2% of the population with medical aid (private health insurance scheme) membership (Department of Health 2011, p. 9). In addition, the privileged few with such medical aid membership also enjoyed a tax break for their contributions to the private health insurance schemes, which was equal to R10.1 billion in 2005 – approximately a third of the government's health spending that year (McIntyre et al. cited in Marais 2011, p. 314).

Since 1994, the Department of Health has – as it readily acknowledges – convened numerous committees of inquiry into the issue of the need for equitable health insurance in South Africa (2011, pp. 13–15). But as Hein Marais observed, 'The [AIDS-related] debacles and fiascos that made headlines on the watch of successive health ministers also denuded them of the political capital they needed to confront the for-profit healthcare sector' (2011, p. 314). The Zuma administration has shed the health policy credibility deficit of his predecessor and former rival. This has enabled his health minister Motsoaledi to pursue the issue much more convincingly.

In August 2011, the government released a 'green paper' (draft policy discussion document) proposing to introduce an NHI scheme in South Africa. The NHI scheme would consist of a national health care financing mechanism (fund) covering the whole South African population so that they could access free health care at the point of service. Owing to the extensive scope of the reform, the government proposes it be phased in over 14 years (Department of Health 2011). Membership of the NHI would be compulsory for all in the country, but individuals would be entitled to purchase additional private health insurance if they so desired, albeit without enjoying a tax rebate for this extra cover (Department of Health 2011, p. 43). South Africa's government plans to simultaneously execute wide-ranging reforms in the management and administration of public health care services. These are necessary to ensure adequate middle-class buy-in to the reform.

There is a great deal of controversy over the putative scheme and some of the main points of contention are:

- Whether it is necessary and will address the underlying causes of the crisis in South Africa's health system.
- How much it will cost and whether the country can afford it.
- The type of tax which should be used to finance it.

Three months after the publication of the NHI green paper, Section 27 (a new NGO incorporating the AIDS Law Project) and the TAC joined civil society allies in the National Health Insurance Coalition (NHIC). This NHI Coalition praised key elements of the proposed scheme, not least its principles that the health system should enhance social solidarity, realize the right to access to services and increase equity and affordability of services (NHIC 2011, p. 2).

The new NHI coalition supported the policy's goal of raising the quality of the services provided in the public sector to match those available in the private sector. The activists were also in agreement with the proposed scrapping of tax subsidies for medical aid contributions, introduction of a mandatory health tax, its emphasis on primary health care and plans to improve the management of health information (NHIC 2011).

By contrast, one of the plan's staunchest critics has been health economist Alex van der Heever, who was previously a Central Advisor to the Council of Medical Schemes. Van der Heever's main line of critique of the Green Paper is that it does not 'provide a rational business case' for the NHI scheme (2011, p. viii). This, he claims, is because the government's green paper has overstated the increases in medical scheme membership dues and specialist costs over a seven-year period. He has added that, in his view, the NHI scheme could circumscribe economic growth by increasing the share of many middle-class people's disposable income which would be transferred to finance public health expenditure. Instead, he argues, people above the taxable threshold should be forced to take out medical aid and the schemes obliged to fund their members' utilization of public sector health services.

The South African Private Practitioner Forum, representing specialists working in the country's private sector, have similarly critiqued the NHI green paper's positing of the two-tier system as the cause of the crisis in the public sector of the health system. Instead, the specialists argue, the private sector is neither 'over-priced' nor 'unsustainable' but rather 'a national asset that should be nurtured' while the public sector is improved (2011, p. 3). They also hold that the proposal 'triggers a number of constitutional concerns', including that it would infringe upon the right to access to health care of the 'current private medical scheme population'; 'service providers' rights to property'; their right to 'freedom of trade, occupation and profession'; and, the 'freedom of association' of medical scheme members (2011, p. 5).

Much more research is required on the fiscal implications on the measure; however, opponents' arguments that the malfunctioning of the public sector of the health system has nothing to do with the functioning of its private sector are disingenuous. South Africa's private sector facilities and medical aid schemes are a fundamental pillar of inequity in the country's health system, as a whole. It is also questionable whether the specialists' arguments that their rights to private property would be infringed by the NHI scheme would hold up in a constitutional challenge on the issue. As the TAC argued in its *amicus* application in the Medicines Act case (outlined in Chapter 5) – South Africa's Constitution contains a Limitation clause (s.36), which means that any right, including that to private property, can be limited by the state as long as the infringements are 'reasonable and justifiable in an open and democratic society based on human dignity, equality and freedom' (Heywood 2001, p. 13). Furthermore, their arguments that more affluent patients' rights to 'access to health care' can only be 'progressively realized' through medical aid membership and their use of private sector facilities are certainly debatable.

Moreover, being attuned to the NHI's equity-promoting potential does not automatically mean one has to be blinkered about the challenges facing the public sector of South Africa' health system. At the time of writing, in March 2012, two provinces – Gauteng and KwaZulu-Natal – had recently delayed payments to the National Health Laboratory Services (NHLS), a company which conducted vital pathology tests, including CD4 tests and pap smears, for government health facilities (COSATU 2012; *The Daily News* 07 February 2012; TAC 2012). The NHLS had, as a consequence, for a period, closed down several of its laboratories in those provinces, with adverse effects in terms of the clinic management of HIV. In recent months, there has also been a spate of infant deaths at Baragwanath hospital, one of the country's largest public-sector, tertiary institutions. These deaths have been attributed to drastic staff shortages in the hospital's maternity ward (IOL 08 February 2012). The NHI scheme will, in all likelihood, not be a magic bullet for all of the problems at South African hospitals and clinics, but it could be used, in tandem with other measures, to promote social justice in the country's health system

Constitutional democracy and socio-economic rights litigation in South Africa

In recent years, some of the TAC founders have widened the focus of their activism to campaign for the advancement of socio-economic rights, in general. The ALP became Section 27 in May 2010, and the new organization's name referred to the clause of South Africa's Constitution dealing with socio-economic rights. Section 27's head, Mark Heywood, sat on a committee advising the Minister of Health on the proposals to introduce the new NHI scheme. Zackie Achmat went on to co-found the Social Justice Coalition (2008) and became Director of the Centre for Law and Social Justice (2009), later renamed *Ndifuna Ukwazi* (Dare to Know) (2011).

The success of the TAC's Nevirapine case – discussed in Chapter 6 – required an independent judiciary willing to order the government to set aside a policy which was irrational and unconstitutional. In that case, the movement forced the government to be accountable to poor and marginalized women and to justify its policies. Many of South Africa's neighbours are not constitutional democracies where there is rule of law: there are comparatively few African countries where judges are able to review and rule against acts of parliament or policies made by the executive branch of government.

At the time of writing, various legal commentators had accused President Zuma of having attacked constitutional democracy when he suggested that there was a need to 'review' the 'powers' of the Constitutional Court and of harbouring a desire to return South Africa's legal system to one of parliamentary sovereignty – a concept described in Chapter 4 (De Vos 2012; Pityana 2012). Fortunately, such a change to the Constitution would require the ruling party to have a 75% majority in the National Assembly, which the ANC does not have at the time of writing. But, it is legitimate to worry that some judges could, in future, give in to political pressure to deliver judgements more palatable to the executive branch of the government. To return to the example of the TAC's Nevirapine case, if the judges had been unable to rule against the policies of the former Health Minister, thousands of poor infants would have died preventable AIDS deaths. Geoff Budlender, the TAC's advocate in its Nevirapine case, has convincingly argued that the courts have often been asked to set aside policies in cases such as that where he acted for the AIDS movement, precisely because parliament has failed to provide effective oversight of executive policy making (2011). Govender's experiences trying to critique the Mbeki administration's AIDS policies during her time as a representative in the National Assembly lend credence to this critique.

Furthermore, if South Africa were to cease having an independent judiciary, it is not as though country's activists could readily fall back on international law or courts to seek accountability from the state for unjust health policies. South Africa has signed, but not ratified, the International Covenant on Economic, Social and Cultural Rights – ICESCR – which enshrines the right to health. This means that the South African government is not obliged to submit regular reports to the UN Committee on Economic, Social and Cultural Rights which monitors its implementation. But even if South Africa were to ratify the treaty, this international Committee could only make *recommendations* to the government on ways it could improve its work to progressively realize the right to health. In a context where the international system provides such weak legal sanctions when countries fail to progressively realize socio-economic rights, there is no multilateral 'Plan b' for 'cause lawyers' in the event that South Africa's judiciary becomes an adjunct of the executive branch of government. Defending South Africa's Constitution will, therefore, for the foreseeable future, remain an urgent task for South African social justice advocates.

Conclusion

In December 2011, TAC Chairperson Khumalo told the world that if donor countries gave adequate aid to the Global Fund their investments would generate 'immeasurable returns in saved human lives'. Khumalo's presence at, and statement to, the British parliamentary committee can be used to highlight important elements of the TAC's domestic political reinventions and the recession-era global challenges it faced. She was the first female chairperson of a much more gender-focused movement. Moreover, the movement she led largely endorsed the Zuma administration's proposal to introduce an NHI scheme. This TAC-supported NHI proposal entailed a monumental restructuring of health care financing and management in South Africa, which was especially pressing, given the Global Fund's dwindling resources. Her invitation to London was a product of the TAC's moral capital in both the international HIV treatment access movement and wider transnational AIDS research and policy networks.

*   *   *

On the wintery World AIDS Day in London, when I heard Khumalo give her address the British parliamentary committee on HIV/AIDS, I could only reflect, as a historian, that older challenges remained very current for transnational HIV treatment activists. Indian patent law had become the fulcrum around which transnational activist campaigns for affordable medicines turned. Given India's status as the pharmacy of the world's poor, the stakes in this fight were higher than ever before, which, generated new questions for me. Looking out of the window on that grey day, I wondered whether the activists in international HIV treatment access movement would be as effective in pressing Novartis to cease their Indian litigation, as they had been in forcing the drug companies to withdraw from suing Mandela in the past, especially in recession-era Europe?

Then, in March 2012, looking back on that afternoon as I wrote this postscript, I wondered whether the time could have been any riper for a reanalysis of the chasm between the international human rights norms enshrined in treaties, and the real, everyday functioning of the UN and the current international system? Was it not, also, still relevant for me to urge my readers to contemplate the gap between South Africa's constitutional values and the lived reality of poor, sick people in the country? Gaps which had been revealingly illuminated by the work of the TAC – a diverse group of former anti-apartheid, gay and women's rights activists from an emerging middle power; an activist group who had also crafted moral authority which they then used to challenge *both* their government's adoption of pseudo-science *and* the international dominance of neoliberal policy approaches to global health. As I contemplated the sheer scale of the unmet, global need for access to medicines, it became clear to me that the changes that the TAC demanded had yet to become internationally entrenched. Still, I could foresee a different future – one made thinkable by the emancipatory moments that the TAC had helped to catalyse. Right there, shimmering on the horizon, I could see the possibilities for a more accountable South African state, a new diplomacy, a different set of international institutions, and, ultimately, a fairer world.

Notes

Introduction: South African AIDS Activism and Global Health Justice

1. This portion of Heywood's speech is recorded in Jack Lewis's 2001 documentary film 'Patient Abuse'.
2. The Department of Health's annual antenatal clinic HIV and syphilis survey found that 22.4% of women who were tested at public facilities around the country were living with the virus (Department of Health 2000).
3. A fuller definition of 'global health' is provided on p. 17.
4. In the book, I use the term 'global North' to describe the wealthier countries to the North of the globe, such as those in North America, Western Europe and Japan. The term 'global South' is used to describe 'developing' countries in Latin and Central America, the Caribbean, Asia and Africa.
5. Many African histories have drawn on oral methods: space constraints only permit me to list those that have directly helped me think about such processes of gathering evidence.
6. A critical exception is a book chapter by Jonathan Wolff which discusses the Soobramoney and TAC cases in brief, but he neither discusses them in historical perspective nor situates the work of the South African activists within that of the international HIV treatment access movement in the manner of this book (2011).

1 Health for All? Healthworker AIDS Activism, 1982–94

1. Historical Papers, University of the Witwatersrand, NAMDA Collection, NAMDA Conference Proceedings and Publications 1985–1990 Box, M. Susser, 'Health, the State of Physical, Mental and Social Well-being', in *Proceedings: Health Priorities for the 1990s: NAMDA 7th Annual National Conference, University of Natal, Durban 13,14, 15 July 1990*, p. 20.
2. Ibid., p. 20.
3. Ibid.
4. Ibid.
5. Ibid.
6. 'The Freedom Charter Adopted at the Congress of the People, Kliptown, on 26 June 1955', http://www.anc.org.za/show.php?id=72, accessed 26 June 2012.
7. Historical Papers, University of the Witwatersrand, National Progressive Primary Health Care Collection, Funding/Finances Box, NPPHCN Letters Etc File, 'National Progressive Primary Health Care Network' (undated). One can reasonably assume it is an early document which dates from before 1991, when the NPPHCN's national AIDS programme office was formally established, as it makes no mention of the AIDS programme.
8. Historical Papers, University of the Witwatersrand, NPPHCN Collection, Discussion Papers Box, Reports File, 'National Progressive Primary Health Care Network – Southern Transvaal Region: Regional Coordinator's Report for September 1988 to September 1989', p. 3.

9. PPHC S. Tvl. Regional Coordinator's report, p. 3.

10. Historical Papers, University of the Witwatersrand, NPPHCN Collection, Funding and Finances Box, Conferences and Meetings File, 'Letter from Malcolm Steinberg to Prax dated 25 March 1989', p. 3.

11. Historical Papers, University of the Witwatersrand, National Progressive Primary Health Care Network Collection, Funding/Finances Box, PPHC Memoranda File, 'AIDS IN PROGRESSIVE PRIMARY HEALTH CARE NETWORK (PPNCN)', p. 2. This document is undated but only lists activities in 1988 and 1989, so was probably produced in 1989–90.

12. Ibid., p. 3.

13. Ibid.

14. Historical Papers, University of the Witwatersrand, NPPHCN Collection, Funding/Finances Box, NPPHCN Discussion Papers File, 'AIDS in South Africa: Experiences and Responses, August 1990: A paper prepared for the ANC presentation to Congressman McDermitt,' p. 8.

15. Historical Papers, University of the Witwatersrand, NPPHCN Collection, Funding/Finances Box, NPPHCN Minutes File, 'PPHC AIDS Working Group – S. Tvl., Sept 1990,' p. 6.

16. Iliffe has also described the country as having had a less advanced epidemic than many other African countries in this period (2006).

17. As late as 1986, Marais Malan would report in the *SAMJ* that there were no female black South African cases: (Malan 1986, p. 119).

18. Historical Papers, University of the Witwatersrand, NAMDA Collection, NEC Minutes Box 1986–91, HIV/AIDS Issue File, 'Declaration on Health in Southern Africa. Maputo, April 15, 1990', p. 1.

19. Ibid., p. 1.

20. 'Maputo Statement on HIV and AIDS in Southern Africa', in Z. Stein and A. Zwi (eds.), *Action on AIDS in Southern Africa: Maputo Conference on Health in Transition in Southern Africa April 1990* (New York, 1990), p. 137.

21. Ibid.

22. Ibid., p. 138.

23. Ibid., p. 139.

24. Ibid., p. 140.

25. Centre for Health Policy Resource Room, University of the Witwatersrand, M. Steinberg, 'NACOSA: South Africa United Against AIDS', *AIDS Bulletin*, 1, 2, December (1992), p. 12.

26. Centre for Health Policy Resource Room, University of the Witwatersrand, M. Galloway, 'Individual Focus: Addressing the Challenge of AIDS: Cheryl Carolus', AIDS Bulletin, 1, 1, August 1992 (1992), p. 5.

27. Ibid.

28. Centre for Health Policy Resource Room, University of the Witwatersrand, M. Steinberg, 'Editorial: Why an AIDS Newsletter?', *AIDS Bulletin*, 1, 1, August 1992 (1992), p. 3.

29. Ibid.

30. Steinberg, 'NACOSA', p. 12.

31. Ibid.

32. Ibid.

33. Ibid.

34. Centre for Health Policy Resource Room, University of the Witwatersrand, A. Fleming, 'Conference of the National AIDS Convention of South Africa

(NACOSA), NASREC Conference Centre, Johannesburg 23–24 October 1992-Report', p. 2.
35. Ibid., p. 2.
36. Ibid.
37. Steinberg, 'NACOSA'.
38. Fleming, 'NACOSA'.
39. 'NACOSA: South Africa United Against AIDS: A National AIDS Plan for South Africa 1994–1995', July (Sunnyside, 1994), p. 3.
40. Ibid.
41. Ibid., p. xii.
42. Ibid., p. xii.
43. Fleming, 'NACOSA', p. 2.
44. Ibid., p. 5.
45. Ibid., p. 5.
46. Steinberg, 'NACOSA'.
47. These regulations were under the Health Act 63 of 1977 and the Admissions of Persons to the Republic Act 59 of 1972. Congress of South African Trade Unions (COSATU) archives, HIV/AIDS Box, C. van Wyk, 'AIDS in the Workplace: Legal Aspects,' in ed. J. de Jongh van Arkel, *Living in AIDS Culture* (Pretoria: UNISA Press, 1991), pp. 30–1.
48. National AIDS Plan, p. 4.
49. Centre for Health Policy Resource Room, Department of Health, *Towards a National Health System: Draft for Discussion* (Pretoria: Department of Health, 1995), p. 99.

2 From Pride to Political Funeral: Gay AIDS Activism, 1990–4

1. This scrap book is now preserved at GALA. GALA, GASA, GASA/GASA 6010 Box: Media Scrap Books, 'Scrap book kept by Leon Eksteen who died in August 1986. He was the 5th Capetonian to die of AIDS.' 'Homosexual disease kills SAA Staff', *Argus,* 4 January 1983.
2. GALA, GASA, GASA/GASA 6010 Box: Media Scrap Books, 'Scrap book kept by Leon Eksteen who died in August 1986. He was the 5th Capetonian to die of AIDS', ' "Gay" plague: More victims?', *Sunday Times,* 9 January 1983.
3. GALA, GASA, GASA/GASA 6010 Box: Media Scrap Books, 'Scrap book kept by Leon Eksteen who died in August 1986. He was the 5th Capetonian to die of AIDS'.
4. GALA, Triangle Project, Box: am2974/Triangle Project C.1.1.1–2; C.1.2.1–2; C.1.3; C.1.4; C.1.5.1.–2., File C.1.5.1: Annual Reports, 'Triangle Project Annual Review 1996', p. 13.
5. Ibid.
6. Ibid.
7. 'Moffie' was a derogatory word used to describe gay men. 'Dyke' was a derogatory term used in South Africa and internationally to describe lesbian women. *Isitabane* and *ungqingili* are *isiZulu* terms which have been considered to be derogatory terms for gay people as they can also be used to describe hermaphrodites and reinforce the homophobic stereotype that all gay people are also intersex or occupy some middle-gender. The term *isitabane* has also been used in a derogatory way against lesbians.

8. GALA GASA, GASA/GASA 6010 Box, Media Scrap Books, 'Scrap Book Kept by Leon Eksteen', Leon Eksteen, Shaun Harris, 'Row brews over "moffie" posters', Unknown newspaper. GALA, GASA, GASA/GASA 6010 Box, Media Scrap Books, Vol. 8.5, 'Gays angry over blood transfusion poster', *The Citizen*, 29 January 1986, p. 15.
9. 'Triangle Project Annual Review, 1996', p. 13.
10. GALA, GASA, Gay Groups Minutes Etc Box, File A: National Gay Groups Minutes- Northern Cape, Eastern Cape, Natal Costal (Durban) and Port Elizabeth 1984– 1985, 'GASA Natal Coast: Chairman's Report 1984/85: Report of the Second AGM held on Friday 19 April 1985 at GASA Natal Coast Office 51 Williams Rd, Congella, Durban', p. 11.
11. Ibid.
12. 'Simon and I', Directed by B. P. Ditsie and N. Newman, 2002, 52 minutes.
13. GALA, Peter Tatchell Collection, AM2715, Peter Tatchell, 'Out and against Apartheid', *HIM*, No 28, p. 12.
14. Tatchell, 'Out and against Apartheid'. GALA, Triangle Project Collection, AM2974, Box B9.1.1-AIDS Consortium- Broader Community Liaison, Minutes, 'AIDS Consortium Meeting: 23rd January 1993: Minutes', p. 2.
15. GALA, 'Interview with Edwin Cameron, *Apostles*', pp. 45–6.
16. 'Interview with Edwin Cameron, *Apostles*', pp. 45–6.
17. This quote is taken from an article by Samantha Power entitled 'Letter from South Africa: The AIDS Rebel', which was published The New Yorker (19 May 2003).
18. GALA, ABIGALE, 'Constitution: Association of Bisexuals, Gays and Lesbians', p. 1.
19. ABIGALE, 'Constitution', p. 1.
20. Ibid.
21. GALA, ABIGALE, 'Strawbs: The Struggle Continues', p. 1.
22. GALA, ABIGALE, 'Mid Year Chairperson's Report', 1–3. This is obviously not an exact statistic, as it would have meant the organization had one and a half white members, but it indicates that its chairman's perception was that an overwhelming number of its members were African or Coloured.
23. This civil litigation was by means of a delictious (tortious) action.
24. GALA, Edwin Cameron Collection, Box A, File B.1: Press Clippings- Local, C. Naidoo, 'World Watches as AIDS Case Drags On', *Sunday Times*, 2 July 1993, p. 4.
25. The judgement was based on the common-law right to privacy as the case pre-dated the adoption of the Constitution of the Republic of South Africa Act 200 of 1993('the Interim Constitution') and the Final Constitution of 1996. Interview with Edwin Cameron, *Apostles*, 6. Jansen van Vuuren and Another NNO v Kruger *(675/91) [1993] ZASCA 145; 1993 (4) SA 842 (AD); [1993] 2 All SA 619 (A) (28 September 1993)*, p. 43.
26. I am referring to s.2.2 of the chapter on Fundamental Rights of the Interim Constitution of 1993 and s9.3 and s.27 of the Bill of Rights of the Final Constitution of 1996. In the case of the Interim Constitution, it only included the right to access to health care under a section on Children's Rights.
27. 'Interview with Edwin Cameron', *Apostles*, p. 29.
28. 'Interview with Edwin Cameron', *Apostles*.
29. Ibid., p. 31.
30. Centre for Health Policy (CHP) Resource Room, University of the Witwatersrand, *The AIDS Consortium Project Bulletin*, 1, August 1992, p. 1.
31. 'Interview with Edwin Cameron', *Apostles*, p. 32.
32. Ibid.

33. Ibid.
34. Ibid.
35. GALA, ABIGALE, 'ABIGALE Newsletter, No 3 March 1993', clipping from article by Mark Gevisser in the *Weekly Mail*, 5–11 March 1993, p. 1.
36. 'ABIGALE Newsletter', p. 1.
37. Ibid.
38. Ibid.
39. Ibid.
40. 'ABIGALE Newsletter, No 3 March 1993', clipping from article by Mark Gevisser in the *Weekly Mail*, 5–11 March 1993, p. 1.
41. 'ABIGALE Newsletter'.
42. GALA, Triangle Project Collection AM2974, Box B9.1.1-AIDS Consortium-Broader Community Liaison, Minutes, 'AIDS Consortium Meeting: 23rd February 1993: Minutes', p. 3; GALA, Triangle Project Collection AM2974, Box B9.1.1-AIDS Consortium- Broader Community Liaison, Minutes, 'AIDS Consortium Meeting: 23rd March 1993: Minutes', p. 10.
43. GALA, Triangle Project Collection AM2974, Box B9.1.1-AIDS Consortium-Broader Community Liaison, Minutes, 'AIDS Consortium Meeting, 28 June 1994,' Item 7: 'Advocacy and rights protection: report back from US trip,' 3.
44. GALA, Triangle Project Collection AM2974, Box B9.1.1-AIDS Consortium-Broader Community Liaison, 'Minutes, AIDS Consortium Meeting', Item 6: 'ACT-UP', p. 2
45. 'Interview with Edwin Cameron', *Apostles*, p. 56.
46. Ibid.
47. 'ABIGALE Newsletter', p. 1.
48. Ibid.
49. GALA, ABIGALE, 'Gay Rights Now!', p. 1.
50. 'Interview with Edwin Cameron', *Apostles*, p. 58.
51. Historical Papers, University of the Witwatersrand, NPPHCN, AG3176, 'Report of the National AIDS Convention of South Africa (NACOSA), NASREC, Johannesburg 23 and 24 October 1992', S. Mellors, 'What is HIV/AIDS', p. 15.

3   Women, Science and Sexism in AIDS Activism in the 1990s

1. Inquest No. KwaMashu CAS 375:12:98, p. 63; Interview with Promise Mthembu.
2. Dlamini Inquest.
3. Centre for Health Policy (CHP), Personal papers, Helen Schneider and Liz Floyd, 'HIV and AIDS in South Africa Today,' in Z. Stein and A. Zwi (eds.), *Action on AIDS in Southern Africa: Maputo Conference on Health in Transition in Southern Africa, April 1990* (New York: CHISA, 1990), p. 86.
4. CHP, Women's Health Project Archive, Manto Tshabalala, 'An overview of Some Considerations in Formulating Policy on Women's Health', Paper presented at the 1990 Maputo conference on women's health, 1.3,27, (1990) p. 2.
5. Similarly, writing during the transition era, Cherryl Walker questioned to what extent the ANC was committed to women's rights for their own sake or simply as a tool to mobilize women (1991, p. xvi).
6. SAHA, 2457 Collection – The Original SAHA Collection – I-Women's Organizations, Wits and UCT Women's Movements and Powa Box, 'Women's Charter for Effective Equality. Adopted at the National Convention convened by the Women's National Coalition, 25–27 February, 1994', p. 7.

7. Shireen Hassim's personal papers: Shireen Hassim, 'Women's health projects in South Africa: A framework for funding, Prepared for Oxfam Canada, January 1992', Unpublished, p. 6.
8. The strategy has also been critiqued by 'independent' left academics because it promoted such policies (Bond 2000; Klein 2007).
9. Promise Mthembu, 'Testimonials Project on HIV/AIDS-related Stigma and Discrimination: Young Women Living with HIV/AIDS Have Rights Too.' Available at http://www.abanet.org/AIDS/testimonials/mthembu.html, date accessed 11 November 2009.
10. Interview with Thabo Cele 25 April 2007; Interview with Jonathan Berger on 10 April 2008.

4   Science and Sexuality in the Formation of the TAC, 1994–2001

1. Historical Papers, ALP Collection, Box: I1.1-I1.4, File: I1.1: Individual file- Zackie Achmat, 'E-mail from Zackie Achmat to all NCGLE affiliates, members, allies and supporters, Re: Letter on HIV dated 27 August 1998'.
2. 'E-mail from Zackie Achmat', p. 1.
3. Ibid.
4. Ibid.
5. Ibid., p. 2.
6. The Consortium still existed at the time of writing, when it was still mentioned on its website, http://www.aidsconsortium.org.za/About.htm, date accessed 12 February 12.
7. Ibid.
8. Historical Papers, CHP, Box D-E- CHP Special Topics and Correspondence, File: D1 CHP Sarafina 2, 'Report in terms of section 8(2) of the public protector Act 23 of 1994. Report No 1 (Special Report) Investigation of the play Sarafina II', p. 3.
9. 'Investigation of the Play Sarafina 2', p. 4.
10. Ibid., p. 46.
11. Historical Papers, University of the Witwatersrand, CHP, 'Media Statement by NACOSA Co-chairs on *Sarafina 2* and the Public Protector's Report, Status: Immediate', Fax dated 8 June 96, pp. 1–2.
12. NACOSA, 'History'. Available at http://www.nacosa.org.za/Column3.php?pageID=10.
13. Historical Papers, University of the Witwatersrand, AIDS Law Project Collection AG3077, Box C3: ALP Confidentiality, File C3.2. (b), M. Colvin, 'Editorial: Should AIDS Be Notifiable?', *SAMJ*, 89, 2 (1999), p. 147.
14. Historical Papers, University of the Witwatersrand, AIDS Law Project Collection: AG3077, File A4.7(a): ALP Correspondence, 'Letter from Nkosazana Zuma to Morna Cornell dated 1998–01–21, Re: Notifiability of AIDS', p. 1.
15. Ibid.
16. Historical Papers, University of the Witwatersrand, AIDS Law Project Collection, Box C5: ALP Criminalisation of HIV, File: C5 (1): Criminalization of HIV to a sex partner 1993–9, 'South African Law Commission Discussion Paper 80: Aspects of the law relating to AIDS: The need for a statutory offence aimed at harmful HIV-related behavior (Closing date for comments: 31 March 1999)', p. 1.
17. Ibid.

18. Historical Papers, University of the Witwatersrand, ALP Collection, Box C5 (1): ALP Criminalization of HIV, File: C5 (1): Criminalization of HIV to a sex partner 1993–1999, 'E-mail from Zackie Achmat to Morna Cornell and others Re: South African Law Commission Meeting Report dated Thursday 3rd June 1999', p. 2.

19. GALA, Triangle Project Collection, Box: AM2974 Triangle Project Box C.2.5.2-C.2.2.8, File: C.2.2.5.2: NAPWA, 'NAPWA SA Statement (dated 3 October 1995)', p. 1.

20. GALA, Triangle Project Collection, Box C2.5.2-C2.2.8, File C.2.2.5.2: NAPWA, 'Letter dated 18 May 1994 from Shaun Mellors', p. 1.

21. Centre for Health Policy Resource Room, Treatment Action Campaign, 'Treatment Action Campaign – An Overview', p. 2.

22. Centre for Health Policy Resource Room, 'Treatment Action Campaign (TAC): Memorandum to Minister of Health: Dr Nkosazana Zuma (dated Friday April 30th 1999)', in, *TAC HIV &AIDS Treatment Action Campaign. A Reading Package for Treatment Action Campaign Volunteers HIV/AIDS: An Activists Guide to Treatment Rights and Literacy. Building a Movement to secure the rights to dignity and access to treatment for people with HIV and AIDS*, p. 7

23. CHP Collection, Box B1–5: Centre for Health Policy, Department of Health, 'Minutes of the National AIDS Programme Meeting 21–22 April 1998, Pretoria', p. 3.

24. 'Minutes of the NAP Meeting, 21–22 April 1998', p. 3.

25. Ibid., p. 3.

26. Ibid.

27. Centre for Health Policy Resource Room, Treatment Action Campaign, 'Treatment Action Campaign – An Overview', p. 2.

28. Ibid.

29. TAC, 'The TAC – An Overview', p. 10.

30. Department of Health, 'HIV/AIDS/STD strategic plan for South Africa 2000–2005'. Available at http://www.queensu.ca/sarc/Projects/AIDS/HASplan.pdf

31. Mark Gevisser's personal papers, 'Letter from Makgoba to Mbeki, Re: Response, undated', p. 3.

32. Ibid.

33. These subsequent claims that Mankahlana died of AIDS are discussed in Nattrass (2007).

34. This is evident in footage of the demonstration in *Patient Abuse*, a 2001 Jack Lewis film.

35. This quote is taken from footage in *Patient Abuse*, a 2001 Jack Lewis film.

36. Ibid. This estimate of the size of the demonstration is taken from ACT-UP, one of the co-organizers (ACT-UP 2000).

37. This quote is taken from footage in *Patient Abuse*, a 2001 Jack Lewis film.

38. Ibid.

39. Ibid.

40. A copy of the speech is available on AIDS dissident website *Virusmyth*. I was there that evening, and it appears that the version posted on the *Virusmyth* website is both true and accurate (Mbeki 2000).

41. This quotation is taken from a recording of Cameron's speech which is in Jack Lewis's film 'Patient Abuse'.

42. Ibid.

43. I am grateful to archivists at the Mandela Foundation for bringing this speech to my attention: N. Mandela, 'Closing address by former President Nelson Mandela,

XIII International AIDS Conference: 14 July 2000, Durban, South Africa', www. actupny.org/reports/durban-mandela, date accessed 13 Feburary 2012.

44. For a refutation of this impression of Mbeki having stumbled across AIDS dissidence on the internet see Myburgh (2007).

45. As late as 2007, it was estimated that over 80% of South Africans had never accessed the Internet (Manta 2007).

5   'Pharma' v Mandela: South African Moral Capital in a Global Movement, 1998–2001

1. 'Pharma' is the acronym for Pharmaceutical Research and Manufacturers of America but it is also used colloquially to refer to the industry in general both in the United States and South Africa.

2. E-mail from James Love to pen-l Progressive Economics List dated 6 March 2001, 'Re: Report on Court Case Over South Africa's Medicines Act', http://www. mail-archive.com/pen-l@galaxy.csuchico.edu/msg53638.html, date accessed 1 September 2010.

3. Love, 'Report on Court Case', p. 6.

4. Love, 'Report on Court Case'.

5. Love, 'Report on Court Case'.

6. TAC Records, Box 15 of 87: A5: AIDS Organizations, File A5.3: AIDS Consortium, 'AIDS Consortium Meeting Minutes 20 April 1999'.

7. Historical Papers, TAC Records, Box 15 of 87: A5 AIDS Organizations, File A5.3: AIDS Consortium, 'Letter from NAPWA-TAC to Brian Collier, CEO, Glaxo Dated April 22, 1999', p. 1.

8. 'Letter from NAPWA-TAC', p. 1.

9. 'Letter from NAPWA-TAC', p. 2.

10. Andrew Natsios famously said that Africans 'don't know what Western time is' and that if asked to take drugs at a particular time they 'do not know what you are talking about'. Quoted in 'Shame on Mr Natsios, Hon. Janice D. Shakowsky of Illinois in the House of Representatives', Wednesday, 20 June 2001, United States of America Congressional Record: Proceedings and Debates of the 107th Congress, Volume 147, Part 8 (Washington DC: United States Government Printing Office, 2001), 11275, http://www.schakowsky.house.gov/index.php?option= com_content&view=article&id=196&catid=17:2001-press-releases&Itemid=35, date accessed 1 September 2010.

11. As described in his autobiography (Obama 2004).

12. TAC, 'TAC – An Overview.'

13. TAC, 'HIV/AIDS: An Activists' Guide', p. 117.

14. TAC, 'HIV/AIDS: An Activists' Guide', p. 118.

15. TAC, 'HIV/AIDS: An Activists' Guide', p. 118.

16. TAC, 'TAC – An Overview', p. 10.

17. TAC, 'TAC – An Overview', p. 11.

18. TAC, 'TAC – An Overview,' p. 11.

19. TAC, 'TAC – An Overview', p. 11.

20. TAC, 'TAC – An Overview', p. 11.

21. TAC, 'TAC – An Overview', p. 11.

22. TAC, 'TAC – An Overview'.

23. TAC, 'TAC – An Overview', p. 11.
24. TAC, 'TAC – An Overview', p. 12.
25. Figure 2, reverse image (page 2).
26. Figure 2, reverse image (page 2).
27. Figure 2, reverse image (page 2).
28. TAC, 'TAC – An Overview', p. 11.
29. TAC, 'TAC – An Overview', p. 13.
30. This argument is based upon S.36 of the Final Constitution's Bill of Rights dealing with the 'Limitation of Rights'.
31. 'Theodora Steele, Replying Affidavit in TAC's Application to Be Admitted As an Amicus Curiae, 01/03/2001', p. 11.
32. James Love, 'Affidavit in the Matter Between the PMA, the President of South Africa and Others and TAC dated April 2001', p. 10.
33. Love, 'Affidavit', p. 10.
34. Love, 'Affidavit', p. 10.
35. Love, 'Affidavit', p. 13. Love refuted elements of the following study: (DiMasi et al. 1991).
36. Love, 'Affidavit', p. 13.
37. Love, 'Affidavit', p. 15.
38. Love, 'Affidavit', p. 20.
39. Love, 'Affidavit', pp. 20–1.
40. Love, 'Affidavit', p. 6.
41. Love, 'Affidavit', p. 24.
42. Eric Goemare, 'Affidavit in the Matter Between PMA and President of South Africa dated April 2001', p. 4.
43. Love, 'Affidavit', pp. 25–6.
44. This excerpt from the programme is reproduced in the Jack Lewis's 2001 documentary *Patient Abuse*.

6   Radical Legitimacy: Rights and 'Reasonableness' in the TAC, 2001–2003

1. Busisiwe Maqungo, 'Affidavit of Busisiwe Maqungo, Submitted in Support of the Applicants', *Minister of Health & Others v Treatment Action Campaign & Others (No 2)* 2002 (5) SA 721 (CC) (S. Afr.) (August 2001) [hereinafter Maqungo Aff.]. Available at http://www.law-lib.utoronto.ca/Diana/TAC_case_study/AffidavitMAQUNGO.html, date accessed 18 August 2011.
2. Ibid.
3. Ibid.
4. Ibid.
5. Ibid.
6. Ibid.
7. Ibid.
8. Section 33 of the Constitution of the Republic of South Africa, 1996 provides for the right to fair, just and reasonable administrative action.
9. 'Treatment Action Campaign and Others v Minister of Health and Others, High Court, Transvaal Provincial Division, Judgement Date 14 December 2002, Case No: 21182/2001, Before C. Botha, Judge', *South African Law Reports* (2002), 4, BCLR 356 (T).

10. 'Treatment Action Campaign High Court Judgment', 14 December 2001.
11. Ibid.
12. This quoted section of the statement is not in square brackets and, therefore, forms part of the original 17 April statement, as indicated in the document (GCIS 2002).
13. Constitutional Court, 'Minister of Health and others v Treatment Action Campaign and others Constitutional Court Judgment 5/7/02', http://www.tac.org.za/Documents/MTCTCourtCase/ConCourtJudgmentOrderingMTCTP-5 July2002.pdf, date accessed 14 February 2012, pp. 74–6.
14. 'Treatment Action Campaign Constitutional Court Judgment', pp. 75–6.
15. Maqungo Aff.
16. Ibid.
17. Ibid.
18. In using this concept of 'recognition' they are clearly referencing the work of philosopher Nancy Fraser (2003).
19. TAC, 'Statement of Complaint in Terms of Section 49(2)(b) of the Competition Act 89 or 1998', p. 5, http://www.section27.org.za/wp-content/uploads/2010/10/TauvGSKevidenceAndLegalSubmissions.pdf, date accessed 5 August 2011.
20. TAC, 'Competition Commission Complaint', p. 5. Discussed in Flynn (2010, p. 463).
21. TAC, 'Competition Commission Complaint'.
22. ©Fred Askew, 'First New York City Vigil', http://www.actupny.org/reports/tac-2-13-03.html, date accessed 24 June 2012.
23. Health GAP, 'Support the Treatment Action Campaign,' http://www.healthgap.org/camp/tac_samp_ltr.html, date accessed 10 August 2011.
24. Clinton's efforts to reach out to Mbeki to convince him to change his views were mentioned in interviews with Stephen Lewis (Interview 26 August 2011) and Jim Yong Kim (Interview 21 November 2011).

7   'The Durban Effect': The TAC's Impact on Global Health Diplomacy and Governance, 2001–2003

1. Joao Biehl has offered a very similar account of these negotiations (2007, p. 77).
2. Technically, the IFP and ANC ruled in a coalition government in this period, but the former remained the dominant partner, especially as the premiership was still help by the IFP (Southall 2003).
3. CHP Resource Room, Michelle Galloway, 'Creating a Sense of Right', *AIDS Bulletin* (Pretoria: Medical Research Council), p. 7.
4. Ibid.
5. Ibid.
6. Ibid.
7. Ibid.

Postscript: Recession and Reinventions

1. South Africa's Finance Minister Pravin Gordhan announced that R121.9 billion would be allocated by the Treasury for health in the R1.06 trillion 2012/2013 budget.

2. According to the WHO, NCDs cause 60% of deaths globally, and 80% of NCD deaths occur in low and middle-income countries (2008, p. 9).
3. 'Siyayinqoba Beat It! 2006 Ep. 11 – Gender based violence – Lorna Mlofana', Dir. Jack Lewis, http://www.beatit.co.za/archive-people/mandla-majola, date accessed 12 August 2011.

Bibliography

Manuscript and archival sources

Historical papers, William Cullen Library, University of the Witwatersrand

AIDS Law Project Collection
Centre for Health Policy Collection
Helen Joseph Papers
National Medical and Dental Association Collection
National Progressive Primary Health Care Network Collection

South African History Archive, William Cullen Library, University of the Witwatersrand

AL2457: The Original SAHA Collection – I – Women's Organizations

Gay and Lesbian Memory in Action (GALA)

Edwin Cameron Collection
Gay Association of South Africa Collection
Simon Nkoli Collection
Association of Bisexuals, Gays and Lesbians (ABIGALE)
Triangle Project Collection

COSATU archives and resource room

HIV/AIDS Box

Activists' private records

Private Collection of Brigid Schutz held at the African Research and Education Puppetry Program.
Private Collection of Mark Gevisser held at his home in Johannesburg.
Private Collection of Shireen Hassim held at her office at the Department of Politics at the University of the Witwatersrand.
Private Collection of Warren Parker held at his home in Johannesburg.
Private Collection of Mandisa Mbali held at her home in Durban.

Research unit records

Centre for Health Policy, University of the Witwatersrand Resource Room.
Centre for Health Policy, University of the Witwatersrand, Personal Papers of Helen Schneider.
Centre for Health Policy, University of the Witwatersrand Resource Room, Women's Health Project Records.

Nelson Mandela Foundation
Speeches given by Nelson Mandela on AIDS.

Printed primary sources

(1990) 'AIDS in South Africa: Government and ANC Response', *AIDS Analysis Africa: Southern Africa Edition*, August/September 1990, 1.

(1991) 'ANC to Test its Exiles for AIDS', *AIDS Analysis Africa: Southern Africa Edition*, 2(2), August/September 1991, 4.

Abdool Karim, Q. (1998) 'Women and AIDS – the Imperative for a Gendered Prognosis and Prevention Policy', *Agenda*, 39, 15–25.

Abdool Karim, Q., S. S. Abdool Karim, B. Singh, R. Short and S. Ngxongo (1992) 'Seroprevalence of HIV Infection in Rural South Africa', *AIDS*, 6(12), 1535–9.

Abdool Karim, Q, S. S. Abdool Karim, K. Soldan and M. Zondi (1995) 'Reducing the Risk of HIV Infection among South African Sex Workers: Socioeconomic and Gender Barriers', *American Journal of Public Health*, 85(11), 1521–5.

Achmat, Z. (2002) 'Message from Zackie Achmat – Treatment Action Campaign (South Africa) to the 14th International AIDS Conference – Barcelona', www.healthgap.com/press_releases/02/071102_TAC_PS_speech_BCN.html, date accessed 11 July 2011.

ACT UP (2000) 'Treatment Access March 09/07/00', available at http://www.actupny.org/reports/durban-TAC.html, date accessed 13 February 2012.

ACT UP (2003) 'Call for Solidarity for AIDS Activists in South Africa', http://www.actupny.org/reports/tac-2-13-03.html, date accessed 10 August 2011.

ACT UP Paris (2001) 'Press Statement: WTO Declaration on TRIPS and Health: People with AIDS 1, Drug Industry 0', 15 January 2001, www.healthgap.org/press_releases/01/111501_AP_PS_Doha_decl.html, date accessed 21 July 2011.

ACT UP Paris (2003) 'Act Up-Paris zappe l'ambassade d'Afrique du Sud, 24 Avril 2003', available at www.actupparis.org/spip.php?article1099, date accessed 23 July 2011.

The AIDS Consortium (1992) 'The HIV & AIDS Charter', http://www.ac.org.za/english.htm, date accessed 20 October 2010.

ANC Health Department (1990) 'Strategies for the Control of AIDS in the African National Congress', in Z. Stein and A. Zwi (eds.) *Action on AIDS in Southern Africa: Maputo Conference on Health in Transition in Southern Africa April 1990* (New York: Committee for Health in Southern Africa), 111–19.

Anonymous (2002) 'Castro Hlongwane, Caravans, Cats, Geese, Foot & Mouth and Statistics: HIV/AIDS and the Struggle for the Humanization of the African, March 2002', http://www.virusmyth.com/aids/hiv/ancdoc.htm, date accessed 14 February 2012.

Attaran, A. and J. Sachs (2001) 'Defining and Refining International Donor Support for Combating the AIDS Pandemic', *The Lancet*, 357, 57–61.

Behforouz, H. L., P. E. Farmer, and J. S. Mukherjee (2004) 'From Directly Observed Therapy to *Accompagnateurs*: Enhancing AIDS Treatment Outcomes in Haiti and in Boston', *Clinical Infectious Diseases*, 38, 429–36.

Bezuidenhout, F., H. J. Bookes, J. Chaveau, M. Colvin, C. Conolly, P. Ditlopo, K. Kelly, J. P. Moatti, D. Anderson Loundou, W. Parker, L. Richter, C. Schwabe, O. Shisana, L. C. Simbayi, D. Stober, Y. Toefy, J. Van Zyl (2002) *Nelson Mandela/HSRC Study of HIV/AIDS: South African National HIV Prevalence,*

Behavioural Risks and Mass Media. Household survey 2002 (Cape Town: Human Sciences Research Council), http://www.hsrcpress.ac.za/product.php?productid=2009&freedownload=1, date accessed 14 February 2012.

Budlender, G. (2011) 'People's Power and the Courts, Bram Fischer Memorial Lecture', http://www.casac.org.za/?wpfb_dl=1, date accessed 9 March 2012.

Bush, G. W., (2003) 'State of the Union Address, Jan 28, 2003', http://www.washingtonpost.com/wpsrv/onpolitics/transcripts/bushtext_012803.html, 3 August 2011.

Busse, P. (2006) 'There Was an Incredible Sense of Excitement and History in the Making', in S. de Waal and A. Manion (eds.) *Pride: Protest and Celebration* (Sunnyside: Jacana), 38–9.

Cameron, E. (1994) 'Unapprehended Felons: Gays and Lesbians and the Law in South Africa', in E. Cameron and M. Gevisser (eds.) *Defiant Desire: Gay and Lesbian Lives in South Africa* (Johannesburg: Raven Press), 89–98.

Cameron, E. (2003) 'The Dead Hand of AIDS Denialism', Edward A Smith Annual Lecture at Harvard Law School's Human Rights Programme, 17 April 2003, http://ww2.aegis.org/news/dmg/2003/MG030410.html, date accessed 13 February 2012.

Cameron, E. (2005) *Witness to AIDS* (Cape Town: I.B. Tauris).

Campbell, C. (1997) 'Migrancy, Masculine Identities and AIDS: the Psychosocial Context of HIV Transmission on the South African Gold Mines', *Social Science and Medicine*, 45(2), 273–81, http://eprints.lse.ac.uk/2820/1/Migrancy,_masculinities_amd_AIDS.pdf, date accessed 10 February 2012.

CIPLA and MSF (2001) 'Joint Statement: February 23, 2001', http://lists.essential.org/pipermail/pharm-policy/2001-February/000717.html>, date accessed 2 August 2011.

Clinton Presidential Center (2003) 'Clinton Foundation Announces Agreement on Major Reduction in Price of AIDS Drugs, October 24, 2003', http://www.clintonpresidentialcenter.org/drug_announcement.html, date accessed 1 August 2011.

Colvin, M. (1999) 'Editorial: Should AIDS be Notifiable?', *South African Medical Journal*, 89(2), 147–8.

COSATU (2012) 'Outsourcing to Blame for NHLS Crisis – COSATU Gauteng, 13 February 2012', http://www.politicsweb.co.za/politicsweb/view/politicsweb/en/page71654?oid=279925&sn=Detail&pid=71654, date accessed 8 March 2012.

Coovadia, H. M. (1988) 'The Case for a National Health Service: A Framework for Discussion', in C. P. Owen (ed.) *Towards a National Health Service: Proceedings of the 1987 NAMDA Annual Conference Held at the University of the Western Cape* (Cape Town: NAMDA), 11–22.

Creamer, T. (2003) 'Deal Opens Way for Cheaper Aids Drugs in SA', *Polity*, 10 December 2003, www.polity.org.za/print-version/deal-opens-way for-cheaper-aids-drugs.-in-sa-2003-12-10 html, date accessed 7 August 2011.

Dancaster J. T. and L. A. Dancaster (1995) 'Confidentiality Concerning HIV/AIDS Status- the Implications of the Appeal Court Decision', *South African Medical Journal* 85(3), 141–4.

Department of Health (2000) 'National HIV and Syphilis Sero-Prevalence Survey of Women Attending Public Antenatal Clinics in South Africa 2000', http://www.doh.gov.za/show.php?id=632, date accessed 17 August 2011.

Department of Health (2002) 'Summary Report: National HIV and Syphilis Sero-prevalence Survey in South Africa 2002' (Pretoria: Department of Health), http://www.doh.gov.za/docs/reports/2002/hiv-syphilis.pdf, date accessed 14 February 2012.

Department of Health (2005) 'National HIV and Syphilis Antenatal Sero-prevalence Survey in South Africa 2005' (Pretoria: Department of Health), http://www.doh.gov. za/docs/reports/2005/hiv.pdf, date accessed 15 February 2012.

Department of Health (2009) *'2008 National Antenatal Sentinel HIV & Syphilis Prevalence Survey: South Africa Report, September 2009'* (Pretoria: Department of Health), 6, http://www.doh.gov.za/docs/index.html, date accessed 1 September 2010.

Department of Health (2011) 'National Health Insurance in South Africa: Policy Paper' (Pretoria: Department of Health), http://www.info.gov.za/view/ DownloadFileAction?id=148470, date accessed 3 March 2012.

De Vos, P. (2012) 'An Unambiguous Attack on Constitutional Democracy', http://constitutionallyspeaking.co.za/an-unambiguous-attack-on-constitutional-democracy/, date accessed 9 March 2012.

DiMasi, J. A., Grabowski, R. W., Lasagna, L. (1991) *Journal of Health Economics*, 10, 2, 107–42.

Donttradeourlivesaway (2011) 'Leaked Text: Draft Chapter of IP India-EFTA FTA', http://donttradeourlivesaway.wordpress.com/2011/11/25/leaked-text-draft-chapter-of-ip-of-india-efta-fta/, date accessed 9 March 2012.

Dorrington, R. D. Bourne, D. Bradshaw, R. Laubscher I. M. Timaeus (2001) *The Impact of HIV/AIDS on Adult Mortality in South Africa: Technical Report* (Cape Town: Medical Research Council), date accessed 12 February 2012, http://www.africa.upenn.edu/ Urgent_Action/apic-101501.html.

Doyle, P. (1993) 'The Demographic Impact of AIDS on the South African Population', in A. Whiteside and S. Cross (eds.) *Facing Up to AIDS: The Socio-economic Impact of AIDS in Southern Africa* (London: Palgrave Macmillan), 87–111.

Enhancing Care Initiative (ECI), (1998) 'Background and Mission', www.eci.harvard. ed/overview/index.html, date accessed 22 July 22 2011.

Fleming, A. F. (1992) 'South Africa and AIDS – Seven Years Wasted', *Current AIDS Literature* 5(11), 425–8.

G8 (2000) 'G8 Communique, Okinawa, 23 July 2000', www.g8.utoronto.ca/summit/ 2000okinawa/finalcom.htm, date accessed 21 July 2011.

Global Fund to Fight AIDS, Tuberculosis and Malaria (2012) 'Pledges', http://www. theglobalfund.org/documents/core/financial/Core_PledgesContributions_List_en/, date accessed 8 March 2012.

Global Fund Observer, (2011) 'Why the Global Fund Cancelled Round 11', Global Fund Observer, 170, 9 December 2011, http://www.aidspan.org/index.php? issue=170&article=1, 8 March 2012.

Global Tuberculosis Community Advisory Board (2012) 'PEPFAR Raided to Meet Global Fund Pledge in President Obama's Fiscal Year 2013 Budget', *TB Online*, 13 February 2012, http://www.tbonline.info/posts/2012/2/13/pepfar-raided-meet-global-fund-pledge-president-ob/, date accessed 8 March 2012.

Gonsalves, G. (2010) 'Emanuel's Neo-Malthusian Views Are Shaping Global Health Policy', http://www.housingworks.org/blogs/detail/critiquing-obamas-global-health-policy/, date accessed 9 March 2012.

Govender, P. (2007) *Love and Courage: A Story of Insubordination* (Sunnyside: Jacana).

Govender, P. (2009) 'Love, Courage, Insubordination and HIV/AIDS Denialism', in K. Cullinan and A. Thom (eds.) *The Virus, Vitamins & Vegetables: The South African HIV/AIDS Mystery* (Sunnyside: Jacana), 36–57.

Government Communication and Information System (2002) 'Lend a Hand in the Campaign of Hope Against HIV/AIDS: An Update on Cabinet's Statement of 17 April 2002 on Fighting HIV/AIDS, 9 October 2002', http://www.info.gov.za/speeches/ 2002/02101011461001.htm, date accessed 14 February 2012.

Government Communication and Information System (2003a) 'Special Cabinet Meeting Statement, 8 August 2003, Enhanced Programme Against HIV and AIDS', http://www.gcis.gov.za/media/cabinet/2003/030808.htm, date accessed 1 February 2009.

Government Communication and Information System (2003b) 'Statement of Cabinet on a Plan for Comprehensive Treatment and Care for HIV and AIDS in South Africa, 19 November 2003', http://www.info.gov.za/speeches/2003/03111916531001.htm, date accessed 1 February 2009.

Guay, L. A., P. Musoke, T. Fleming, D. Bagenda, M. Allen, C. Nakabiito, J. Sherman, P. Bakaki, C. Ducar, M. Desvve, L. Emel, M. Mirochnick, M. G. Fowler, L. Mofenson, P. Miotti, P. Dransfield, D. Bray, F. Mmiro and J. B. Jackson (1999) 'Intrapartum and Neonatal Single-dose Nevirapine Compared with Zidovudine for Prevention of Mother-to-Child transmission of HIV-1 in Kampala, Uganda: HIVNET 012 Randomised Trial', *Lancet*, 354(9181), 795–802.

Harnbridge, M. (1995) 'A Profile of the Minister of Health Dr Nkosazana Dlamini Zuma', *AIDS Analysis Africa: Southern Africa Edition*, 5(6), 3.

Harvard Faculty (Individual Members), (2001) 'Consensus Statement on Antiretroviral Treatment for AIDS in Poor Countries', www.cid.harvard.edu/cidinthenews/pr/consensus_aids_therapy.pdf, date accessed 23 June 2011.

Hassan, F. (2010) 'Re: Request for Urgent Forensic Investigation into Prima Facie Allegations of an Abuse of Public Funds', Letter dated 8 March 2004 addressed to Auditor General from AIDS Law Project on behalf of TAC', http://www.tac.org.za/, date accessed 20 October 2010.

Health GAP (2003), 'Support the Treatment Action Campaign', http://www.healthgap.org/camp/tac_samp_ltr.html, date accessed 10 August 2011.

Health GAP and TAC (2000) 'Treatment for All…Now! Global Manifesto, Durban South Africa, 9 July 2000', http://www.actupny.org/reports/durban-access.html, date accessed 28 February 2012.

Heywood, M. 'Debunking "Conglomo-talk": A Case Study of the Amicus Curiae as an Instrument for Advocacy, Investigation and Mobilisation'. Unpublished Paper presented at 'Health, Law and Human Rights: Exploring the Connections, An International, Cross-disciplinary Conference Honoring Jonathan Mann', 9 September–1 October 2001, Philadelphia, Pennsylvania, http://www.ldd.org.za/index.php?option=com_zine&view=article&id=179%3Adebunking-conglomotalk-a-case-study-of-the-amicus-curiae-as-an-instrum&Itemid=14,   date accessed 13 February 2012.

Hogan, B. (2008) 'Speech by the Minister of Health Ms Barbara Hogan at the HIV Vaccine Research Conference: Cape Town ICC; 13 October 2008', available at http://www.tac.org.za/community/node/2421, date accessed 9 March 2012.

Hudson, C. J. Saba, G. Haverkamp, G. Gray, J. McIntyre, F. Mmiro, C. H. Ndungura, H. M. Coovadia, J. Moodley, C. H. Kilewo, A. Massawe, P. Kituuka, P. Okong, H. von Briesen, J. Goodsmit, G. Biberfield, A. Grulich, G. J. Weverling, J. M. A. Lange (2002) 'Efficacy of Three Short-course Regimens of Zidovudine and Lamivudine in Preventing Early and Late Mother to Child Transmission of HIV-1 in Tanzania, South Africa and Uganda (Petra study): A Randomized, Blind, Placebo-controlled Trial', *Lancet*, 359, 1178–86.

International Treatment Preparedness Coalition (2011) 'Concerns About Process, Principles of Medicines Patent Pool and the Licence, 11 October 2011', http://www.petitionbuzz.com/petitions/mppunitaid, date accessed 9 March 2012.

IRIN (2003) 'SOUTH AFRICA: National AIDS Conference Opens', http://www.irinnews.org/printreport.aspx?reportid=45298, date accessed 14 February 2012.

IRIN (2011) 'Swaziland: Funding Fiasco Leaves Country Short of Lab Supplies', http://www.plusnews.org/PrintReport.aspx?ReportID=94209, date accessed 8 March 2012.

Joint Working Group (2007) 'Summary Report on Levels and Trends of Hate Victimisation of Lesbian, Gay, Bisexual and Transgendered (LGBT) Persons in the Gauteng, KwaZulu-Natal and Western Cape Provinces, South Africa', http://www.jwg.org.za/component/option,com_remository/Itemid,40/func,startdown/id,24/, date accessed 6 March 2012.

Kaiser Network (2002) 'United States and Africa: Protestors Make Powerful Impact During US Health Secretary's Speech', *Kaiser Network*, 10 July 2002.

Khumalo, N. (2011) 'Bail Out Global Health – Message from Nonkosi Khumalo, TAC Chairperson', http://www.tac.org.za/community/node/3215, date accessed 5 March 2012.

Lubinski, C. (2011) 'Updated: Budget Deal Takes Hit at PEPFAR and NIH', *Science Speaks: HIV and TB News*, 13 February 2012, http://sciencespeaksblog.org/2011/04/12/fiscal-year-2011-budget-deal-takes-hit-at-pepfar-and-nih/, date accessed 8 March 2012.

Lubinski, C. (2012) 'PEPFAR Raided to Meet Global Fund Pledge in President Obama's Fiscal Year 2013 Budget', *Science Speaks: HIV and TB News*, http://sciencespeaksblog.org/2012/02/13/pepfar-raided-to-meet-global-fund-pledge-in-president-obama%E2%80%99s-fiscal-year-2013/, date accessed 8 March 2012.

Makgoba, M. W. (1997) *Mokoko – The Makgoba Affair: A Reflection on Transformation* (Johannesburg: Vivlia).

Malan, M. (1986) 'Letter to Editor: AIDS in the USA and RSA – An Update', *South African Medical Journal*, 70, 119.

Mann, J. (1990) 'Global AIDS: Revolution, Paradigm and Solidarity', *AIDS*, 4 (Suppl. 1), S247–50.

Manta SEO Blog (2007) 'SA Internet Growth – Many South Africans Unaccounted For', http://www.mantaseosolutions.com/blog/2007/sa-internet-growth-many-south-africans-unaccounted-for/, date accessed 13 June 2012.

Mbeki, T. (1999) 'Address to the National Council of the Provinces, Cape Town, 28 October 1999', http://www.anc.org.za/ancdocs/history/mbeki/1999/tm1028.html, date accessed 2 March 2009.

Mbeki, T. (2000) '13th International AIDS Conference Durban, Speech of the president of South Africa at the opening session of the conference, Office of the Presidency 9 July 2000', http://www.virusmyth.com/aids/news/durbspmbeki.htm, date accessed 13 February 2012.

Medicines Patent Pool (2011) 'Current Licences', http://www.medicinespatentpool.org/LICENSING/Current-Licences, date accessed 9 March 2012.

Médicins Sans Frontierès (2012) 'EU-India Trade Deal Could Cut Medicines Lifeline for People in Developing Countries', http://www.msfaccess.org/about-us/media-room/press-releases/eu-india-trade-deal-could-cut-medicines-lifeline-people, 9 March 2012.

Milano, M. (2006) 'Persona Perspective: Zapping for Drugs', *AIDS Community Research Initiative of America*, 15(4), Fall, 12–13.

Mkhize, N, J. Bennett, V. Reddy and R. Moletsane (2011) *The Country We Want to Live in: Hate Crimes, Homophobia and the Lives of Black Lesbian South Africans* (Cape Town: HSRC Press).

Matlala, M. (1993) 'Don't Take Out Your Condom in a Taxi', *SPEAK*, 55, 33.

Mthembu, P. (1998) 'A Positive View', *Agenda*, 39(1998), 26–9.

National Health Insurance Coalition (2011) 'The Green Paper on National Health Insurance: Civil Society Discussion Document, November 2011', http://www.section27.org.za/wp-content/uploads/2011/12/NHI-Coalition-Discussion-Paper.pdf, date accessed 5 March 2012.

Nkoli, S. (2006) 'Quote from Opening Address to the People Assembled for the First Gay and Lesbian Pride March, Johannesburg, 13 October 1990', in S. de Waal and A. Manion (eds.) *Pride: Protest and Celebration* (Sunnyside: Jacana), 37.

Organization of African Unity (OAU), 'Abuja Declaration on HIV/AIDS, Tuberculosis and Other Related Infectious Diseases', http://www.uneca.org/adf2000/abuja%20declaration.htm, date accessed 4 August 2011.

Over, M. (2008) 'Prevention Failure: The Ballooning Entitlement Burden of U.S. Global Treatment Spending and What to Do About It, Center for Global Development Working Paper 144, April 2008', http://www.cgdev.org/files/15973_file_Presidential_AIDS_Policy_FINAL.pdf, date accessed 9 March 2012.

Pan-African HIV Treatment Access Movement (PATAM) (2002) 'Pan-African HIV Treatment Access Movement: Declaration of Action, 25 August 2002', http://www.tac.org.za/community/node/2480, date accessed 16 February 2012.

Panda, T. (1992) 'Gay and Proud', *SPEAK*, December 1992, 11.

Pegge, J. V. (1994) 'Living with Loss the Best Way We Know How: AIDS and Gay Men in Cape Town', in M. Gevisser and E. Cameron (eds.) *Defiant Desire: Gay and Lesbian Lives in South Africa* (New York and London: Routledge), 301–10.

Pendry, B. (1998) 'The Links Between Gender Violence and HIV/AIDS', *Agenda*, 39, 30–3.

Pityana, S. M. (2012) 'Don't Snuff Out Our Guiding Light', *Mail & Guardian*, 24 February 2012.

Plotz, D. (1999) 'Gore Promises Clintonism With a Chastity Belt', *Slate*, 16 June 1999, http://www.slate.com/id/1003019/, date accessed 1 September 2010.

Rebe, K., G. de Swardt, H. Struthers, J. A. McIntyre (2011) 'Conference Report: Top2Btm Symposium on Health Care for Men who have Sex with Men (MSM)', *Southern African Journal of HIV Medicine*, 12, 3, http://www.sajhivmed.org.za/index.php/sajhivmed/article/view/749/591, date accessed 7 March 2012.

Republic of South Africa (1993) 'Constitution of the Republic of South Africa Act 200 of 1993', http://www.info.gov.za/documents/constitution/index.htm, date accessed 20 October 2010.

Republic of South Africa (1996) 'Constitution of the Republic of South Africa, 1996', http://www.info.gov.za/documents/constitution/index.htm, date accessed 20 October 2010.

Retief, G. (1994) 'Keeping Sodom Out of the Laager: State Repression of Homosexuality in Apartheid South Africa', in M. Gevisser and E. Cameron (eds.) *Defiant Desire: Gay and Lesbian Lives in South Africa* (Johannesburg: Ravan), 99–111.

Sachs, A. (2006) 'Message from Albie Sachs, Then a Member of the ANC's National Executive Committee, in Support of Pride 1990', in S. de Waal and A. Manion (eds.) *Pride: Protest and Celebration* (Sunnyside: Jacana), 14.

Sachs, J. (2000) 'HIV Non-intervention: A Costly Option. A New Framework for Globalization Presentation at Durban International AIDS Conference', http://academiccommons.columbia.edu/catalog/ac:124089, date accessed 15 February 2012.

Safai, B., J. E. Groopman, M. Popovic, M. G. Schübach, M. G., Sarngadharan, K. Arnett, A. Sliski and R. C. Gallo (1984) 'Seroepidemiological Studies of Human T-Lymphotropic Retrovirus Type III in Acquired Immune Deficiency Syndrome', *The Lancet*, 323(8392), 1438–40.

Sawyer, E. (2002) 'An ACT UP Founder "Acts up" for Africa's Access to AIDS', in B. Shephard and R. Hayduk (eds.) *From ACT UP to the WTO* (London and New York: Verso), 92.

Schaay, N. (1992) 'The AIDS Program of the National Progressive Primary Health Care Network', *AIDS Bulletin*, 1(2), December, 1.

Schoub, B. D., A. N. Smith, S. F. Lyons, S. Johnson, D. J. Martin, G. McGillivray, G. N. Padayachee, S. Naidoo, E. L. Fisher and H. S. Hurwitz (1988) 'Epidemiological Considerations of the Present Status and Future Growth of the Acquired Immunodeficiency Syndrome Epidemic in South Africa', *South African Medical Journal*, 74, 153–7.

Shaffer, N., R. Chuachoowong, P. A. Mock, C. Bhadrakom, W. Siriwasin, N. L. Young, T. Chotpitayasunondh, S. Cheraskul, A. Roongpisunthipong, P. Chinayon, J. Karon, D. Mastro, R. J. Simonds and Bangkok Collaborative Perinatal HIV Transmission Study Group (1999) 'Short-course Zidovudine for Perinatal HIV-1 Transmission in Bangkok, Thailand: A Randomized Controlled Trial', *Lancet*, 353, 773–80.

Sher, R. (1989) 'HIV Infection in South Africa 1982–1989 – A Review', *South African Medical Journal*, 76, 314–8.

Shilts, R. (1987) *And the Band Played On: Politics, People and the AIDS Epidemic* (New York: St Martin's Press).

Smith, C. (2001) *Proud of Me: Speaking Out Against Sexual Violence and HIV* (London: Penguin).

South African Private Practitioners' Forum (2011) 'National Health Insurance in South Africa: SAPPF Submissions on the Green Paper on National Health Insurance', http://www.hsf.org.za/projects/health-reform/national-health-insurance-project-developments/nhi-useful-resources/responses-to-national-health-insurance-green-paper, date accessed 6 March 2012.

SPEAK, (1991) 'Enough is Enough: Joburg Women March to Stop Violence Against Women', *SPEAK*, 34, 11.

SPEAK, (1992) 'Educating around AIDS', *SPEAK*, 38(July 1992), 25.

SPEAK, (1993) 'I Learned the Hard Way', *SPEAK*, 38, 14.

Strebel, A. (1992) ' "There's Absolutely Nothing I Can Do, Just Believe in God": South African Women with AIDS', *Agenda*, 12, 50–62.

Tallis, V. (1992) 'Lesbians and AIDS', *Agenda*, 69–80.

Treatment Action Campaign (2001a) 'TAC Call for Global Day of Action 5 March 2001 and Generic Antiretroviral Provision', http://www.thefreelibrary.com/March+5%3a+%22Global+Day+of+Action+against+Drug+Company+Profiteering%2c%22+as+...-a070202020, date accessed 24 October 2010.

Treatment Action Campaign (2001b) 'TAC Welcomes Harvard Consensus Statement on Antiretroviral Treatment for AIDS in Poor Countries', www.tac.org.za, date accessed 1 July 2011.

Treatment Action Campaign (2002) 'Urgent Joint Statement on Global Fund Allocation to KwaZulu-Natal, 1 August 2002', http://lists.essential.org/pipermail/ip-health/2002-August/003385.htm, date accessed 22 July 2011.

Treatment Action Campaign (2003a), 'TAC Appeal for International Solidarity for March to Opening of Parliament on 14 February 2003', http://www.healthgap.org/camp/tac.html, date accessed 3 August 2011.

Treatment Action Campaign (2003b) 'Dying for Treatment: TAC Briefing Document on Civil Disobedience Campaign – March 2003', http://www.tac.org.za/Documents/CivilDisobedience/briefingdocument.htm, date accessed 14 February 2012.

Treatment Action Campaign (2003c) 'Stand Up For Our Lives!', http://www.actupny.org/reports/tac-2-13-03.html, date accessed 10 August 2011.

Treatment Action Campaign (2003d) 'TAC NEC Resolution 29 April 2003', http://www.africaaction.org/docs03/acc0304b.htm, date accessed 10 August 2011.

Treatment Action Campaign (2008) *Treatment Action Campaign Diary 2008* (Cape Town: Treatment Action Campaign).

Treatment Action Campaign (2012) 'TAC Electronic Newsletter, 10 February 2012: Gauteng Department of Health Working in Crisis Mode' (Cape Town: Treatment Action Campaign).

Treatment Action Campaign and Health Global Access Project (2000) 'Memorandum: Global Manifesto to Save 34 Million Lives: Measures Needed to Rapidly Expand Access to Essential Treatments for HIV/AIDS: Health Before Profits!', http://www.actupny.org/reports/durban-access.html, date accessed 13 February 2012.

UNAIDS (1998) 'AIDS Epidemic Update: December 1998' (Geneva: UNAIDS).

UNAIDS (1999) 'AIDS Epidemic Update: December 1999' (Geneva: UNAIDS).

UNAIDS (2000) 'AIDS Epidemic Update: December 2000' (Geneva: UNAIDS).

UNAIDS (2010) 'UNAIDS Report on the Global AIDS Epidemic' (Geneva: UNAIDS).

UN General Assembly (2001) 'Declaration of Commitment on HIV/AIDS', www.unaids.org/en/media/contentassets/dataimport/publications/irc-pub03/aidsdeclaration_en.pdf, date accessed 22 July 2011.

van der Heever, A. (2011) 'Evaluation of the Green Paper on National Health Insurance, 20 December 2011', http://www.hsf.org.za/projects/health-reform/national-health-insurance-project-developments/nhi-useful-resources/responses-to-national-health-insurance-green-paper, date accessed 6 March 2012.

Van Harmelen, J., R. Woodman, M. Lambrick, E. P. Rybicki, A. Williamson and C. Williamson (1997) 'An Association Between HIV-1 Subtypes and Mode of Transmission in Cape Town, South Africa', *AIDS*, 11(1), 81–7.

Vetten, L. and K. Bhana (2001) *Violence, Vengeance and Gender. A Preliminary Investigation into the Links Between Violence Against Women and HIV/AIDS in South Africa* (Johannesburg: Centre for the Study of Violence and Reconciliation).

Vilmer, E., C. Rouzioux, F. Venizet Brun, A. Fischer, J. C. Chermann, F. Barre-Sinoussi, C. Ganzengel, C. Dauguet, P. Manigne, C. Griscelli and L. Montagnier (1984) 'Isolation of New Lymphotropic Retrovirus from Two Siblings with Haemophilia B, One with AIDS', *The Lancet*, 323 (8380), 753–7.

Whiteside Alan and Jack van Niftrik (1990) 'AIDS in South Africa: Government and ANC Response', *AIDS Analysis Africa: Southern Africa Edition*, August/September, 1.

WHO (1978) 'Declaration of Alma-Ata, International Conference on Primary Health Care, Alma-Ata, USSR, 6–12 September 1978', www.who.int/hpr/NPH/docs/declaration_almaata.pdf, date accessed 9 February 2012.

WHO (1983) *Apartheid and Health: Report of an International Conference Held in Brazzaville, People's Republic of the Congo* (Geneva: World Health Organisation).

WHO (2008) '2008–2013 Action Plan for the Global Strategy for the Prevention and Control of Noncommunicable Diseases', http://whqlibdoc.who.int/publications/2009/9789241597418_eng.pdf, date accessed 10 March 2012.

World Bank, Africa Region (1999) 'Intensifying Action Against HIV/AIDS in Africa: Responding to a Development Crisis' (Washington, DC: World Bank, 1999), http://siteresources.worldbank.org/AFRICATEXT/Resources/aidstrat.pdf, date accessed 1 September 2010.

Zuma, N. (1997) 'South Africa's New National Drug Policy', *Journal of Public Health Policy*, 18(1), 98–105.

Zwi, A. and D. Bachmayer (1990) 'HIV and AIDS in South Africa: What Is an Appropriate Public Health Response?', *Health Policy and Planning*, 5(4), 316–26.

Interviews with key informants

Interview with Quarraisha Abdool Karim on 18 October 2006 at her offices at the Nelson R. Mandela Medical School, University of KwaZulu-Natal. She was an epidemiologist who was the Director of the government's AIDS programme from 1995–6.

Interview with Salim Abdool Karim on 15 September 2003 at the Nelson R. Mandela School of Medicine at the University of KwaZulu-Natal in Durban. Abdool Karim was a member of NAMDA in Durban in the 1980s and went on to become an epidemiologist. He was one of the main organizers of the 2000 International AIDS Conference in Durban and spoke out against Mbeki's adoption of AIDS dissidence.

Interview with Jonathan Berger on 10 April 2008 at Exclusive Books, Sandton City, Johannesburg. Berger was an activist in the NCGLE, the TAC and the ALP.

Interview with Sindi Blose on 11 July 2011 at my home in Durban. Blose was a volunteer with TAC and then held the positions of Treatment Project coordinator and District Organizer.

Interview with Deborah Bonin on 2 February 2006 at Yossi's restaurant in Durban. Bonin was a co-founder of the feminist journal *Agenda*, which began to cover the issue of AIDS in the early 1990s.

Interview with Brian Brink on 27 February 2007 at Anglo American's offices in Central Johannesburg. Brink was a doctor who worked for Anglo American. He conducted early studies on AIDS in the mining industry and later went on to design and implement the company's program providing antiretrovirals for its employees.

Interview with Edwin Cameron in 4 October 2004 at his home in Johannesburg. Cameron was a human rights lawyer and gay rights and AIDS activist. He founded the AIDS Consortium (1992), the ALP (1993), and co-authored the Charter of Rights for People Living with HIV. In 1995, he became a High Court judge. He revealed his HIV status at the hearings of the Judicial Services Committee. He became a judge of the Supreme Court of Appeals in 2000 and was an outspoken opponent of Mbeki's AIDS dissidence.

Interview with Cheryl Carolus on 7 May 2007 at Peotona Holdings in Rivonia in Johannesburg. Carolus was a UDF activist who was also involved in the ESG. In the transition-era she became one of the ANC's spokespersons on health.

Interview with Thabo Cele on 25 April 2007 at the Treatment Action Campaign's Provincial Offices in Durban. Cele was a NAPWA member who joined the Gugu Dlamini Action Committee and later the TAC in Durban.

Interview with Jerry Coovadia on 3 September 2003 at the Nelson R. Mandela School of Medicine at the University of KwaZulu-Natal in Durban. Coovadia was an anti-apartheid paediatrician who belonged to NAMDA. He was one of the main organizers of the 2000 International AIDS Conference in Durban and later spoke out against Mbeki's AIDS dissidence and in favour of antiretrovirals for PMTCT.

Interview with Morna Cornell on 28 March 2007 at the School of Public Health at the University of Cape Town's Medical School. Cornell was the AIDS Consortium's Coordinator and its main spokesperson for most of the 1990s.

Interview with Mary Crewe on 18 October 2006 in her office at the Centre for the Study of AIDS at the University of Pretoria. Crewe researches AIDS and belonged to the AIDS Consortium and participated in its drafting of the Charter of Rights for People Living with HIV and the 1994 National AIDS Plan. She was also close friends with Peter Busse.

Interview with Jeremy Cronin on 30 March 2007 at his offices in Parliament in Cape Town. Cronin was an SACP activist who knew an early proponent of elements of

AIDS dissidence in the ANC in the late 1980s. He was an ANC MP from 1999 and senior SACP office bearer over the period.

Telephonic interview with Lynn Dalrymple on 18 October 2006. Dalrymple founded DramAidE, which was part of the Beyond Awareness Coalition.

Interview with Bev Ditsie on 14 September 2006 at her home in Johannesburg. Ditsie was a gay rights activist who was a co-chair of GLOW and a member of the Township AIDS Project. She became a film maker in the early 2000s.

Interview with Lihle Dlamini on 8 April 2008 at the Treatment Action Campaign's offices at 320 West Street in Durban. Dlamini became a TAC activist during the movement's Civil Disobedience Campaign.

E-mail interview with Peter Doyle on 17 January 2007. Doyle was an Actuarial scientist at Metropolitan Life who produced important early predictions on future HIV prevalence.

Telephonic interview with Jennifer Flynn on 24 May 2011. Flynn was an activist with Health GAP in New York City.

Interview with Peter Folb at the Baxter Theatre on 17 January 2006 at the Baxter Theatre in Cape Town. Folb was a NAMDA supporter and professor of Internal Medicine and Pharmacology at the University of Cape Town. He was a member of the MCC in the 1980s and its president during the Virodene controversy.

Interview with Janet Giddy on 15 September 2003 at McCord's Hospital in Durban. Giddy was involved in the ECC and worked as a doctor in Bethesda in rural Zululand in the 1980s. She went on to become an HIV specialist at McCord's Hospital in Durban.

Telephonic interview with Eric Goemaere on 20 December 2010. Goemaere was a Belgian physician who established an MSF clinic providing combination antiretroviral therapy in Khayalitsha township in Cape Town.

Interview with Gregg Gonsalves on 19 May 2011 at my office at Yale. Gonsalves was involved in ACT UP's Treatment and Data group and worked for the Treatment Action Group (TAG) and Gay Men's Health Crisis (GMHC) in New York City. He helped the TAC design its treatment literacy program.

Interview with Pregs Govender on 28 March 2007 at her office in Muizenburg, Cape Town. Govender was a founder of Natal Organization of Women (NOW) and participated in the WNC. She served as an ANC MP and chairperson of the Joint Parliamentary Committee on the Quality of Life and Status of Women. She offered a feminist critique of Mbeki's AIDS dissidence.

Interview with Mark Harrington on 20 May 2011 at the offices of the Treatment Action Group (TAG) in New York City. Harrington assisted TAC in designing its early treatment literacy programs.

Interview with Fatima Hassan on 16 March 2008 at the AIDS Law Project's Offices in Cape Town. Hassan worked as a lawyer at the ALP in the late 1990s and early 2000s.

Interview with Shireen Hassim on 19 September 2006 at the Wits Institute for Socioeconomic Research at the University of the Witwatersrand in Johannesburg. Hassim is a feminist political scientist who produced an early paper on women and AIDS.

Interview with May Hermanus on 15 February 2007 at the Centre for Sustainability in Mining and Industry at the University of the Witwatersrand. Hermanus served as the NUM's Health and Safety Officer in the late 1980s and early 1990s.

Interview with Mark Heywood on 15 April 2008 at the AIDS Law Project Offices in Braamfontein, Johannesburg. Heywood became friends with Zackie Achmat in the 1980s as both were Trotskyites. Both went to work at the ALP in 1994 and were founder members of the TAC in 1998.

Interview with Nokhwezi Hloboyi on 10 November 2010. Hloboyi was the District Coordinator of the Ekhurhuleni Branch of the TAC.

Telephonic interview with Alan Jaffe 2 May 2007. Jaffe pioneered AIDS awareness programs at Bethesda Hospital in rural Zululand in the 1980s.

Interview with Mazibuko Jara on 26 March 2007 at the Olympia Café in Muizenberg, Cape Town. Jara was a staff member of the NCGLE and went on to become a founder member of the TAC. He was also its chairperson for the first year of its existence.

Interview with Rachel Jewkes on 16 April 2007 at the Medical Research Council's office in Pretoria. Jewkes produced research on violence against women and participated in a pioneering epidemiological study on links between the phenomenon and the transmission of HIV.

Interview with Karen Jochelson on 7 November 2007 at the King's Fund's offices in London. As a Sociology graduate student Jochelson participated in producing an early study around AIDS on the mines and in surrounding communities in the late 1980s and early 1990s.

Telephonic Interview with Jim Yong Kim on 21 November 2011. Kim was a Harvard-trained physician who specialized in infectious diseases. He co-founded Partners in Health with Paul Farmer and was the Director of the WHO's HIV/AIDS Department, where he drove the 3×5 initiative.

Interview with Barbara Klugman on 24 October 2007 at the Ford Foundation's offices in New York City. Klugman was a women's health activist and feminist who worked at the Women's Health Project at the University of the Witwatersrand.

Interview with Steven Knight and Coral Vinsen on 11 April 2007 at Vestige Restaurant in Durban. Knight is a public health physician who worked at Bethesda Hospital in the 1980s. Vinsen was a medical technologist at the Department of Virology in Durban. Both participated in an early AIDS committee at the Natal University Medical School.

Interview with Jean Leger on 19 February 2007 at Vesco Plastics in Denver, Johannesburg. Leger was a collaborated with Karen Jochelson in producing a controversial study on AIDS on the mines and in surrounding communities at the University of the Witwatersrand in the late 1980s and early 1990s.

Interview with Jack Lewis on 22 January 2007 at the offices of the Community Health Media Trust in Cape Town. Jack Lewis is a film-maker and gay rights and human rights activist. He was formerly Zackie Achmat's partner and has extensively documented the Treatment Action Campaign's activities from the movement's formation.

Interview with Stephen Lewis on 26 August 2011 at Grand Central Station in New York City. Lewis was a Canadian politician appointed by UN Secretary General as Special Envoy on AIDS in Africa.

Interview with Leslie London on 15 January 2007 at the Health Sciences Campus of the University of Cape Town. Leslie London was an anti-apartheid and trade union doctor who participated in the Maputo Conference.

Interview with Prudence Mabele on 22 November 2006 at her home in Johannesburg. Mabele was a member of NAPWA, a founder member of the TAC and a founded the Positive Women's Network.

Interview with Mandla Majola on 3 April 2008 at the Treatment Action Campaign's offices in Khayalitsha, Cape Town. Majola was a PAC-aligned activist who joined the TAC in 1999. He later went on to become its Western Cape Provincial Coordinator in 2000.

Interview with Thoko Makhanya on 13 September 2007 at her home in Durban. Makhanya was a qualified midwife and AIDS activist who volunteered with the PPHC and sat on its committee in Durban with Coral Vinsen and Stephen Knight.

Interview with William Malegapuru Makgoba on 7 September 2007 at the Westville Campus of the University of KwaZulu-Natal in Durban. Makgoba was an immunologist who privately and publicly advocated for the Mbeki administration to adopt mainstream scientific approaches to addressing the AIDS epidemic.

Interview with James McIntyre on 19 February 2007 at the Perinatal HIV Research Unit at Baragwanath Hospital in Soweto, Johannesburg. McIntyre was an obstetrician and gynaecologist who with Glenda Gray co-founded the HIV clinic at Baragwanath Hospital. He also researched mother-to-child transmission and volunteered as an activist with NACOSA and the AIDS Consortium.

Interview with Shamim Meer and Karen Hunt on 10 February 2006 at Shamim Meer's home in Johannesburg. Meer and Hunt were part of the editorial team of *SPEAK* magazine in the 1980s and early 1990s.

Interview with Phumzile Mthethwa on 15 April 2008 at the Equality Project's offices in Yeoville, Johannesburg. Mthethwa worked for the ALP and volunteered with the NCGLE and was a co-founder of the TAC.

Interview with Promise Mthembu on 29 August 2003 at the Gender AIDS Forum in Smith Street, Durban. Mthembu volunteered for the NACOSA network, was a member of NAPWA and a founder member of the Gugu Dlamini Action Committee. She also worked for the Young Positive Living Ambassadors Committee and went on to become a member of the TAC's NEC.

Interview with Peter Mugyenyi on 28 March 2011 in my office at Yale. Mugyenyi was a Ugandan paediatrician and AIDS specialist who played a critical role in the design of PEPFAR.

Interview with Warren Parker on 31 January 2007 at the Centre for AIDS Development Research's offices in Johannesburg. Parker worked as a consultant to the AIDS Directorate of the National Department of Health.

Telephonic interview with Peter Piot on 7 October 2011. Piot was a Belgian physician, microbiologist and public health expert who worked at the WHO's Global Program on AIDS and went on to become to head of UNAIDS.

Interview with Eleanor Preston-Whyte on 1 February 2006 at her offices at the School of Development Studies at the University of KwaZulu-Natal in Durban. Preston-Whyte was an anthropologist who researched AIDS and gender and was also Deputy Vice-Chancellor of the University of Natal in the late 1990s.

Interview with Shan Ramburuth on 28 February 2007 at his home in Johannesburg. Ramburuth worked at the AIDS Centre of the SAIMR, was a member of the PPHC and was an NGO representative in the NACOSA network.

Interview with Helen Rees on 7 February 2007 at the offices of the Reproductive Health Research Unit in Hillbrow, Johannesburg. Rees was an anti-apartheid physician who co-chaired the ANC's Women's Health Policy committee with Manto Tshabalala in the transition era. She went on to become the chair of the Medicines Control Council and became the Executive Director of the Reproductive Health Research Unit at the University of the Witwatersrand.

Interview with Nikki Schaay on 11 January at her home in Cape Town. Schaay worked for the AIDS program of the PPHC.

Interview with Helen Schneider on 7 April 2008 at the School of Public Health at the University of Cape Town's Medical School. Schneider was an anti-apartheid physician and public health specialist based at the University of the Witwatersrand's

Centre for Health Policy. She produced an expert affidavit for the TAC's Nevirapine court case.

Interview with Brigid Schutz on 7 February 2007 at the AIDS Research, Education and Puppetry Program (AREPP) offices in Sydenham, Johannesburg. Schutz was a theatre for development practitioner based at AREPP, which was affiliated to the AIDS Consortium.

Interview with Judy Seidman on 4 December 2006 at her home in Johannesburg. Judy Seidman was an anti-apartheid activist and artist who produced several early AIDS awareness posters for the PPHC. Seidman was also a member of NAPWA.

Interview with Ruben Sher on 30 January 2007 at his home in Johannesburg. Sher was an immunologist who played a vital role in diagnosing the first AIDS cases in South Africa and in the AIDS Advisory Group.

Interview with Olive Shisana on 27 March 2007 at the Human Sciences Research Council's offices in Cape Town. Shisana was Director-General of the South African national Department of Health from 1995–8.

Interview with Elinor Sisulu on 31 January 2007 at her home in Pretoria. Sisulu was a Zimbabwean married to Max Sisulu of the famous ANC family. In the early 1990s, she played a key role in encouraging the staff at *SPEAK* magazine to cover AIDS.

Telephonic interview with Rose Smart on 5 March 2007. Smart was a nurse who had worked for the Pietermaritzburg Chamber of Commerce on its programs around AIDS in the workplace in the early 1990s. After 1994, she worked for the AIDS Directorate and became its head in 1997.

E-mail interview with Charlene Smith on 26 March 2008. Smith was a journalist at the *Mail & Guardian* who spoke out about being raped and the difficulties she experienced in accessing antiretrovirals for use in PEP in 1999.

Interview with Zena Stein on 18 October 2007 at her offices at Columbia University in New York. Stein was an adherent of the primary health care model promoted by Sidney and Emily Kark. She played an important role in advocating for the development and implementation of AIDS-related, feminist epidemiological research agendas. She was a co-organizer of the Maputo Conference, particularly its sessions dealing with the AIDS.

Interview with Mervyn Susser on 7 August 2003 at McCord's Hospital in Durban. Susser was an anti-apartheid physician who also followed the primary health care model promoted by Sidney and Emily Kark. While holding an Epidemiology Chair at Columbia in New York City, he alerted NAMDA and the ANC to the likelihood that a massive HIV epidemic would develop in post-apartheid South Africa. Also, as a founder of CHISA, he was a co-organizer of the Maputo Conference.

Interview with Ivan Toms on 11 January 2007 at the Cape Town Civic Centre. Toms was an anti-apartheid physician and activist with the ECC who founded the SACLA clinic in Crossroads, Cape Town. He was sentenced to imprisonment as a conscientious objector in a trial where his sexual orientation was raised by the prosecution. Toms also experienced AIDS-related discrimination in a smear campaign orchestrated by the security forces during his trial and while imprisoned. On his release he became active in the PPHC.

Interview with Lisa Vetten on 21 February at the Tswaranang Legal Advocacy Centre in Braamfontein, Johannesburg. Vetten was a feminist AIDS activist who promoted research and activism around the links between violence against women and AIDS.

Interview with Eddie Webster on 25 September 2006 at Spiro's Coffee Shop in Mellville, Johannesburg. Webster was a Sociologist at the University of the

Witwatersrand. He became embroiled in the controversy around Karen Jochelson's research around AIDS on the mines in the early 1990s.

Telephonic interview with Alan Whiteside on 21 September 2007. Whiteside was an economist who researched labour migration who became interested in AIDS in the late 1980s. He founded the newsletter *AIDS Analysis Africa* and produced a number of critical early scholarly articles dealing with the economic impact of the epidemic. He also sat on the AIDS advisory committee from 1996 to 2000.

Newspaper articles

'794 New HIV Cases in W Cape', *Cape Times*, 21 October 1994.

Achmat, Z. 'The Long Walk to Civil Disobedience', *Mail & Guardian*, 10 April 2003.

'AIDS Millions in the Balance', *The Daily News*, 11 April 2003.

Althenroxel L., and Reuters, 'Mbeki's Aids Stance Stuns US Government', *The Star*, 20 April 2000.

Amla, I. 'Heterosexual Aids Cases on the Increase', *Natal Witness,* 26 March 1992.

Armstrong, S., 'AIDS Myths in Black and White', *Democracy in Action*, 15 July 1994.

Athenroxel, L. 'AIDS Money for KZN Still in Limbo', *The Star*, 9 September 2002.

Babcock C. R, and C. Connolly, 'AIDS Activists Badger Gore Again', *Washington Post*, 18 June 1999.

Barber, S. 'Detractors hound Gore over AIDS drugs', *Business Day*, 30 June 1999.

Barrell, H. and S. Hess, 'Zuma Defends AZT Policy', *Mail & Guardian*, 16 October 1998.

Barrell, H. 'Would the Real AIDS Dissident Please Declare Himself?', *Mail& Guardian*, 19 April 2002.

Battersby, J. 'Mbeki Backs Dr No on KZN Aids Funding', *The Star*, 26 July 2002.

Bechoo, I. 'Plans to Get HIV Notifiable', *The Daily News*, 21 April 1999.

Bechoo, I. 'Drugs Case Judge Rules in Favour of Aids Activists', *The Daily News*. 7 March 2001.

'Beetroot But No Blushes', *Economist*, 24 August 2006, http://www.economist.com/node/7843324, date accessed 8 March 2012.

Beresford, B. 'No New Law on Deliberate HIV Infection', *Mail & Guardian*, 28 September 1999.

Bezuidenhout, J., S. Msomi, C. Keeton, 'Mandela's joy at Aids Decision', *Sunday Times*, 10 August 2003.

Bhengu, C. and M. Vincent, 'Lobbyists Appeal to Govt to Improve Aids Policy', *The Sowetan*, 26 June 2002.

Bisseker, C. 'AIDS: The Perils of Making It a Notifiable Disease', *Financial Mail*, 30 April 1999.

Bissecker, C. 'Row Over AIDS Money', *Financial Mail*, 14 June 2002, www.hst.org.za/news/row-over-aids-money, date accessed 7 July 2011.

Blustein, P. 'Activists Hail President's Call for More Funding to Fight AIDS', *Washington Post*, 29 January 2003.

Brink, A. 'AZT: A Medicine from Hell', *The Citizen*, 17 March 1999.

Brummer S. and L. Gledhill, 'Virodene's Unanswered Questions', *Weekly Mail & Guardian,* 13 March 1998.

Caelers, D. 'Officials Helped Draft Aids Plan', *Cape Argus*, 18 February 2003.

Caelers D. and P. Cardwell, 'Sign Aids Agreement or Else, Says TAC', *Saturday Weekend Argus*, 15 February 2003.

Chuenyane, G. 'Drug Companies "Likely to Withdraw Court Case" ', *The Sowetan*, 19 April 2000.

Clarke, L., 'Don't Believe Aids Is Only a "Gay" or "Black" Disease, Warn Experts', *Sunday Tribune*, 2 June 1988.
Cullinan, K., N. Kalideen, J. Green, 'Gift of Life to Millions Living with HIV/Aids', *The Star*, 20 November 2003.
Daily News Correspondent, 'Hope for Aids Babies', *The Daily News*, 17 February 1999.
Daily News Correspondent, 'I Have Aids: Judge', *The Daily News*, 20 April 1999.
Day, J. 'Virodene "Cruel Trick" ', *Weekly Mail & Guardian*, 28 February 1997.
'Deadlock Over HIV/AIDS Grant Looms', *Mail & Guardian*, 12 July 2002.
Deene, N. 'TAC to Charge Ministers over Aids Deaths', *Mail & Guardian* 27 March 2003.
De Waal, S. 'Censors "Don't Ban Films" ', *Weekly Mail*, 28 October 1993.
'Do It Now, Mbeki', *The Star*, 20 February 2002.
Dwyer, P. 'SOUTH AFRICA: "Dying to Fight" for Treatment', *Green Left Weekly*, www.greenleft.org.au/node/2939, date accessed 24 July 2011.
'Editorial: A Wrong Turn on Aids', *Business Day*, 5 July 2000.
Edmunds, M. 'Government Aims to "own" Aids Drug', *Weekly Mail &Guardian*, 31 January 1997.
'Frightening Twist to Spread of Aids', *Sunday Express*, 9 January 1983.
'Gay activist Nkoli in US', *The Sowetan*, 28 August 1988.
Gaye Stolberg, S. 'AIDS Fund Falls Far Short of Goal and US is Given Some Blame', *The New York Times*, 13 February 2002.
Gevisser, M. 'Finally, The State Gets Serious about AIDS', *Weekly Mail & Guardian*, 28 July 1994.
Gledhill, L. 'Virodene May Activate Aids Virus', *Weekly Mail & Guardian*, 20 March 1998.
Granelli, M. 'Mbeki Favours HIV Disclosure', *The Star*, 22 April 1999.
Granelli, M. and P. Singh, 'Aids Activists Lash Mbeki Stand', *Pretoria News*, 22 April 1999.
Greenwald J. and E. Love, 'The Harvard Debt Doctor's Controversial Cure', *TIME*, 6 November 1989.
Heywood, M. 'Aids Council Carries Hopes of Millions', *The Sowetan*, 25 January 2000.
'HIV/Aids Protests to Go Global', *Sunday Times*, 30 March 2003.
Hlongwa, W. 'TAC Aiming to Strengthen Its AIDS Struggle', *City Press*, 3 August 2003.
Holden, S. 'AIDS Tests for Returning Exiles are "Not Viable" ', The Herald 23 August 1990.
'Honorary Degree for TAC Leader, *Natal Witness*, 7 March 2003.
Horler V. and L. Athenroxel, 'Treatment with New Aids Drug on Hold', *Pretoria News*, 25 January 1997.
'I Won't Let Government Kill Me', *The Star*, 5 August 2003.
IRIN, "South Africa: Global Fund Money Becomes Available," IRIN, 7 August 2003.
Jepson, G. 'TAC Moved the Nation, Says Graca', *This Day*, 7 October 2003.
Jubasi, M. 'Poor to Get Aids Drugs first', *Sunday Times*, 3 November 2002.
ka Mathe, T. 'Selfless Spirit and Champion in the Struggle against AIDS', *City Press*, 7 July 2002.
Kalideen, N. 'Mandela Backtracks on Aids Row', *Pretoria News*, 20 February 2002.
Karon, T. 'South African AIDS Activist Zackie Achmat', *TIME*, April 19, 2001, http://www.time.com/time/nation/article/0,8599,106995,00.html, date accessed 1 September 2010.
Keeton, C. 'Experts at Odds Over Aids Plan', *The Sowetan*, 3 May 1999.
Keller, B. 'Apartheid's Gone, and Anything Goes' *The New York Times*, 28 December 1994.

Khumalo, N. 'TAC's Aids March in Step with People's Wishes', *Pretoria News*, 11 February 2003, p.11.

Khumalo, S. 'To Some the Only Safe Sex Is No Sex at ALL!', *City Press*, 7 August 1996.

'Leading Figures on AIDS Panel', *The Star*, 5 May 2000.

'Legal Prostitution "Not Considered" ', *The Citizen*, 28 May 1991.

Lekota, I. 'Cosatu's U-turn on Aids', *The Sowetan*, 28 February 2003, p.1.

Mabasa, T. 'TAC Plans March', *The Citizen*, 14 January 2003.

'Madiba to Put Aids Activist's Case to Mbeki', *Sunday Times*, 28 July 2002.

Mahlangu, D. and M. Makhabela, "Protest Over Act for Cheaper Medicine," *City Press*, 4 March 2001.

Mantjiu, M. 'We Can Save Those Babies', *Sunday Tribune*, 6 December 1998.

Martin, D. J. 'AZT: A Medicine from Heaven', *The Citizen*, 31 March 1999.

'Mbeki: The Big Debate', *Sunday Times*, 19 July 2000.

'MCC Again Refuses Testing of Virodene', *The Citizen*, 3 February 1998.

McGreal, C. 'Dying for Drugs: South Africa's Sick Wait for Judgment Day: Multinationals Go to Court Today Over a Law Aimed at Cutting the Cost of Medicines', *The Guardian*, 5 March 2001.

McGreal, C. 'ANC Urged to Make Aids Drugs Available: As Pharmaceutical Companies Cave in, South Africans Call on the State to Exploit Victory and Distribute Medicines', *The Guardian*, 20 April 2001.

McGreal, C. 'Mandela Hits Again at President's AIDS Policy: Message is Pressed Home at a Meeting with Dying HIV Activist in His Strongest Stand Yet', *The Guardian*, 29 July 2002.

McGreal, C. 'Mandela Breaks Taboo on Aids: Ex-president Becomes First ANC Member to Say Publicly That He Has Lost Family to Virus', *The Guardian*, 26 August 2002.

Meldrum, A. 'HIV/AIDS in Africa: Free Treatment for All', *The Observer*, 23 November 2003.

Menakar, D. 'Spread of AIDS Threatens Transition in South Africa', *The Dallas Morning News*, 25 September 94.

Michaels, J. 'Aids Ads a Wish List, Says TAC', *Cape Argus*, 24 March 2003.

Munsamy, R. 'Stop Aids Nonsense', *Sunday Times*, 17 February 2002.

Naidoo, C. 'Campaigning Gore Is Hit by Pro-SA AIDS Activists', *Sunday Times*, 20 July 1999.

Naidu, D. 'TAC Call Attention to Govt. Delay in AIDS Help', *Leader*, 31 January 2003.

Ndaba, B. 'Hate Crimes against Lesbians Slated', IOL, 13 July 2007. http://www.iol.co.za/news/south-africa/hate-crime-against-lesbians-slated-1.361821, date accessed 6 March 2012.

'NGOs in Plea for AIDS, TB Funding', *The Star*, 11 February 2012.

Nolen, S. 'A Victory for South Africa's Martyr-in-chief', *Globe and Mail*, 13 September 2003.

'Not Much Comfort on Social Issues', *Sunday Times*, 4 November 1993.

Own correspondent, 'Government's Decision to on AZT to Be Reviewed', *The Star*, 30 June 1999.

Pagani, S. 'Global War Chest Opened in Fight Against AIDS', *Toronto Star*, 21 July 2001.

Peer, N. 'I'm No Martyr, Says Achmat', *Cape Times*, 1 August 2002.

Power, S. 'Letter from South Africa: The AIDS Rebel', *The New Yorker*, 19 May 2003.

'Pretoria Declines Thai Offer for Free HIV Medicine', *Mail & Guardian*, 18 January 2002.

'R14,7m AIDS Musical Probe', *Eastern Province Herald*, 14 February 1996.

Redvers, L. 'Swazi AIDS Response in Cash Crisis', *Mail & Guardian*, 27 February 2011, http://mg.co.za/article/2012-02-27-swazi-aids-response-in-cash-crisis/, date accessed 8 March 2012.

'Resolve Status of Virodene – Zuma', *Weekend Saturday Argus*, 7 December 1997.

Richter, M. 'A New Feminism', *Mail & Guardian*, 9 December 2005, http://www.aegis.com/news/DMG/2005/MG051206.html, date accessed 8 March 2012.

Ripley, A. 'What Makes a Hero?', *TIME*, 28 April 2003.

Roberts C. and P. Barnes, 'Most new Aids Sufferers Are Heterosexuals', *The Star*, 20 August 1990.

'SAA Disapproves of Homosexuality', *The Citizen*, 8 January 1983.

SAPA, 'W. Cape Hospitals to Give AZT Drug', *The Citizen*, 20 February 1999.

SAPA, 'Mbeki Is Wrong: AZT Is Safe, Says Glaxo', 28 October 1999, www.virusmyth.com/aids/news/sapambeki.htm, date accessed 13 February 1012.

SAPA, "HIV/AIDS Drug Deal to Be Signed on Friday," 27 November 2000, http://www.iol.co.za/general.news/newsprint/php?art_id=qw9758862119F425&sf, date accessed 1 September 2010.

SAPA, 'Thousands of Aids Activists to March on Parliament', *Cape Times*, 14 February 2003.

SAPA, 'Financial Crisis, Funding Shortage Hit TAC', *The Citizen*, 30 November 2008, http://www.citizen.co.za/index/article.aspx?pDesc=84223,1,22, date accessed 1 September 2009.

SAPA, 'Judge Appointed to Resolve KZN Lab Crisis', *The Daily News*, 7 February 2012, http://www.iol.co.za/dailynews/news/judge-appointed-to-resolve-kzn-lab-crisis-1.1229285, date accessed 8 March 2012.

SAPA, 'South Africa's First R1 Trillion Budget', *The Sowetan*, 22 February 2012, http://www.sowetanlive.co.za/news/business/2012/02/22/south-africa-s-first-r1-trillion-budget, date accessed 6 March 2012.

Schoofs, M. and M. Waldholz, 'Price War Breaks Out Over AIDS Drugs in Africa as Generics Present Challenge', *Wall Street Journal*, 7 March 2001.

Segar, S. 'Govt Won't Change Aids Policy', *Natal Witness*, 5 April 2001.

'Sisulu's Name on Fake "Aids" Leaflet', *Weekly Mail*, 5 October 1990–11 October 1990.

'South Africa: Deputy President Zuma Opens AIDS Conference in Durban' BBC Summary of World Broadcasts, 3 August 2003.

'South Africa: Government to Sign US$41 mil Deal with Global Fund' *BuaNews*, 6 August 2003.

'S. Africans Demand More Money from G7 for Fight Against AIDS', Xinhua, 9 October 2002.

Smetherham, J. A. 'No Anti-retrovirals for Me', *The Star*, 4 July 2002.

Smetherham, J. A. 'Worldwide Support for TAC Protest Campaign', *Cape Times*, 17 March 2003.

Smetherham, J. A. 'Doctors Show Their Colours on Aids Drugs', *Cape Times*, 6 May 2003.

Smetherham J. A. and J. Ancer, 'Aids Activist Achmat and TAC Nominated for Nobel Peace Prize', *Cape Times*, 3 December 2003.

Sole, S. 'AIDS: The Battle Is Over – and We Lost', *Sunday Tribune*, 29 March 1998.

Sole, S. 'Government Bungling Gridlocks Issue of HIV/AIDS', *Sunday Independent*, 29 October 2000.

Sowetan correspondent, 'Aids Team Get a Reprimand', *The Sowetan*, 27 February 1997.

Staff Reporter, 'Women Bear the Brunt of Aids in SA', *The Star*, 22 November 1996.

Sternberg, S. 'AIDS Advocates Praise Bush's $15 billion Proposal', *USA TODAY*, 30 January 2003.

Stucky, C. 'AZT: 'If They Wanted Guns, They Would Find the Money', *Sunday Independent*, 24 January 1999.

Strachan, K. 'University to Probe AIDS Researchers' "Breach of Practice" ', *Business Day*, 24 January 1997

St. Leger, C. 'Legalise Prostitution Call to Control Aids', *Sunday Times*, 25 May 1991.

Stuart, B. 'More Spent on Defence Than on Aids', *The Citizen*, 10 May 2000.

Sulcas, A. 'Aids Will Be Driven Underground', *Sunday Tribune*, 25 April 1999.

Swarns, R. L. 'Drug Makers Drop South Africa Suit Over AIDS Medicine', *The New York Times*, 20 April 2001, http://query.nytimes.com/gst/fullpage.html?res=9F00E6DE1330F933A15757C0A9679C8B63&sec=&spon=&pagewanted=2, date accessed 1 September 2010.

Taitz, L. 'Activists Threaten to Boycott SA Aids Talks', *Sunday Times*, 31 January 1999.

Taitz, L. and C. Paton, 'Mbeki: Wise Man or Fool?', *Sunday Times*, 7 May 2000.

Terreblanche, C. 'Minister Withholds Details of HIV/Aids Treatment Options', *Cape Times*, 14 May 2003.

Thom, A. 'Alarm Over Aids-babies Toll', *The Star*, 26 June 1998.

Thom, A. 'Aids Activists Lie Down for Better Care', *The Star*, 22 March 1999.

Thom, A. 'Aids Activists Lambast Drug Companies', *Sunday Independent*, 14 May 2000.

Thom, A., 'The Fight Goes On', *Cape Argus*, 1 November 2000.

Thom, A., 'Bara Baby Crisis', IOL, 8 February 2012, http://www.iol.co.za/lifestyle/family/baby-toddler/bara-baby-crisis-1.1229791?ot=inmsa.ArticlePrintPageLayout.ot, date accessed 8 March 2012.

'Transfer of KwaZulu Money Bedevils UN AIDS Fund Deal', *Business Day*, 11 April 2003.

Tshabalala-Msimang, M. 'The State *has* an Aids Plan', *Mail & Guardian*, 6 March 2003.

Underhill, G. 'Sister's Anguish Over Achmat's Stand', *Cape Times*, 2 August 2002.

Van Zilla, L. 'Mandela Rallies HIV Troops', *Cape Times,* 13 December 2002, p.4

Viall, J. 'Can We Afford Not to Use AZT?', *Cape Argus*, 16 October 1998.

Vulliamy, E. 'How Drug Giants Let Millions Die of Aids', *The Observer*, 19 December 1999, http://www.guardian.co.uk/uk/1999/dec/19/theoberserver.uknews6, date accessed 1 September 2010.

'What's Going On at the AIDS Council', *Mail & Guardian*, 27 September 2002.

Whiteside, A. 'AIDS Battle Should Involve All', *Business Day*, 10 December 1998.

'Women Urge Rapists be Tested for AIDS', *The Citizen*, 27 November 1995.

World Trade Organization (2001) 'Doha Declaration on the TRIPS Agreement and Public Health', 14 November 2001, www.wto.org/english/thewto_e/min01_e/minded_trips_e.htm, date accessed 22 July 2011.

Documentary films

'Patient Abuse', Directed by J. Lewis, 2001, 58 minutes.

'Siyayinqoba Beat It! 2006 Ep. 11 – Gender Based Violence – Lorna Mlofana', Dir. Jack Lewis, available at http://www.beatit.co.za/archive-people/mandla-majola, date accessed 12 August 2011.

'Simon and I', Directed by B. P. Ditsie and N. Newman, 2002, 52 minutes.

'It's My Life', Directed by D. Tilley, 2001, 72 minutes.

Secondary sources

Abu-Lughod, L. (2008) *Writing Women's Worlds: Bedouin Stories* (Berkeley, Los Angeles and London: University of California Press).

Adebayo, A. (2010) *The Curse of Berlin: Africa After the Cold War* (New York: Columbia University Press).

Adusei, P. (2010) 'Regulatory Diversity as Key to the "Myth" of Drug Patenting in Sub-Saharan Africa', *Journal of African Law*, 54(1), L26–50.

aids2031 Costs and Financing Working Group (2010) *The Long-Term Costs of HIV/AIDS in South Africa* (Washington, DC: Results for Development Institute).

Akintola, O., (2004) 'The Gendered Burden of Home-based Care-giving, Policy Brief', http://www.dec.org/pdf_docs/PNADB615.pdf, date accessed 11 January 2012.

Albertyn, C. and S. Meer (2008) 'Citizens or Mothers? The Marginalization of Women's Reproductive Rights in the Struggle for Access to Health Care for HIV-positive Pregnant Women in South Africa', in M. Mukhopadhyay and S. Meer (eds.) *Gender, Rights and Development: A Global Sourcebook* (Amsterdam: Royal Tropical Institute), 27–56.

Altman, D. (1973) *Homosexual Oppression and Liberation* (New York: Avon).

Anand S. and K. Hanson (2004) 'Disability-Adjusted Life Years: A Critical Review', in S. Anand, F. Peter and A. Sen (eds.) *Public Health, Ethics and Equity* (Oxford: Oxford University Press), 183–200.

Appiah, K. A. (1992) *In My Father's House: Africa in the Philosophy of Culture* (Oxford and New York: Oxford University Press).

AVERT (2012) South Africa: HIV & AIDS Statistics', http://www.avert.org/safricastats.htm, date accessed 14 February 2012.

Baldwin-Ragaven, L., J. de Gruchy and L. London (1999) *An Ambulance of the Wrong Colour: Health Professionals, Human Rights and Ethics in South Africa* (Rondebosch: University of Cape Town Press).

Ballard, R., A. Habib and I. Valodia (2006) 'Conclusion: Making Sense of Post-apartheid SA's Voices of Protest', in R. Ballard, A. Habib and I. Valodia (eds.) *Voices of Protest: Social Movements in Post-apartheid South Africa* (Scottsville: University of KwaZulu-Natal Press), 397–418.

Barak-Erez, D. and A. M. Ross (2007) 'Introduction: Do We Need Social Rights? Questions in the Era of Globalisation, Privatisation, and the Diminished Welfare State', in A. M. Gross (ed.) *Exploring Social Rights: Between Theory and Practice* (Oxford and Portland: OR Hart Publishing), 1–20.

Barnes, A. and G. W. Brown (2011) 'The Global Fund for Fight AIDS, Tuberculosis and Malaria: Expertise, Accountability and the Depoliticisation of Global Health Governance', in S. Rushton and O. Williams (eds.) *Partnerships and Foundations in Global Health Governance* (Houndsmills and New York: Palgrave Macmillan, 2011), 53–75.

Bayly, C. A., S. Beckert, M. Connelly, I. Hofmeyr, W. Kozol, P. Seed (2006) 'AHR Conversation: On Transnational History', *The American Historical Review*, 111(5), 1441–64.

Beauchamp, T. L. and J. F. Childress (2008) *Principles of Biomedical Ethics*, 6th edition (Oxford: Oxford University Press).

Behrman, G. (2004) *The Invisible People: How the U.S. Has Slept Through the Global AIDS Pandemic, the Greatest Humanitarian Catastrophe of Our Time* (New York, London, Toronto, Sydney: Free Press).

Beinart, W. (2010) 'Popular Politics and Resistance Movements in South Africa' in W. Beinart and M. C. Dawson (eds.) Popular Politics and Resistance Movements in South Africa, (Johannesburg: Wits University Press), 1–30.

Benatar, S. and G. Brock (2011) 'Introduction' in S. Benatar and G. Brock Global Health and Global Health Ethics (Cambridge: Cambridge University Press), 1–10.

Benatar, S. R., A. S. Daar and P. A. Singer (2003) 'Global Health Ethics: The Rationale for Mutual Caring', *International Affairs* 79(1), 107–38.

Benjamin, S. (2007) 'The Feminization of Poverty in Post-apartheid South Africa: A Story Told by the Women of Bayview, Chatsworth', *Journal of Developing Societies* 23(1–2), 175–206.

Bentham, J. (2003) 'An Introduction to the Principles of Morals and Legislation', in M. Warnock (ed.) *Utilitarianism and On Liberty: Including Mill's 'Essay on Bentham' and Selections from the Writings of Jeremy Bentham and John Austin* (Malden, MA and Oxford: Blackwell), 17–51.

Berger, J. (2008) 'Getting to the Constitutional Court on Time: A Litigation History of Same-sex Marriage', in M. Judge and A. Manion (eds.) *To Have and to Hold: The Making of Same-sex Marriage in South Africa* (Sunnyside: Jacana, 2008), 17–28.

Berlin, I. (2002) 'Two Concepts of Liberty', in H. Hardy (ed.) *Liberty* (Oxford: Oxford University Press), 166–217.

Biehl, J. (2007) *Will to Live: AIDS Therapies and the Politics of Survival* (Princeton and Oxford: Princeton University Press).

Biko, S. (1996) *I Write What I Like* (Johannesburg: Ravan Press).

Bilchitz, D. (2002) 'Giving Socio-economic Rights Teeth: The Minimum Core and Its Importance, *South African Law Journal*, 119, 484–501.

Birn, A. E., Y. Pillay and T. H. Holtz (2009) *Textbook of International Health: Global Health in a Dynamic World* (Oxford: Oxford University Press).

Bond, P. (2000) *Elite Transition: From Apartheid to Neoliberalism in South Africa* (Scottville: University of Natal Press).

Bond, P. (2001) *Against Global Apartheid: South Africa meets the World Bank, IMF and International Finance* (Cape Town: University of Cape Town Press).

Bozzoli, B. And N. Nkotsoe (1991) *Women of Phokeng: Consciousness, Life Strategy, and Migrancy in South Africa, 1900–1983* (Portsmouth, NH: Heinemann).

Brier, J. (2009) *Infectious Ideas: U.S. Political Responses to the AIDS Crisis* (Chapel Hill, NC: University of North Carolina Press).

Brock, D. W. (2004) 'Ethical Issues in the Use of Cost Effectiveness Analysis for the Prioritisation of Health Care Resources', in S. Anand, F. Peter and A. Sen, (eds.) *Public Health, Ethics and Equity* (Oxford: Oxford University Press), 201–24.

Bromley Chan, K. (2006) 'From Legal Universalism to Legal Pluralism: Expanding and Enhancing the Human Rights Approach to HIV/AIDS', *South African Journal on Human Rights*, 22, 191–203.

Brown, C. (2007) *Moral Capital: Foundations of British Abolitionism* (Chapel Hill, NC: University of North Carolina Press).

Brown, T., M. Cueto and E. Fee, (2006) 'The World Health Organization and the Transition from 'International' to 'Global' Public Health', *American Journal of Public Health*, 96(1), 62–72.

Budlender, D. (1996) 'South Africa: The Women's Budget', *Southern Africa Report*, (1996) 12, 1, http://www.africafiles.org/article.asp?ID=3865, date accessed 10 February 2012.

Budlender, D. (2001) 'The South African Women's Budget Initiative: What does it tell us about Poverty Alleviation', in F. Wilson, W. Kanji and E. Braathen (eds.)

Poverty Reduction: What Role for the State in Today's Globalized Economy (London and New York: Zed Books), 327–40.

Bush, G. W. (2010) *Decision Points* (New York: Crown, 2010).

Butler, J. (1999), *Gender Trouble* (London and New York: Routledge).

Calland, R. (2006) *Anatomy of South Africa: Who Holds the Power?* (Cape Town: Zebra Press).

Campbell, J. L. (2005) 'Where Do We Stand? Common Mechanisms in Organizational and Social Movement Research', in G. F. Davis, D. McAdam, W. R. Scott, M. N. Zaid (eds.) *Social Movements and Organizational Theory* (Cambridge: Cambridge University Press), 41–68.

Chauncey, G. (1995) *Gay New York: Gender, Urban Culture and the Making of the Gay Male World* (New York: Basic Books).

Chigwedere, P., G. R. Seage, S. Gruskin, T. H. Lee, M. Essex (2008) 'Estimating the Lost Benefits of Antiretroviral Drug Use in South Africa', *Journal of Acquired Immune Deficiency Syndrome*, 49(4), 410–5.

Clifford, J. (1988) *The Predicament of Culture: Twentieth-Century Ethnography, Literature, and Art* (Cambridge MA and London: Harvard University Press)

Cohen, J. and A. Arato (1992) *Civil Society and Political Theory* (Cambridge: MIT Press).

Comaroff, J. L. and J. Comaroff (1992) *Ethnography and the Historical Imagination* (Boulder CO and Oxford: Westview Press).

Comaroff, J. L. and J. Comaroff (1997) *Of Revelation and Revolution: The Dialectics of Modernity on a South African Frontier* (Chicago and London: University of Chicago Press).

Connor, C. and M. Mbali (2007) 'South African AIDS Activism: A Feminist View', in C. Clark, A. Holmes, L. VeneKlasen and E. Win (eds.) *Women Navigate Power: Stories About Reclaiming Our Rights* (London: ActionAid International), 49–74.

Cross, C. and M. Friedman (1997) 'Women and Tenure: Marginality and Left-hand Power', in S. Meer (ed.) *Women, Land and Authority: Perspectives from South Africa* (Cape Town and Oxford: David Phillip and Oxfam), 17–34.

Croucher, S. (2002) 'South Africa's Democratization and the Politics of Gay Liberation', *Journal of Southern African Studies*, 28(2), 315–30.

Curtin, P. D. (1969) 'Oral Traditions and African History', *Journal of the Folklore Institute*, 6(2/3), 137–55.

Daniels, N. (2011) 'International Health Inequalities and Global Justice: Towards a Middle Ground', in S. Benatar and G. Brock (eds.) *Global Health and Global Health Ethics* (Cambridge: Cambridge University Press), 97–107.

Daum, C. (2009) 'Deciding under the Influence? The 'One Hit Wonders' and Organizational Interest Participation in U.S. Supreme Court Litigation', in S. Barclay, M. Bernstein and A. M. Marsall (eds.) *Queer Mobilizations: LGBT Activists Confront the Law* (New York and London: New York University Press, 2009), 72–102.

Davis, D. (2006) 'Adjudicating Socio-economic Rights in the South African Constitution – Towards a Deference Lite?', *South African Journal of Human Rights*, 22, 301–27.

Denny, C. C. and E. Emanuel (2008) 'US Health Aid Beyond PEPFAR: The Mother & Child Campaign', *Journal of the American Medical Association*, 300(17), 2048–51.

De Waal, S. and Manion A. (2006) 'Introduction', in S. de Waal and A. Manion (eds.) *Pride: Protest and Celebration* (Sunnyside: Jacana), 6–18.

Diani, M. (2003) 'Introduction: Social Movements, Contentious Actions and Social Networks: "From Metaphor to Substance?" ', in M. Diani and D. McAdam (eds.) *Social Movements and Networks: Relational Approaches and Collective Action* (Oxford: Oxford University Press), 1–19.

278   *Bibliography*

Digby, A. (2008) 'From Racial Segregation towards Transformation', in A. Digby, H. Phillips, H. Deacon and K. Thomas (eds.) *At the Heart of Healing: Groote Schuur Hospital, 1938–2008* (Sunnyside: Jacana), 103–34.

Draper, J. A. (2003) 'Script, Subjugation, and Subversion: An Introduction', in J. A. Draper (ed.) *Orality, Literacy and Colonialism in Southern Africa* (Pietermaritzburg: Cluster Publications), 1–9.

Dugard, J. (2004) 'Twenty Years of Human Rights Scholarship and Ten Years of Democracy', *South African Journal of Human Rights*, 20, 345–54.

Dutfield, G. (2008) 'Delivering Drugs to the Poor: Will the TRIPs Amendment Help?' *American Journal of Law & Medicine* 34, 107–24.

Epprecht, M. (2004) *Hungochani: The Story of a Dissident Sexuality in Southern Africa* (Kingston: McGill-Queen's University Press).

Epstein, H. (2007) *The Invisible Cure: Africa, the West and the Fight Against AIDS* (New York: Farrar, Strauss and Giroux, 2007).

Epstein, S. (1996) *Impure Science: AIDS, Activism and the Politics of Knowledge* (Berkeley, Los Angeles and London: The University of California Press, 1996).

Farmer, P. (2001) *Infections and Inequalities: The Modern Plagues* (Berkeley and Los Angeles: University of California Press).

Fassin, D. (2007) *When Bodies Remember: Experiences and Politics of AIDS in South Africa,* Transl. A. Jacobs and G. Varro (Berkeley, Los Angeles and London: University of California Press).

Finnemore, M. (1996) *National Interests in International Society* (Ithaca and London: Cornell University Press).

Flynn, S. M. (2010) 'Using Competition Law to Promote Access to Knowledge', in G. Krikonan and A. Kaczynski (eds.) *Access to Knowledge in the Age of Intellectual Property* (New York: Zone Books, 2010), 451–74.

Fraser, N. (2003) 'Social Justice in the Age of Identity Politics: Redistribution, Recognition and Participation', in N. Fraser and A. Honneth (eds.) Transl. J. Golb, J. Ingram and C. Wilke, *Redistribution or Recognition? A Political-Philosophical Exchange* (London and New York: Verso), 8–109.

Friedman, S. and S. Mottiar (2005) 'A Rewarding Engagement? The Treatment Action Campaign and the Politics of HIV/AIDS', *Politics and Society*, 33, 511–65.

Geffen, N. (2010) *Debunking Delusions: The Inside Story of the TAC* (Sunnyside: Jacana).

Gevisser, M. (1994) 'A Different Fight for Freedom: A History of South African Lesbian and Gay Organization from the 1980s-1990s', in M. Gevisser and E. Cameron (eds.) *Defiant Desire: Gay and Lesbian Lives in South Africa* (New York and London: Routledge), 14–86.

Gevisser, M. (2007) *Thabo Mbeki: The Dream Deferred* (Johannesburg: Jonathan Ball).

Gilpin, R. G. (1986) 'The Richness of the Tradition of Political Realism', in R. O. Keohane (ed.) *Neorealism and Its Critics* (New York: Columbia University Press), 301–21.

Gostin, L. O. and A. L. Taylor (2008) 'Global Health Law: A Definition and Grand Challenges' *Public Health Ethics*, 1(1), 53–63.

Gouws, A. (2005a) 'Introduction', in A. Gouws (ed.) *(Un)thinking Citizenship: Feminist Debates in Contemporary South Africa* (Aldershot: Ashgate), 1–20.

Gouws, A. (2005b) 'Shaping Women's Citizenship: Contesting the Boundaries of State and Discourse', in A. Gouws (ed.) *(Un)thinking Citizenship: Feminist Debates in Contemporary South Africa* (Aldershot: Ashgate), 71–90.

Grebe, E. (2008) 'Transnational Networks of Influence in South African AIDS Treatment Activism', http://www.cssr.uct.ac.za/sites/cssr.uct.ac.za/files/pubs/WP222.pdf, date accessed 27 February 2012.

Gumede, W. M. (2007) *Thabo Mbeki and the Battle for the Soul of the ANC* (Johannesburg: Struik).

Gunner, L. (2004) 'Africa and Orality', in F. A. Irele and S. Gikandi (eds.) *The Cambridge History of African and Caribbean Literature: Volume 1* (Cambridge: Cambridge University Press), 1–18.

Habib, A. (2003) 'State-civil Society Relations in Post-apartheid South Africa', in J. Daniel, A. Habib and R. Southall (eds.) *State of the Nation: South Africa 2003–2004* (Cape Town: HSRC Press), 227–41.

Hall, J. J. and R. Taylor (2003) 'Health for All Beyond 2000: the Demise of the Alma-Ata Declaration and Primary Health Care in Developing Countries', *The Medical Journal of Australia*, 178(1), 17–20.

Harms, R. (1987) *Games Against Nature: An Eco-Cultural History of the Nunu of Equatorial Africa* (Cambridge: Cambridge University Press).

Harries, P. (1994) *Work, Culture and Identity: Migrant Labourers in Mozambique and South Africa, c.1860–1910* (Johannesburg: Heinemann).

Harrison, M., (2004) *Disease and the Modern World* (Cambridge: Polity Press).

Harvey, D. (2005) A Brief History of Neoliberalism (Oxford: Oxford University Press).

Hassim, S. (2004) 'Voices, Hierarchies and Spaces: Reconfiguring the Women's Movement in Democratic South Africa', www.ukzn.ac.za/ccs, date accessed 10 February 2012.

Hassim, S. (2006) *Women's Organizations and Democracy in South Africa: Contesting Authority* (Scottsville: University of KwaZulu-Natal Press).

Hein, W. L. Kohlmorgen and S. Bartsch (2007) 'Introduction: Globalization, HIV/AIDS and the Rise of Global Health Governance', in W. L. Hein, L. Kohlmorgen and S. Bartsch (eds.) *Global Health Governance and the Fight Against HIV/AIDS* (Houndsmills: Palgrave Macmillan), 1–17.

Heywood, M. (2003) 'Current Development: Preventing Mother-to-child Transmission in South Africa: Backgrounds, Strategies and Outcomes in the Treatment Action Campaign case against the Minister of Health', *South African Journal on Human Rights*, 19, 278–303.

Heywood, M. (2004) 'The Price of Denial', *Development Update: From disaster to Development: HIV & AIDS in Southern Africa*, 5(3), 93–122.

Hoad, K., K. Martin and G. Reid (2005) *Sex and Politics in South Africa* (Cape Town: Double Storey).

Hofmeyr, I. (2004) *The Portable Bunyan: A Transnational History of The Pilgrim's Progress* (Princeton and Oxford: Princeton University Press).

Hollis A. and T. Pogge (2008) *Health Impact Fund: Making New Medicines Accessible For All* (New Haven: Incentives for Global Health).

Hunter, D. and A. J. Dawson (2011) 'Is There a Need for Global Health Ethics? For and Against', in S. Benatar and G. Brock (eds.) *Global Health and Global Health Ethics* (Cambridge: Cambridge University Press), 77–88.

Hunter, M. (2002) 'The Materiality of Everyday Sex: Thinking Beyond Prostitution', *African Studies*, 61(1), 99–120.

Hunter, M (2010) *Love in the Time of AIDS: Inequality, Gender and Rights in South Africa* (Bloomington, IN: Indiana University Press).

Iliffe, J. (2007) *Africans: The History of a Continent* (Cambridge: Cambridge University Press).

Iliffe, J. (2006) *The African AIDS Epidemic: A History* (Oxford: James Currey).

Iriye, A. (2004) 'Transnational History', *Contemporary European History*, 13(2), 211–22.

Jones, P. (2004) 'When Development' Devastates: Donor Discourses, Access to HIV/AIDS Treatment in Africa and Rethinking the Landscape of Development', *Third World Quarterly*, 25(2), 385–404.

Kapczynski, A. (2009) 'Harmonization and its Discontents: A Case Study of TRIPS Implementation in India's Pharmaceutical Sector' *California Law Review*, 97, 1571–651.

Kapczynski, A. and J. M. Berger (2009) 'The Story of the TAC Case: The Potential and Limits of Socio-Economic Rights Litigation in South Africa', in D. R. Hurwitz, M. L. Satterthwaite and D. Ford (eds.) *Human Rights Advocacy Stories* (New Delhi: Foundation Press, 2009), available at http://papers.ssrn.com/sol3/papers.cfm?abstract_id=1323522, date accessed 18 August 2011.

Kark, S. and E. Kark (1999) *Promoting Community Health: From Pholela to Jerusalem* (Johannesburg: Witwatersrand University Press).

Keck, M. E. and Sikkink K. (1998) *Activists Beyond Borders: Advocacy Networks in International Politics* (Ithaca, N.Y.: Cornell University Press).

Keswa B. and S. Wieringa (2005) 'Chapter Six', in R. Morgan and S. Wieringa (eds.) *Tommy Boys, Lesbian Men and Ancestral Wives: Female Same-sex Practices in Africa* (Sunnyside: Jacana), 199–230.

Klein, N. (2007) *The Shock Doctrine: The Rise of Disaster Capitalism* (London: Metropolitan Books/Henry Holt).

Klotz, A. (1995) *Norms in International Relations: The Struggle Against Apartheid* (Ithaca, NY: Cornell University Press).

Klugman, B. (2011) 'Effective Social Justice Advocacy: A Theory-of-Change Framework for Assessing Challenges', *Foundation Review*, 19(38), 146–62.

Lawson, L. (2008) *Side effects: The story of AIDS in South Africa* (Cape Town: Double Storey).

Leon, T. (2008) *On the Contrary: Leading the Opposition in a Democratic South Africa* (Johannesburg: Jonathan Ball).

Locke, J. (2003) '*Two Treatises of Government*: The Second Treatise: An Essay Concerning the True Original, Extent, and End of Civil Government', in I. Shapiro (ed.) *Two Treatises of Government and a Letter Concerning Toleration* (New Haven and London: Yale University Press), 100–210.

Louw, R. (2001) 'Mkhumbane and New Traditions of Un(African) Same-sex Weddings', in R. Morrell (ed.) *Changing men in Southern Africa* (Pietermaritzburg: University of Natal Press), 287–96.

Lowry, C. and U. Schüklenk (2009) 'Two Models in Global Health Ethics', *Public Health Ethics*, 2(3), 276–84.

Luirink, B. (2000) *Moffies* (Cape Town: David Philip).

MacGregor H. and E. Mills (2011) 'Framing Rights and Responsibilities: Accounts of Women with a History of AIDS Activism', *BMC International Health and Human Rights*, 11(Suppl. 3), S7, 53–7.

Mamdani, M. (1996) *Citizen and Subject: Contemporary Africa and the Legacy of Late Colonialism* (Princeton: Princeton University Press).

Manchester, J. (2004) 'Hope, Involvement and Vision: Reflections on Positive Women's Activism around HIV', *Transformation*, 54, 85–103.

Marais, H. (2000) *To the Edge: AIDS Review 2000* (Pretoria: Centre for the Study of AIDS, University of Pretoria).

Marais, H. (2011) *South Africa Pushed to the Limit: the Political Economy of Change* (Cape Town: University of Cape Town Press).

Mbali, M. (2004) 'AIDS Discourses and the South African State: Government Denialism and Post-apartheid AIDS Policy-making', *Transformation*, 54, 104–22.

Mbembe, A. (1992) 'Provisional Notes on the Postcolony', *Africa: Journal of the International African Institute*, 62(1), 3–37.

McAdam, D. (1982) *Political Processes and the Development of Black Insurgency, 1930–1970* (Chicago and London: University of Chicago Press).

McNeely, I. F. (2002) *Medicine on a Grand Scale: Rudolf Virchow, Liberalism and the Public Health* (London: Wellcome Trust Centre for the History of Medicine at UCL).

Mill, J. S. (2003) 'On Liberty', in M. Warnock (ed.) *Utilitarianism and On Liberty Including Mill's Essay on Bentham and Selections from the writings of Jeremy Bentham and John Austin* (Oxford and Malden MA: Blackwell, 2003), 88–180.

Mindy, D. (2001) 'Nongovernmental Organizations, "Grassroots," and the Politics of Virtue', *Signs*, 26(4), 1187–211.

Moodie, T. D, V. Ndatshe and B. Sibuye (1988) 'Migrancy and male sexuality on the South African Gold Mines', *Journal of Southern African Studies*, 14(2), 228–56.

Moyn, S. (2010) *The Last Utopia: Human Rights in History* (Cambridge MA: The Belknap Press of Harvard).

Msimang, S. (2003) 'HIV/AIDS, Globalisation and the International Women's Movement', *Gender and Development*, 11(1), 109–13.

Mugyenyi, P. (2008) *Genocide by Denial: How Profiteering from HIV/AIDS Killed Millions* (Kampala: Fountain Publishers).

Nattrass, N. (2007) *Mortal Combat: AIDS Denialism and the Struggle for Antiretrovirals in South Africa* (Scottsville: University of KwaZulu-Natal Press).

Nel, J. A. And M Judge (2008) 'Exploring Homophobic Victimisation in Gauteng, South Africa: Issues, Impacts and Responses', *Acta Criminologica*, 21(3), 19–36.

Nosyk, B. And J. S. G. Montaner (2012) 'The Evolving Landscape of the Economics of HIV Treatment and Prevention', *PLoS Medicine*, http://www.plosmedicine.org/article/info:doi/10.1371/journal.pmed.1001174, date accessed 9 March 2012.

Nozick, R. (1974) Anarchy, Society and Utopia (New York: Basic Books).

Nunn, A. (2009) *The Politics and History of AIDS Treatment in Brazil* (New York: Springer).

Nussbaum, M. C. (2010) *From Disgust to Humanity: Sexual Orientation and Constitutional Law* (Oxford: Oxford University Press).

Obama, B. (2004) *Dreams from My Father: A Story of Race and Inheritance* (New York: Three Rivers Press).

O'Brien, P. (2006) 'Historiographic Traditions and Modern Imperatives for the Restoration of Global History', *Journal of Global History*, 1, 3–39.

Oppenheimer, Gerald M. and Ronald Bayer (2007) *Shattered Dreams? An Oral History of the South African AIDS Epidemic* (Oxford: Oxford University Press).

Orbinski, J. (2008) *An Imperfect Offering: Dispatches from the Medical Frontline* (London: Ebury).

Passy, F. (2003) 'Social Networks Matter. But How?', in M. Diani and D. McAdam (eds.) *Social Movements and Networks: Relational Approaches to Collective Action* (Oxford: Oxford University Press), 21–48.

Patton, C. (1990) *Inventing AIDS* (London and New York: Routledge).

Peacock, D., T. Budaza, T. and A. Greig, (2008) ' "Justice for Lorna Mlofana": The Treatment Action Campaign's AIDS and Gender Activism', in A. Ndinga-Muvumba and R. Pharoah (eds.) *HIV/AIDS and Society in South Africa* (Scottsville: University of KwaZulu-Natal Press), 85–102.

Pieterse, M. (2004) 'Coming to Terms with Judicial Enforcement of Socio-economic Rights', *South African Journal of Human Rights*, 20, 383–417.

Pogge, T. (2002) *World Poverty and Human Rights: Cosmopolitan Responsibilities and Reforms* (London: Polity).

Porter, D (1999) *Health, Civilization and the State: A History of Public Health from Ancient to Modern Times* (Abingdon and New York: Routledge 1999).

Posel, D. (2005) 'Sex, Death and the Fate of the Nation: Reflections on the Politicization of Sexuality in Post-apartheid South Africa', *Africa*, 75(2), 125–53.

Price, M. (1989) 'Explaining Trends in the Privatization of Health Services in South Africa', *Health Policy and Planning*, 4(2), 121–30.

Ramphele, M. (1995) *Across Boundaries: The Journey of a South African Woman Leader* (New York: The Feminist Press at CUNY).

Ramphele, M. (1996) 'Political Widowhood in South Africa: The Embodiment of Ambiguity', Daedalus, 125, 1, 99–117.

Reddy, V., T. Sandfort and L. Rispel (2009) 'Introduction', in V. Reddy, T. Sandfort and L. Rispel (eds.) *From Social Silence to Social Science: Same-Sex Sexuality, Gender & HIV/AIDS in South Africa* (Cape Town: HSRC Press), xi–xxxiii.

Reid, G. and T. Dirsuweit (2002) 'Understanding Systematic Violence: Homophobic Attacks in Johannesburg and its Surrounds', *Urban Forum*, 13(3), 99–126.

Reid, R. (2008) *A History of Modern Africa: 1800 to the Present* (Oxford: Blackwell).

Robins, S. L. (2008) *From Revolution to Rights in South Africa: Social Movements, NGOs and Popular Politics After Apartheid* (Oxford: James Currey).

Rosen, G. (1993) *A History of Public Health* (Baltimore, MD: Johns Hopkins University Press).

Ruger, J. P. (2009) *Health and Social Justice* (Oxford: Oxford University Press).

Rushton, S. and O. D. Williams (2011) 'Private Actors in Global Health Governance', in S. Rushton and O. D. Williams (eds.) *Partnerships and Foundations in Global Public Health* (London: Palgrave Macmillan, 2011), 1–29.

Sachs, J. (2005) *The End of Poverty: Economic Possibilities for Our Time* (New York: Penguin).

Saunier, P. Y. (2008) 'Learning by Doing: Notes about the Making of the *Palgrave Dictionary of Transnational History*', Journal of Modern European History, 6(2), 159–80.

Sen, A. (1999) *Development as Freedom* (Oxford: Oxford University Press).

Shamir, R. (2005) 'Corporate Responsibility and the South African Drug Wars: Outline of a New Frontier for Cause Lawyers', in A. Sarat and S. A Scheingold (eds.) *The Worlds That Cause Lawyers Make: Structure and Agency in Legal Practice* (Stanford: Stanford University Press), 37–62.

Smith R. A. and Patricia D. Siplon (2006) *Drugs into Bodies: Global AIDS Treatment Activism* (Westport Connecticut and London: Praeger).

Smith, R. D. C. Correa and C. Oh (2009) 'Trade, TRIPs and Pharmaceuticals', *Lancet* 373, 684–91.

Snow, D. A. (2004) 'Framing Processes, Ideology and Discursive Fields', in D. A. Snow, S. A. Soule and H. Kriesi (eds.) *The Blackwell Companion to Social Movements* (Oxford, Malden, VA and Victoria: Blackwell), 380–412.

Southall, R. (2003) 'The State of Party Politics: Struggles Within the Tripartite Alliance and the Decline of Opposition', in J. Daniel, R. Southall and A. Habib (eds.) *State of the Nation: South Africa 2003–4* (Cape Town: HSRC Press, 2003), 53–77.

Steinberg, C. (2006) 'Can Reasonableness Protect the Poor? A Review of South Africa's Socio-economic Rights Jurisprudence', *South African Law Journal*, 123(2), 264–79.

Steinberg, J. (2008) *Three-letter Plague: A Young Man's Journey through a Great Epidemic* (Johannesburg and Cape Town: Jonathan Ball).

Stephen, J. (2009) 'Saints and Sinners: The Treatment Action Campaign', in K. Cullinan and A. Thom (eds.) *The Virus, Vitamins & Vegetables: The South African HIV/AIDS Mystery* (Sunnyside: Jacana), 157–74.

Stocking, G. W. (1992) *The Ethnographer's Magic and Other Essays in the History of Anthropology* (Madison: University of Wisconsin Press)

Susser, I. (2002) 'Health Rights for Women in the Age of AIDS', *International Journal of Epidemiology*, 31, 45–8.

Susser, I. (2009) *AIDS, Sex and Culture: Global Politics and Survival in Southern Africa* (Malden and Oxford: Blackwell).

Susser, M. (1999) 'Foreword', in S. Kark and E. Kark (eds.) *Promoting Community Health: From Pholela to Jerusalem* (Johannesburg: Witwatersrand University Press), v–x.

Susser, M. (2006) 'A Personal History: Social Medicine in a South African Setting, 1952–5. Part I: The Shape of Ideas Forged in the Second World War', *Journal of Epidemiology and Community Health*, 60, 554–7.

Takiff, M. (2010) *A Complicated Man: The Life of Bill Clinton as Told by Those Who Know Him* (New Haven and London: Yale University Press).

Tarrow, S. (1998) *Power in Movement: Social Movements and Contentious Politics* (Cambridge: Cambridge University Press).

Tarrow, S. (2005) *The New Transnational Activism* (Cambridge: Cambridge University Press).

Thelen, D. (1999) 'The Nation and Beyond: Transnational Perspectives on United States History', *The Journal of American History*, 86(3), 965–75.

't Hoen, E. (2009) *The Global Politics of Pharmaceutical Monopoly Power* (Diemen: AMB).

Thoreson, R. R. (2008) 'Somewhere over the Rainbow Nation: Gay, Lesbian and Bisexual Activism in South Africa', Journal of Southern African Studies, 34 (3), 679—97.

Thorn, H. (2006) *Anti-apartheid and the Emergence of a Global Civil Society* (Basingstoke and New York: Palgrave).

Tilly, C. (2004) *Social Movements 1768–2004* (London: Paradigm).

Treichler, P. (1999) *How to Have a Theory in an Epidemic: Cultural Chronicles of AIDS* (Durham and London: Duke University Press).

Tyrell, I. (1991) 'American Exceptionalism in an Age of International History', *The American Historical Review*, 96(4), 1031–55.

Walker, C. (1991) *Women and Resistance in South Africa* (Cape Town and Johannesburg: David Philip).

Walsh, D. (2009) 'Citizenship, Gender and Civil Society in South Africa', in H. Britton, J. Fish and S. Meintjes (eds.) *Women's Activism in South Africa: Working across Divides* (Scottsville: University of KwaZulu-Natal Press), 44–63.

Waltz, K. N. (1986) 'Anarchic Orders and Balances of Power', in R. O. Keohane (ed.) *Neorealism and Its Critics* (New York: Columbia University Press), 98–130.

Waning, B., E. Diedrichsen, S. Moon (2010) 'A Lifeline to Treatment: the Role of Indian Generic Manufacturers in Supplying Antiretroviral Medicines to Developing Countries', *Journal of the International AIDS Society*, 13, 35, http://www.jiasociety.org/content/13/1/35, date accessed 9 March 2012.

Waning, B., W. Kaplan, A. C. King, D. A. Lawrence, H. G. Leufkens and M. P, Fox (2009) 'Global Strategies to Reduce the Price of Antiretroviral Medicines: Evidence from Transactional Databases', *Bulletin of the World Health Organization*, 87, 520–528.

Wendt, A. (1999) *Social Theory of International Politics* (Cambridge: Cambridge University Press).

Wesson, M. (2004) '*Grootboom* and Beyond: Reassessing the Socio-economic Jurisprudence of the South African Constitutional Court', *South African Journal of Human Rights*, 20(2004), 284–308.

Wiredu, K. (1998) 'How Not to Compare African Thought with Western Thought', in E. C. Eze (ed.) *African Philosophy: An Anthology* (Oxford and Malden, MA: Blackwell), 193–9.

Wolff, J. (2011) 'The Human Right to Health', in S. Benatar and G. Brock (eds.) *Global Health and Global Health Ethics* (Cambridge: Cambridge University Press), 108–18.

Unpublished theses and papers

Abdool Karim, Q. (2000) 'Women and AIDS: Epidemiology and gender barriers to prevention in KwaZulu-Natal, South Africa' (Univ. of Natal PhD thesis).

Carson, T. (2008) 'Black Trade Unions and Consumer Boycotts in the Cape Province, South Africa 1978–1982' (Univ. of Oxford DPhil thesis).

Messac, L. (2011) 'Lazarus at America's Doorstep: Elites and Framing in Federal Appropriations for Global AIDS Relief', Unpublished paper.

Myburgh, J. (2007) 'The African National Congress under the Presidency of Thabo Mbeki, 1997–2002' (Univ. of Oxford DPhil thesis).

Noble, V. (2005) 'Doctors Divided: Gender, Race and Class Anomalies in the Production of Black Medical Doctors in Apartheid South Africa' (Univ. of Michigan PhD thesis).

Schneider, H. (2001) 'The AIDS Impasse in South Africa', Paper prepared for AIDS in Context Conference, History Workshop, 4–6 April 2001', (2001), Unpublished.

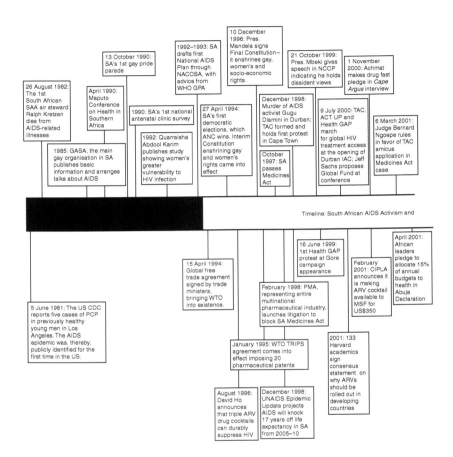

26 August 1982: The 1st South African SAA air steward Ralph Kretzen dies from AIDS-related illnesses

April 1990: Maputo Conference on Health in Southern Africa

13 October 1990: SA's 1st gay pride parade

1990: SA's 1st national antenatal clinic survey

1992–1993: SA drafts first National AIDS Plan through NACOSA, with advice from WHO GPA

10 December 1996: Pres. Mandela signs Final Constitution – it enshrines gay, women's and socio-economic rights.

21 October 1999: Pres. Mbeki gives speech in NCOP indicating he holds dissident views

1 November 2000: Achmat makes drug fast pledge in *Cape Argus* interview

1985: GASA, the main gay organisation in SA publishes basic information and arranges talks about AIDS

1992: Quarraisha Abdool Karim publishes study showing women's greater vulnerability to HIV infection

27 April 1994: SA's first democratic elections, which ANC wins. Interim Constitution enshrining gay and women's rights came into effect

December 1998: Murder of AIDS activist Gugu Dlamini in Durban; TAC formed and holds first protest in Cape Town

October 1997: SA passes Medicines Act

9 July 2000: TAC, ACT UP and Health GAP march for global HIV treatment access at the opening of Durban IAC; Jeff Sachs proposes Global Fund at conference

6 March 2001: Judge Bernard Ngoepe rules in favor of TAC amicus application in Medicines Act case

Timeline: South African AIDS Activism and

5 June 1981: The US CDC reports five cases of PCP in previously healthy young men in Los Angeles. The AIDS epidemic was, thereby, publicly identified for the first time in the US.

15 April 1994: Global free trade agreement signed by trade ministers, bringing WTO into existence.

16 June 1999: 1st Health GAP protest at Gore campaign appearance

February 2001: CIPLA announces it is making ARV cocktail available to MSF for US$350

April 2001: African leaders pledge to allocate 15% of annual budgets to health in Abuja Declaration

February 1998: PMA, representing entire multinational pharmaceutical industry, launches litigation to block SA Medicines Act

January 1995: WTO TRIPS agreement comes into effect imposing 20 pharmaceutical patents

August 1996: David Ho announces that triple ARV drug cocktails can durably suppress HIV

December 1998: UNAIDS Epidemic Update projects AIDS will knock 17 years off life expectancy in SA from 2005–10

2001: 133 Harvard academics sign consensus statement on why ARVs should be rolled out in developing countries

19 April 2001: PMA drops lawsuit against Mandela administration; Achmat named *TIME* magazine's person of the week

5 July 2002: Constitutional Court finds in TAC's favor in Nevirapine case

14 February 2003: 10,000 TAC supporters march to parliament

December 2002: Mandela visits MSF/TAC clinic in Khayalitsha

30 April 2003: TAC suspends its civil disobedience campaign after meeting with Jacob Zuma

October 2003: Competition Commission finds in TAC's favour forcing BI and GSK into negotiations to settle.

18 August 2001: TAC launches Constitutional Court challenge for wider state provision of Nevirapine for PMTCT

September 2002: TAC launches Competition Commission complaint against BI and GSK

20 March 2003: TAC launches 'Dying for Treatment', its 2nd civil disobedience campaign

8 August 2003: SA's cabinet decides Dept. of Health should develop an 'operational plan' to roll out ARVs

19 November 2003: Cabinet announces that Tshabalala-Msimang has presented the Operational Plan to it

Global Health Politics

June 2002: AIDS-ill Achmat delivers taped address to Barcelona IAC; reports KZN Global Fund grant blocked by national govt.

November 2002: American AIDS activists march on White House calling for presidential AIDS Initiative

13 February 2003: ACT UP, Health GAP, GMHC and African Services Committee protest outside SA consulate in NYC

March 2003: ITPC formed at conference held by TAC, TAG and GMHC

22–4 August: TAC hosts founding meeting of PATAM in Cape Town

April 2002: Global Fund starts offering large grants

28 January 2003: Bush unveils US$15 bil for AIDS relief

25–27 June 2001: 1st UN GA Special Session on AIDS

14 November 2001: Doha Declaration clarifiesTRIPS flexibitilies.

Index

Printed and bound in Great Britain by
CPI Antony Rowe, Chippenham and Eastbourne

CL

362.
196
979
200
968
MBA